PSYCHOANALYSIS
SCIENTIFIC METHOD
AND PHILOSOPHY

PSYCHOANALYSIS

SCIENTIFIC METHOD

AND PHILOSOPHY

EDITED BY SIDNEY HOOK

Routledge
Taylor & Francis Group
LONDON AND NEW YORK

Originally published in 1959 by New York University Press.
Published 1990 by Transaction Publishers

Published 2019 by Routledge
2 Park Square, Milton Park, Abingdon, Oxon OX14 4RN
52 Vanderbilt Avenue, New York, NY 10017

First issued in hardback 2019

Routledge is an imprint of the Taylor & Francis Group, an informa business

Library of Congress Catalog Number: 89-48554

Library of Congress Cataloging-in-Publication Data

New York University Institute of Philosophy (2nd: 1958)
Psychoanalysis, scientific method, and philosophy: a symposium/edited by Sidney Hook.
p. cm.
"Proceedings of the second annual New York University Insitute of Philosophy, held at Washington Square, New York, March 28-29, 1958" – T.p. verso.
Reprint. Originally published: New York: New York University Press, 1959.
Includes bibliographical references.
ISBN 0-88738-834-5
1. Psychoanalysis–Congresses. I. Hook, Sidney, 1902- II. New York University. III. Title.
BF173.N44 1958b
150.19'5–dc20 89-48554
CIP

ISBN 13: 978-1-138-53103-1 (hbk)
ISBN 13: 978-0-88738-834-7 (pbk)

Table of Contents

Introduction

IT HAS become a commonplace observation that the distinctive culture of the twentieth century has been profoundly influenced by the ideas of three towering figures—all born in the nineteenth century—Einstein, Marx and Freud.

The consequences of Einstein's ideas should bring home to the most philistine the truth of John Dewey's remark that ideas are the most practical things in the world. They have vastly transformed man's place in nature and potentially his natural home. They have extended the reach of human power to a point where men may before long aspire to the role of the Olympian deities. The power of these deities was great but not infinite, and their wisdom was not commensurate with their power. As men stand poised today in bewilderment at what their minds and hands have wrought, they realize that no advance in power over nature can by itself resolve problems of human nature and society. Perhaps even more important than the increases in power won by the triumphs of modern physics is the intellectual revolution associated with the development of its basic concepts. One aspect of this revolution, its bearings upon the concepts of chance, causality, and determinism, was explored at the First Annual Meeting of the New York Institute of Philosophy and published under the title of *Determinism and Freedom in the Age of Modern Science* (New York, 1958).

The liberation of nuclear energy has made the existence of human life and society problematic. This is comprehensible not as a consequence of a theory of natural science but as a consequence, for the most part, of a social philosophy derived historically, even if not logically, from the social doctrines of Marx.

For good or ill, it is in Marx's name and in the name of those who have declared themselves his disciples that the most formidable challenge to the society of the free world has been made. It is safe to say that the history of physics would have been pretty much the same even if Marx had never lived, or if his ideas had remained without influence. It is almost as certain that the history of human society in the twentieth century would have been enormously different if the Russian October Revolution, engineered by Lenin and Trotsky, had not occurred.

In considering the influence of Freud, we are moving to an unmapped terrain of culture in which it is very difficult to assess the consequences of his ideas. Certainly, the work of Freud and those whom he has influenced has led to a revolution in the way we *talk* about ourselves and others, independently of what stock we put in the validity of his ideas. A large part of the Freudian vocabulary has become an integral part of common usage, at least in America and West European countries. There have not been lacking claims that *potentially* the Freudian theory of man is more far-reaching than all others precisely because it concerns the human mind and behavior, because it offers the central key to understanding the choices and decisions men make or fail to make. After all, it is human choice and the decisions to which it leads that will determine whether we are going to have a world or not, or rather whether or not we are going to continue to live in the physical world whose dimensions have been enormously expanded by the gigantic strides of modern science. Once we have found ways of living peacefully together within the world, other human choices and other decisions will ultimately determine whether the world society gradually emerging out of conditions made possible by the discoveries of scientific technology will be free or totalitarian.

In the light of the foregoing, it should not be hard to understand the selection of the theme for the Second Annual Meeting of the New York University Institute of Philosophy. Our concern, however, was not with the therapeutic implications, individual or social, of psychoanalysis or of any other theory of psychology, but solely with psychoanalysis as a scientific theory. American philosophy is distinguished from philosophies current in other countries by virtue of its intense interest in the methodology and philosophy of science. It seemed, therefore, all the more appropriate, particularly since claims have been made that philosophy is not a subject matter but a series of misdirected inquiries which themselves invite the illumination of the psychoanalytic probe, to focus philosophical interest on the scientific status of psychoanalysis. Whatever else philosophy does, it ought to be able to clarify, or to make less obscure, discourse in any domain where there seems to be a failure of communication between human beings who are otherwise intelligent. I doubt that anyone will deny that psychoanalytical discourse, whether it be the discourse of Freud or of any of his disciples and critics within the psychoanalytical tradition, can profit by clarification.

So far as I am aware, this is the first time in the United States that a distinguished group of psychoanalysts has met with a distinguished group of philosophers of science in a free, critical interchange of views on the scientific status of psychoanalysis. Some psychologists and psychiatrists were present who were not psychoanalysts. The reader must judge for himself whether the interchange proved fruitful. In the nature of the case, the printed record cannot capture the spirit of the proceedings and the liveliness and humor of the discussion. Particularly noteworthy was the sense of absorption and intellectual excitement among the participants, which was sustained from the first moments of the opening session to the closing words of the last session. As a seat-calloused veteran of innumerable conferences and institutes, I have never experienced its like before. In the end, however, it is not the evanescent qualities of the discussion, agreeable as they are, that count most but the contributions made. We submit them, confident that they will not only instruct the reader but enkindle his interest in joining our community of inquiry.

Because of my absence abroad in pursuit of the philosophical and cultural "wisdom of the Orient," the technical details involved in seeing this volume through the press were entrusted to Dr. Raziel Abelson of the Department of Philosophy, University College, New York University. Both the editor and the contributors owe him a debt of gratitude.

SIDNEY HOOK

PART I

PSYCHOANALYSIS AND SCIENTIFIC METHOD

1.

Psychoanalysis As a Scientific Theory

HEINZ HARTMANN, M.D.
Former President
International Society for Psychoanalysis

WHEN some forty-five years ago Freud (12) wrote for the first time about the philosophical interest in analysis, his main point was that philosophy could not avoid taking fully into account what he then called "the hypothesis of unconscious mental activities." He also mentioned that philosophers may be interested in the interpretation of philosophical thought in terms of psychoanalysis—adding, though, here as elsewhere, that the fact that a theory or doctrine is determined by psychological processes of many kinds does not necessarily invalidate its scientific truth. Since then, the knowledge of human behavior and motivation we owe to analysis has greatly increased, has become much more comprehensive but also more specific; and this development has certainly influenced not only social science, anthropology, and medicine, but also philosophy in a broad sense. This does not, though, necessarily mean that analysis can "answer" what one usually calls philosophical problems; it usually means that it leads to looking at them from a new angle. Some of its potentialities in this respect have been made use of only rather scantily so far. I am thinking, for example, of its possible contribution toward a better understanding of ethical problems. The interest psychoanalysis may have for philosophers has clearly two aspects: it resides partly in the new psychological findings and theories of analysis, but also in certain ques-

References in this section are to the bibliography, which begins on page 35.

tions of methodology raised by Freud's and other psychoanalysts' approach to the study of man.

In speaking of psychoanalysis one often refers to a therapeutic technique. One may also refer to a method of psychological investigation whose main aspects are free association and interpretation; or, finally, to a body of facts and theories (Freud, 13). In this last sense, we would certainly consider as psychoanalytical any knowledge gained directly by Freud's method of investigation; but many of us would today consider analysis to include related procedures such as the application of psychoanalytic insights to data of direct child observation, a field which has grown in importance in the last two decades. Of the three aspects just mentioned, it is the method of exploration that has undergone the least change; it is commonly used in a situation defined by a certain set of rules and referred to as the psychoanalytic situation or the psychoanalytic interview. The therapeutic technique has been repeatedly modified, and psychoanalytic theory has gone through a series of more or less radical modifications, by Freud and by others. I want to emphasize that the interrelations among these three aspects are, in analysis, a central topic—though in the context of this presentation I can refer to them only occasionally.

The theories of psychoanalysis follow principles of systematization, as do theories in other fields. Freud, however, did not speak of analysis as a "system," but rather accentuated its unfinished character, its flexibility, and the tentative nature of a considerable part of it. Actually, adjustments and reformulations of various aspects of theory have repeatedly become necessary. There are chapters such as the psychology of the dream, of libidinal development, of anxiety, and of symptom formation, that have been more systematically worked out than others. Psychoanalysis is obviously far from being a closed system of doctrines, though it has sometimes been represented as such. Also, though some fundamental tenets of psychoanalysis are accepted by all (Freudian) analysts, agreement on all of them is obviously lacking.

There is in analysis a hierarchy of hypotheses as to their

closeness to observation, their generality, and the degree to which they have been confirmed. It appears that a neater classification as to these points and a higher degree of systematization (considering the different levels of theorizing) than exist today would not only facilitate my task in discussing psychoanalysis as a scientific theory but also clarify the standing of analysis as a scientific discipline. Promising efforts in this direction have been made and are being made by analysts and also by nonanalysts, but as yet no complete and systematical outline drawn from this angle is available; a recent work by David Rapaport (30), soon to be published, may come close to performing this task. This is probably the reason, or one of the reasons, that in more or less general presentations of psychoanalysis references to its history abound, and the reader will forgive me if they do in this paper too, at least in its first part. I shall mostly refer to the work of Freud, because most of the more general theories of analysis have their origin in it, and because he is in many ways more representative of psychoanalytic thinking than anybody else.

Often historical explanations are substituted for system; an attempt is made to clarify the function of propositions in their relation to others by tracing their place in the development of analysis. Also, without such historical reference it happens over and over again that analytical hypotheses are dealt with on one level, so to say, which belong to different phases of theory formation, and some of which have actually been discarded and replaced by others. Again, because of the comparatively low level of systematization, I think it is true that even today a thorough knowledge of at least some chapters of analytic theory cannot be acquired without knowledge of its history (Hartmann, 16).

From the beginning, explanations of human behavior in terms of propositions about unconscious mental processes have been an essential part and one characteristic feature of psychoanalysis. I may, then, start by introducing Freud's concepts of unconscious processes. He makes a distinction between two forms of unconscious mental activity. The one, called preconscious, functions more or less as conscious activities do. It is not conscious, in a descriptive sense, but can become conscious without having to overcome powerful counterforces. Where such overcoming of resistances is necessary, as is the case with repressed material, we speak of unconscious processes in the stricter, the dynamic, sense of the word. The dynamic impact of these latter unconscious processes on human behavior—and not only in the case of mental disease—is one main tenet of Freud's theory of unconscious mental activities.

There is rather wide agreement that conscious data are insufficient for the explanation of a considerable part of behavior, and particularly of those aspects that were first studied in analysis. However, its critics have repeatedly claimed that the introduction of unconscious processes is superfluous. The explanation needed could be stated, or should be sought for, in terms of the more reliable data of brain physiology. The question here is not just whether, and why, explanations based on such data would be per se more reliable, nor why psychological hypotheses about mental processes ought not to be introduced in explaining human behavior. We have also to consider the fact that, given the actual state of brain physiology, many and even comparatively simple aspects of behavior of the kind we are dealing with in analysis cannot be explained. To rely on brain physiology alone would mean to renounce explanation of the greatest part of the field that psychoanalysis has set out to explain. Or, if one should insist on attempting an explanation on physiological grounds, the resultant hypotheses would of necessity be considerably more tenuous and more speculative even than psychoanalytic hypotheses are suspected to be by its critics today.

Freud, well trained in the anatomy and physiology of the brain, actually started out by attempting to devise a physiological psychology that could provide him with concepts and hypotheses to account for his clinical insights. But beyond a certain point this approach proved of no use. He was thus led to replace it by a set of psychological hypotheses and constructs; and this step represents probably the most important turning point in the history of psychoanalysis. It was the beginning in analysis of psychological theory, the heuristic value of which he found to be greatly superior—a point that, I think, has been corroborated by its subsequent development.

But it is true that even after this radical turn in his approach Freud held on to the expectation, shared by many analysts, that one day the development of brain physiology would make it possible to base psychoanalysis on its findings and theories. He did not think this would happen during his lifetime, in which he proved to be right. In the meantime certain, though limited, parallels between analytic propositions and discoveries in the physiology of the brain have become apparent. Also, the usefulness of some psychoanalytic hypotheses for their field has been recognized by at least some representatives of brain research (Adrian, 1). As to the psychology of unconscious processes, I think it can be said that Freud in developing that part of analysis was much less interested in the ultimate "nature" or "essence" of such processes—whatever this may mean—than in finding a suitable conceptual framework for the phenomena he had discovered.

While Freud, after the first years of his scientific work, relinquished the attempt to account for his findings in terms of physiology, it is nevertheless characteristic of some of his psychoanalytic theorizing that he used physiological models. He was guided by the trend in German physiology which has been designated as the physicalist school (Bernfeld, 5), whose representatives were, among others, Helmholtz and Bruecke, the latter being one of Freud's teachers. Certain aspects of the psychology of neurosis, for example, led him to introduce into psychoanalysis the concept of regression (to earlier stages of development), which had been used in the physiology of his day; this concept, though, acquired new meaning in the context in which he used it. Also, in making "function" the criterion for defining what he called the mental systems (ego, id, superego), Freud used physiology as a model. But this no longer implies any correlation to any specific physiological organization (Hartmann, Kris, Loewenstein, 21). The value of such borrowings or analogies has, of course, to be determined in every single instance by confronting their application with tested knowledge (data and hypotheses). Physiological models (also occasionally physical models, as is obvious, for instance, in Freud's concept of a "mental apparatus") have been used also by other psychoanalysts (see Kubie in a recent lecture) in order to illustrate certain characteristics of mental phenomena or to suggest a new hypothesis. The use even of metaphors need not of necessity lead into muddled thinking once their place in theory has been clearly delineated. The danger that earlier implications of those model concepts might impair their fruitful use in the new context of psychoanalysis has on the whole been successfully avoided (Hartmann-Kris-Loewenstein).

The broadening of the scope of psychology that came about as the consequence of the inclusion of propositions about unconscious mental processes meant, first of all, that many aspects of a person's life history that had never been explained before—and that, as a matter of fact, one had not even tried to explain—could be accounted for in terms of the individual's experience and dispositions. Causation in the field of personality is traceable only at its fringes without this broadening of theory. Freud was a strict determinist and often stated that to fill that gap in earlier psychological approaches, partly because of which the study of personality had been unsatisfactory, was one of his primary aims in developing analytic theory. More recently it has been said, by the mathematician von Mises (29), that the observations correspond rather to statistical than to causal relations. I may mention at this point that this interest in the causation of mental phenomena included, quite naturally, also the interest in what we call the genetic viewpoint, since Freud's attention had been drawn to many facts of early childhood which had been unknown, and regularities in the relationships between early childhood situations and the behavior of the adult had become apparent. With Freud, the investigation of highly complex series of experience and behavior, extending over long periods of time, soon moved into the center of interest. Developmental research was to become equally important for psychoanalytic theory and practice. It is significant that the reconstructive approach in analysis led not only to the discovery of a great wealth of childhood material in every individual case, but also to the ascertainment of typical sequences of developmental phases. The genetic approach has become so pervasive, not only in psychopathology but also in psychoanalytic psychology in general, that in analysis phenomena are often grouped together, not according to their descriptive similarities but as belonging together if they have a common genetic root (oral character, anal character). It was only much later that this predominance of a genetic conceptualization was counterbalanced by a sharper distinction between genesis and function, to which I shall shortly return in speaking of the structural point of view.

Here I want to add that while I just spoke of the study of the individual's "life history," it would be misleading (though it actually has been done) to classify this aspect of analysis as an historical discipline. This misinterpretation may be traceable to its comparison with archaeology, which Freud occasionally uses. It is true that most analytical knowledge has been gained in the psychoanalytic interview and that the concern with developmental problems refers primarily to the history of individuals. But this should not obfuscate the fact that the aim of these studies is (besides its therapeutic purpose) to develop lawlike propositions which then, of course, transcend individual observations.

At this point I should like briefly to summarize the role of psychoanalysis as a psychology of motivation, bearing in mind that nowadays psychoanalysis takes into consideration the interaction of the individual with his environment, as well as his so-called "inner-psychic" processes. The study of these psychic processes constitutes what, in analysis, we call "metapsychology," a term that signifies not (as it might seem) that which is beyond psychology altogether, but simply those psychological investigations that are not limited to conscious phenomena, and that formulate the most general assumptions of analysis on the most abstract level of theory. Metapsychology is concerned with the substructures of personality, with the ego, the id, and the superego which are defined as units of functions. The id refers to the instinctual aspect, the ego to the reality principle and to the "centralization of functional control" (to borrow a term from brain physiology). The superego has its biological roots in the long dependency on the parents and in the helplessness of the human child; it develops out of identifications with the parents; and it accounts for the fact that moral conflict and guilt feelings become a natural and fundamental aspect of human behavior. The theoretical and clinical advantage of the structural formulations, referring to the distinction of ego, id, superego, has several reasons. The most important is probably that the demarcation lines of the three systems, ego, id, superego are geared to the typical conflicts of man: conflicts with the instinctual drives, with moral conscience, and with the outside world. The paramount importance on neurotic *and* normal development of these conflicts, and of the ways to solve them, was one of the earliest discoveries of Freud and has remained central in psychoanalytic practice and theory ever since.

Critics of analysis often tend to underrate the wealth of individual data on which it is built. But on the other hand, it also happens that the theoretical nature of concepts like libido is not fully realized; for example, libido is often identified with sexual experience, or as a mere generalization of some observable connections.

In the beginnings of psychoanalysis (even after the importance of unconscious processes had been realized), Freud still adhered more or less strictly to associationism. But when he found conflict to be a primary motivating force of behavior, and specifically an important etiological agent in neurosis, he gradually developed the concept of mental tendencies and purposive ideas. Psychoanalysis became a psychology of motivation, the motives being partly, but not generally, considered in analogy with those consciously experienced. There originated the idea of wishes, in certain circumstances, warded off by defensive techniques. He discovered the role of repression and later of other defense mechanisms, like projection, isolation, undoing, and so on. The consideration of mental processes from this angle of synergistic or antagonistic motivating forces is what has been known since as the dynamic aspect of psychoanalysis. The systematic and objective study of conflict has remained one of its essential aspects and has proved a necessary and fruitful avenue to the explanation of human behavior. This was a second bold step in the development of psychoanalysis. The importance of "conflict" had, of course, been known in religious and philosophical doctrines and in literature, but scientific psychology before Freud had had no means to approach the subject.

The dynamic factors involved in both sides of a conflict were, for some time, rather poorly defined. It was, then, again primarily data of analytical observation that led to the realization of the dominance of the instinctual drives among the motivating forces. I am referring here to Freud's discovery of infantile sexuality. This discovery was, at the time, considered by many as the product of revolting imagination; today, it can easily be confirmed in every nursery.

Even at the period when instinctual motivation seemed to be pretty much ubiquitous, the basic fact of conflict was not overlooked. Self-preservative instinctual drives were, at the time, thought of as the opponents of sexuality. Besides this, the concept of overdetermination, referring to the multiple motivation of all human behavior, continued also through the phase in which motivation was, on the level of general theory, nearly always considered instinctual.

Again, to fit it to his field of observation Freud had to modify the concept of "instinct" commonly used in other fields. His term, in German, *Trieb,* in English, "instinctual drive," or "drive," is certainly not identical with what one refers to in speaking of the instincts of lower animals. His concept of drives had to prove its usefulness with respect to human psychology. Here, the sources of the drives are of much less importance than their aims and their objects. The lesser rigidity of the human drives, the comparatively easy shift of the aims, the freeing of many activities from a rigid connection with one definite instinctual tendency, the comparative independence from and variety of possible response to outer and inner stimuli have to be taken into account in considering the role of the drives in human psychology. Still, the psychoanalytic theory of instinctual drives is broad enough to show also many impressive parallels with the findings of a modern school of zoologists (ethologists).

The concept of a continuity of this driving force allows the consideration of a great variety of mental acts from the angle of their investment with drive energy. Also in this way it is possible to understand the close relationship of many mental processes which, looked at from the surface, would appear to be entirely heterogeneous. The capacity for displacement or transformation into various kinds of human activities; also the motivational role traceable through and specific on all levels of man's growth from birth to maturity; their central role in typical conflicts; and the fact that they involve relations to human objects—these are some of the psychologically essential aspects of the psychoanalytic concept of human drives. According to Freud, sexuality and aggression are, among all the drives one could describe, those that come closest to fulfilling the demands psychoanalysis makes on a concept of drives.

The concept of mental energy was then elaborated in the sense that it is the drives that are the main sources of energy in what Freud calls the "mental apparatus." However, a strictly speaking quantifying approach to these energic problems has so far not been developed. Or rather: while it is possible to speak of a greater or lesser degree of, let's say, a resistance (against the uncovering of some hidden material), we have no way of measuring it. To account for the difference in the unconscious and the conscious (and preconscious) processes Freud postulated two forms of energy distribution, conceptualized as, respectively, primary and secondary processes. The primary processes represent a tendency to immediate discharge, while the secondary processes are guided by the consideration of reality. This distinction is again both theoretically significant and clinically quite helpful. The thesis that behavior is to be explained also in terms of its energic cathexis is what we call, in analysis, the economic viewpoint.

The regulation of energies in the mental apparatus is assumed to follow the pleasure principle, the reality principle (derived from the pleasure principle under the influence of ego-development), and a tendency to keep the level of excitation constant or at a minimum. There are parallels to this in hypotheses formulated by others, and again the use of physical and physiological models played a role in the Freudian concepts.

The three aspects of psychoanalytic theory I have mentioned so far—the topographical (conscious–preconscious–unconscious), the dynamic, and the economic (energic)—represent Freud's first approach to what he called "metapsychology." It is postulated that a satisfactory explanation of human behavior includes its consideration in relation to all aspects of metapsychology. The "meta" in this term points to a theory going "beyond" the investigation of conscious phenomena. The word, generally accepted in psychoanalysis, has proved misleading for many outside analysis. Actually, "metapsychology" is nothing but a term for the highest level of abstraction used in analytic psychology.

A fourth aspect of metapsychology, called structural, was explicitly stated considerably later, though it was implicit in earlier theoretical thinking on mental conflicts. The forces opposing the drives in typical conflict situations, warding them off and forcing them to compromise formations (of which the neurotic symptom may serve as an example), are today conceptualized as an essential aspect of what we call the ego. At the core of this concept formation is the recognition of the relevant differences between instinctual tendencies which strive for discharge, and other tendencies that enforce postponement of discharge and are modifiable by the influence of the environment. This means, of course, that the dynamic and economic viewpoints can no longer be limited to the vicissitudes of instinctual drives. The original concept of a defensive ego had to be broadened to include in the ego those nondefensive functions of the mental apparatus that are noninstinctual in character. Many of these are not, or not necessarily, part of the conflictual set-up; we call them today "the nonconflictual sphere of the ego" (Hartmann, 15). Here belong (though they too may be involved in conflict, without, however, originating in it) perception, thinking, memory, action, and so on. It is likely that in man not only instinctual factors are in part determined by heredity, but also the apparatus of the ego underlying the functions just mentioned. We speak of the primary autonomous functions of the ego. It is true that analysis is, due to its method, directly dealing with environmental factors and with reactions to them, but this has never implied a denial, on principle, of heredity. It is in this sense that we speak of a drive constitution, and today also of constitutional elements in the ego, and of the role of maturational factors in the typical sequence of developmental phases.

To those noninstinctual functions that we attribute to the ego belongs also what one can call the centralized functional control which integrates the different parts of personality with each other and with outer reality. This function (synthetic function or organizing function) is in a way similar to what, since Cannon, we call homeostasis, and may represent one level of it.

The ego is, then, a substructure of personality and is defined by its functions. The instinctual aspect of personality is today conceptualized as the id. Through the development of the ego it becomes possible that the pleasure principle, dominant with the instinctual drives, can be modified to that consideration of reality, in thinking and action, that makes adaptation possible and is termed, as I said before, the reality principle. Through recent work, the relation between adaptation to outer reality and the state of integration of inner reality has become more accessible. This development in psychoanalytic theory has thus led to an improved understanding of man's relations to his environment, and to the most significant part of it, his fellowmen—which is, however, not to say that the socio-cultural aspects of mental functions and development had been overlooked in earlier analysis. Psychoanalysis, in contradistinction to some other schools of psychology, has never considered "inner-psychic" processes only, but also, and not only accidentally, includes the consideration of the individual's interactions with the environment. At any rate, the study of object relations in human development has more recently become one of the most fruitful centers of analytic interest ("new environmentalism," Kris, 25). Ego psychology represents a more balanced consideration of the biological and the social and cultural aspects of human behavior. We may say that in analysis cultural phenomena are often studied in their biological context and significance, and biological phenomena in relation to the sociocultural environment (Hartmann, 19). But this aspect will be discussed more fully later.

Some of the functions of the ego have, in the course of development, to be wrested from the influence of the drives. Gradually, they then reach, through a change of function, a certain degree of independence from instinctual origins and of resistance against reinvolvement with the drives (secondary autonomy—see Hartmann, 15, 17). A similar concept, though less specific in relation to psychoanalytic propositions, has been introduced by G. Allport, (2). This relative independence of the ego is also energically conceptualized, with respect to the sources of energy at the disposal of ego functions. The necessity to distinguish function from genesis more clearly is one of the main implications of the structural viewpoint.

The third unit of functions, considered a substructure of personality, is called the superego. To it we attribute the functions of self-criticism, conscience and the formation of ideals. The acceptance of moral standards is considered a natural step in ontogenesis. Moral conflict, and the guilt feelings that are an expression of it, are, from the time when the superego has been instituted, one fundamental aspect of human behavior. The superego has a biological root in the comparatively long dependency and helplessness of the child of the human species, which also means increased importance of the parents for its development. The superego develops out of identification with them, to which, in subsequent layers of development, identifications with others are added. Also obvious in its genesis is a socio-cultural factor, which accounts for an important segment of tradition formation. The acceptance of certain moral demands, the rejection of others, the degree of severity of the superego and its capacity to enforce its demands can very frequently be traced in clinical investigation.

Structural hypotheses are in many ways more comprehensive,

but also, if I may say so, more elegant than earlier formulations of partly the same problems. They have also a considerable value in clinical thinking, because they are particularly fit to account for what has remained dominant in clinical work, that is, the various forms of typical conflict situations. Actually, the demarcation lines of those units of functions, or systems, or substructures of personality are so drawn that they correspond to the main conflicts of man, which we now describe as conflicts between ego and id, superego and ego, and ego and reality. It was in this respect that Freud found the older topographical model, the layer model (conscious–preconscious–unconscious), rather disappointing, though in other respects it still retains a certain degree of significance. Defenses as well as drives can be unconscious; thus differences between conscious and unconscious processes cannot be used to account for these conflicts.

I thought it advisable to begin by giving a picture of certain fundamentals of psychoanalytic theory, and of the degree of its comprehensiveness, by indicating at least some of its dimensions, and also the relations between different parts of these theories. Its comprehensiveness means also its actual or potential importance in many neighboring fields. My survey shows also at least some of the points at which questions can be raised from the viewpoint of a philosophy of science. There would have been an alternative to the way of presentation I chose. I could have shown how, in the analysis of a symptom or a dream, our observations lead to anticipations, and how the various levels of our conceptual tools are brought to bear on them; also, how in this process theoretical thinking is constantly brought back to the observables. But this alternative would inevitably demand the introduction of a great number of variables and a discussion of the analytic method and the analytic situation much broader than I am able to give here. Of course, a sector of psychoanalytic propositions can be tested outside analysis, and some have been tested in this way; but it is still true that it is, in the field of analysis, extremely difficult to assay the suitability of the hypotheses for the purposes for which they have been primarily devised without the use, in the analytic situation, of the analytic method.

Since its beginnings analysis has struggled for a system of concepts fit to account for the peculiarities of the subject matter it had to deal with. Freud spoke of his endeavor to "introduce the right abstract ideas" and said, "We are constantly altering and improving them." This work has continued, and still not all concepts used are equally well defined. The distinction between independent, intervening, and dependent variables is often not clearly drawn. Also the different degrees of confirmation of the various parts of the complex network of psychoanalytic hypotheses are frequently not made apparent in analytical writings. Actually, there are many reasons for the lack of methodological strictness we often find in analysis. Some of them are encountered in every theoretical approach to the central aspects of personality. In addition, there is the fact that for psychoanalytical research there were no traditional methodological models available that could be used in its service; the differences in content as well as in method prevented a borrowing in this respect. To quote Freud again from a letter about Einstein who had paid him a visit: "He has had the support of a long series of predecessors from Newton onward, while I had to hack every step of my way through a tangled jungle alone."

Freud had a firsthand knowledge of experimental method and was thoroughly steeped in the philosophy of science of the great *Naturforscher* of his day. He was fascinated by the theories of evolution, which left their imprint on his thinking, and, of course, there must have been other factors in the intellectual climate of his "formative years" that influenced his development as a scientist. The heuristic character and value of hypotheses was well known to him, as well as the role of basic concepts and postulates. Though Freud was certainly not primarily interested in the philosophy of science, it is still true, and it has often been said by psychoanalysts and recently also by others (Frenkel-Brunswik, 10) that his "sophistication" in this respect was much greater than early reactions to his work would let one realize. But we have to consider that logical clarification is not usually found in the early development of a science and is often not the work of the great explorers (Hartmann, Kris, Loewenstein, 21). It is only more recently that it has become, for the case of analysis, a subject of particular interest to a great number of workers.

Psychoanalysis was, of course, "new" not only because of its conceptual language, its method, and the methodological problems it posed, but "new" also as to content. The reorganization of commonly accepted knowledge, as a consequence of new data having been found and new modes of thinking having been introduced and of the replacement of old scientific, or old commonsense, or socialized, "truths" by the new ones, is mostly a slow and often a difficult process. In analysis, such new insights, which do not only add to our knowledge but also force upon us a revision of old ways of thinking, abound. There is also the additional difficulty that some (not all) of its discoveries could be made only under specific conditions (the analytic situation); and known facts often appeared in confrontation with such discoveries in a different light. On the other hand, looking at these discoveries from outside analysis, it seemed difficult to "place," if I may say so, these unexpected and apparently improbable insights, their real connections with other factors being hardly understood. Attitudes toward demands for reconsideration of what had appeared to be safely anchored knowledge do not of course always observe the lines of logical thinking. Psychoanalysis has systematically studied—has, indeed, to study in every single clinical case—this problem, that is, the conditions for the capacity or incapacity to observe new phenomena in the realm of psychology and to think rationally about them. At any rate, once the shock the content of Freud's discoveries had represented to his contemporaries had somewhat subsided, people started to take them more seriously and even to attribute to them a certain amount of scientific standing. This process of rehabilitation of analysis was then fortified by the confirmation of psychoanalytic findings in medicine or child psychology, and through the proven usefulness of analytic hypotheses in these fields, as well as in anthropology, and in other social sciences. This, naturally, led to a different evaluation of the psychoanalytic method, too, which was at the origin of these discoveries, and of the psychoanalytic theories of which these hypotheses were a part.

That the newness and the scope of the psychoanalytic findings and theories made changes of concepts and the introduction of new hypotheses imperative, does not seem surprising. In his tentative formulations, Freud occasionally did not even disdain to take models of motivation from common-sense psychology. But to these common-sense elements, confronted with new facts and subjected to analytic conceptualization, mostly rather uncommon sense has accrued. It also seems, from the perspective of a few decades of empirical work, that quite a few methodologically questionable formulations have proved their heuristic value. Given the state of the psychology of personality, risks as to the development of the method, as well as of hypothesis formation, had to be taken. One could not limit the field to those parts that could already be handled in an unobjectionable way. Knowing the inherent difficulties of the subject matter, one may well be inclined to postdict that without the courage and impetus of a genius this most comprehensive attack on the explanation of human behavior that we call analysis could hardly have come about.

I said before that even today some logical uncertainties persist. This may in part be due to the lack of trained clarifiers, as E. Kris (24) has said. We have also to consider that the methodological demands made on science, the signposts which indicate which routes are open and which prohibited, which ways are likely to lead to dead ends, are generally geared to the logically best-developed branches of science. These we rightly admire as models of methodological clarity (which is not to deny that even there methodological controversies arise). Progress in physics, or in biology, has repeatedly led to demands on psychoanalysis for reformulation of its theories in accordance with these developments in other sciences. There is no reason of principle that such borrowings could not enrich the tools or the clarity of analytic thinking, as has happened with other models. But this question is less one of the theory of science, than of the, we could say, "practical" needs of a specific science—the empirical question of the fitness of certain elements of logically well-structured sciences for other less developed fields. There is also, of course, the question of the necessarily different consideration of different fields. There is the need to outline a fruitful methodological approach to the less systematized sciences, to allow maximal productivity on a given level of insight into the relations between fact and hypothesis and according to the degrees of formal organization.

Before discussing in a more general way the relations between data and theories in psychoanalysis, I next shall speak of one of the inherent difficulties of our field. Every psychologist is confronted with the problem of how knowledge of the mental processes of others can be achieved. (I am not speaking here of the possibility of knowing another person's subjective experience.) As to our own mental processes some do—and some don't—refer to "self-experience." For those who do, a further difficulty is introduced if, as is the case in psychoanalysis, self-experience is accepted on principle, but its cognitive value remains in doubt. That is, it is a question of further investigation as to what is the indicative value of a given element of self-perception in terms of mental process. Looked at from this angle, analysis can be termed a systematic study of self-deception and its motivations. This implies that thinking about our own mental processes can be found to be true or false. There is in analysis, as you know, the concept of "rationalization," to give you an example. While self-experience is obviously an important element in analysis, its theories, as I said before, transcend this level of discourse.

The lawlike propositions of metapsychology are not formulated on the level of self-experience. Generally, Freud's views on introspection have not always been clearly appreciated. They are, though, evident already in the kind of psychoanalytic thinking that is comparatively close to observational data, as in Freud's ideas on the psychopathology of everyday life. In a slip of the tongue, for instance, when, in place of a word we consciously intended to use, another one, not consciously intended, appears, we use the behavioral aspect in evaluating the psychological situation—we use it, that is, in taking the word actually spoken as an indication of an unconscious motivation that takes precedence over the conscious one.

The data gathered in the psychoanalytic situation with the help of the psychoanalytic method are primarily behavioral data; and the aim is clearly the exploration of human behavior. The data are mostly the patient's verbal behavior, but include other kinds of action. They include his silences, his postures (F. Deutsch, 7), and his movements in general, more specifically his expressive movements. While analysis aims at an explanation of human behavior, those data, however, are interpreted in analysis in terms of mental processes, of motivation, of "meaning"; there is, then, a clear-cut difference between this approach and the one usually called "behavioristic," and this difference is even more marked if we consider the beginnings of behaviorism, rather than its more recent formulations.

As to the data, it is hard to give, outside the analytic process itself, an impression of the wealth of observational data collected in even one single "case." One frequently refers to the comparatively small number of cases studied in analysis and tends to forget the very great number of actual observations on which we base, in every individual case, the interpretations of an aspect of a person's character, symptoms and so on.*

By keeping certain variables in the analytic situation, if not constant, as close to constancy as the situation allows, it becomes easier to evaluate the significance of other variables that enter the picture. The best-studied example of this is what is called the "passivity" of the analyst, in contradistinction to the considerably more pronounced activity of the psychotherapist. This is not to claim that psychoanalysis is an experimental discipline. However, there are situations where it comes close to it. At any rate, there is sufficient evidence for the statement that our ob-

* Thus every single clinical "case" represents, for research, hundreds of data of observed regularities, and in hundreds of respects.

servations in the psychoanalytic situation, set in the context of psychoanalytic experience and hypotheses, make predictions possible—predictions of various degrees of precision or reliability, but as a rule superior to any others that have been attempted in the psychology of personality. Due to the emphasis on the genetic viewpoint, many predictions are what has been called "predictions of the past," (Hartmann, Kris, 20) that is, reconstructions of the past which can often be confirmed in astonishing detail (Bonaparte, 6). One obvious limitation of our predictive potential is, of course, the great number of factors determining, according to psychoanalytic theory, every single element of behavior—what Freud has termed "overdetermination." Still, our technique is constantly directed by tentative predictions of the patient's reactions. Also, studies in developmental psychology by means of direct child observation, such as have been conducted by E. Kris and other psychoanalysts (M. Kris, 26), are guided by the formulation of expectations and their checking in individual cases. Here I just want to point to one way in which psychoanalytic hypotheses can be used vis-à-vis individual cases and how they may be confirmed in clinical experience. I may mention here that problems of validation of psychoanalytic hypotheses ought not to be equated, as has too often been done, with the problem of therapeutic success.

A further difficulty results from the fact that psychoanalytic theory has also to deal with the relation between observer and observed in the analytic situation. There are personality layers, if you will excuse this term, that in the average case the observed cannot reach without the help of the observer and his method of observation. But the insight of the observer ought not to be confused with the insight of the observed. Some of these problems belong in a theory of psychoanalytic technique. But there is also the problem of the "personal equation" (Hartmann, 18; Kris, 25). The field of observation includes not only the patient, but also the observer who interacts with the former ("participant observation"). The interaction of analyst and analysand are accounted for in the theories of transference and countertransference. As to the potential handicaps of observations traceable to the mental processes of the observer, they are subject to the constant scrutiny of the analyst. Some such handicaps of psychological observation can certainly be eliminated by the personal analysis of the observer, and this is one of the reasons that a didactic analysis is an essential element in the training of our students of analysis. Thus, what I want to say here is not that in the psychology of personality objectivity is impossible. It is rather that psychoanalysis has discovered potential sources of error and found a way to combat them.

Distortions of self-observation as well as of observations of others that occur as consequences of instinctual pressure are clinically easily traceable, and can be accounted for by analytic theory. To one aspect of this problem we find a close analogy in the behavior of animals: the "world" of the hungry animal is different from the "world" of the same animal in heat. In man, following structure formation, the situation is more complex. How much we can perceive psychologically with respect to ourselves and others, and how we perceive it, is also determined by defensive and other functions we attribute to the ego; and the superego, too, can influence our perceptive range and lead to distortions. The influence of central personality factors—needs, desires, affective states—on perception in general (not just in the psychological field) has also been experimentally demonstrated; and how, despite this, "objective" perception is possible is an object of special study (G. Klein, 23). The questions of objectivation and of "testing of reality," as Freud called it, are also accounted for in psychoanalytic theory and lead again to the concept of degrees of ego autonomy that I mentioned before.

The body of analytic theories on the "mental apparatus" must include, as an essential sector, hypotheses fit to explain the distortions of psychological observation. No doubt this involvement of the observer, and the potential sources of error of his perception and judgment, represent an added difficulty in analytic clinic and research. But it is well known that even in other fields, and often in a troubling degree, this problem plays a role. However, this complication we are confronted with in analysis is an essential feature of certain aspects of human behavior rather than a result of imperfections of the state of psychoanalytic theory. There is, as I have said, also a psychologically fruitful side to these same complexities that have led to some methodological discontent. Correction of at least some distortions of psychological observation and thinking are within the reach of our method. In the so far most comprehensive study of Freud's development, his biography by Ernest Jones, the role of his self-analysis in the unfolding of his thought has been emphasized. Now, self-analysis has this function only in exceptional cases; but we have similar experiences in great numbers from the analysis of others. In a more diluted way, this correction of blind spots can even occasionally be achieved outside analysis, as a consequence of changing attitudes toward certain factors that are essential for a psychology of personality.

It is very likely that in the work of Freud and other analysts such unaccountable insights have occurred. If so, it is clear that, certainly with Freud, his striving for scientific discipline, his patient accumulation of observational data, and his search for conceptual tools to account for them have reduced their importance to a stimulus factor in the formation of psychoanalytic theories. Many subjects approached in analysis, had, before Freud, been studied by so-called intuitive psychology only. But he was wont to oppose psychoanalytic psychology to intuitive psychology and the development psychoanalysis has taken bears out this point. Still the relation between data and theory is no doubt a rather complex one in psychoanalysis. There are the cases in which, mostly in the beginning, he approached a problem with what he called "a few psychological formulae," that is tentative hypotheses, whose heuristic value must be determined. To give you one example: certain clinical observations on hysterical patients had been made by Breuer before Freud, and also by Janet. But these discoveries were viewed from the angle of dynamic unconscious processes of conflict and defense only by Freud. It was with him and not with the others who had made similar observations that they opened the way to the understanding of mental conflict in general, which was later found to be an essential factor in normal and abnormal development. Here the introduction of fruitful hypotheses was decisive for the scientific momentum of a discovery (Hartmann). It led to an integration of the observed facts and also to the discovery of new facts. It is true in psychoanalysis as elsewhere that theories cannot be considered as mere summaries of observations. Actually, "the storehouse of pre-existing knowledge influences our expectations" and often "preconscious expectations . . . direct the selection of what is to be registered as observation and what seems to require explanation" (Hartmann, Kris, Loewenstein). It is also obvious in psychoanalysis that the psychoanalytic investigator "must know that every step of his progress depends on his advances in the sphere of theory, and on the conceptual consistency, breadth and depth reached herein" (K. Lewin).

In dealing with new observations and often new hypotheses it has become unavoidable to redefine the meaning of many concepts in analysis and to add new ones. Some concepts that have meaningfully been used, let's say, in studying the psychology of lower animals in experimental situations are less fit if we deal with human behavior. Also, concepts common in everyday usage, in medicine, in philosophy, had to be redefined for psychoanalytic purposes. I mention this here, because it has sometimes made interdisciplinary communication more difficult. Thus, as I said before, the concept of instinctual drives has been radically modified. And there are redefinitions, in analysis, also of the concepts of libido, of anxiety and others. To this, I may quote W. Heisenberg's statement that "the transition . . . from previously investigated fields to new ones will never consist simply of the application of already known laws to these new fields. On the contrary, a really new field of experience will always lead to the crystallization of a new system of scientific concepts and laws."

The fact that the analyst's observations are made in a clinical setting has clearly, in more ways than one, determined the development of the scientific aspect of psychoanalysis. The psychological object is studied in a real-life situation: the patient comes to another person, the analyst, in the hope of being freed from limitations of his capacity for work and his enjoyment of life, imposed by changes in his personality that are considered pathological but remediable. This means readiness for hundreds of hours of work and for being confronted with his life history, with parts of his personality that have been repressed, and, generally, with many surprising and often unpleasant insights into his mental processes. In the therapeutic situation, motivations are mobilized that help to combat the natural resistance against objective scrutiny of one's self. Such motivations can hardly be expected to be available outside a real-life situation; actually the many attempts outside of analysis to create, for purposes of investigation, situations meant to mimic situations of real life, have not led very far. This point, then, refers chiefly to the superiority of analysis in making data available and creating a readiness for their observation.

On the other hand, it is good to remember Freud's reactions when after years of experimental work he decided to follow his research interests in the clinical field (and the quite similar reactions we meet today in young scientists turning to psychoanalysis). "He (Freud) confessed to a feeling of *discomfort.* He who had been trained in the school of experimental sciences was writing what read like a novel. Not personal references, he said, but the subject matter forced such a presentation on him" (Kris, 24). He was confronted with a mostly unexplored field, with human motivations, human needs and conflicts. "Everywhere," he said later, "I seemed to discern motives and tendencies analogous to those of everyday life." Some concepts of common-sense psychology which, as I said before, were tentatively applied, had to be redefined, though the terms were sometimes retained. Thus common-sense psychology soon proved insufficient; nor could the scientific psychology of his day and its methodology be of great help. Freud had only what he called a "few psychological formulae," or hypotheses, to guide him. But it was only after the special and the more general theories of analysis had been developed that the full meaning could be extracted from the clinical data he had gathered.

There is always something ambiguous about the meaning of "clinical research" in general. There exists, so far as I know, no really satisfactory presentation of the subject in terms of the philosophy of science. I just want to say here a word about Freud's case histories, whose style of thinking is, however, unique and has hardly ever been successfully imitated. Every one of his comprehensive case histories is at the same time a study in psychoanalytic theory. I mention them at this point because they show the constant mutual promotion of observation and hypothesis formation, the formation of definite propositions which make our knowledge testable, and the attempts to validate or invalidate them.

Another aspect of the clinical origins of psychoanalytic theory is the fact that more was found, in the beginning, about pathological than about normal behavior. The etiology of neurosis was studied before the etiology of health, though psychoanalysis has, on principle, always aimed at a comprehensive general psychology. Also, as I mentioned, more became known, in the first attempts to deal with the field, about the instinctual drives, especially about sexuality and its development, than about the forces opposing the drives in the typical ego–id conflicts. This, however, has changed in the last two or three decades, and analysis thus has today come closer to what it always was intended to be, though not every aspect and not every implication of its very comprehensive conceptual frame has so far been actually developed.

In clinical work, one is used to being guided by signs and symptoms in forming an opinion on the presence or absence of a pathological process. But the question of the significance and the use of signs for purposes of explanation is, of course, logically of much wider relevance. Different meanings can be attributed to the terms sign, signal, expressive sign, symbol, and so on, and these differences are important also in psychoanalysis. However, I don't propose to deal with this problem here. Suffice it to say that a considerable part of psychoanalytic work can be described as the use of signs—a series of associations, a dream, an affect vis-à-vis the analyst—as indications of mental processes. In this sense one speaks of the psychoanalytic method as a method of interpretation (Hartmann, 14; Bernfeld, 4; Loewenstein, 28). This has both a cognitive and a therapeutic aspect. They partly coincide, that is, in so far as a therapeutic agent of foremost significance in analysis is making the patient aware of, and capable of integrating, previously unconscious and, through defense, split-off processes. Some of those signs, for example, some of the symbols we find in dreams, have a rather ubiquitous meaning, while the interpretation of others requires a closer scrutiny of the individual under observation. At any rate, there are many situations in which the relation between a sign and what it signifies becomes easily recognizable, for instance in the associations immediately following the observation of some detail of behavior. In others, various levels of theory have to be introduced to explain the connection. Such sign systems are used today not only in the psychoanalytic situation, but also in the study by analysts, by means of direct observation, of child development. Many childhood situations of incisive significance for the formation of the adult personality have a low probability of direct manifestation. One tries to learn about the sign function of data of child behavior for a recognition of the central, and often unconscious, development that we know from the psychoanalytic interview (Hartmann, 18). At this point it is possible, or even likely, that a misunderstanding may occur of what I have said about a low probability of manifestation outside analysis of certain processes investigated in analysis. I want, then, to add explicitly that this was not meant to be a general statement. Many phenomena first studied in the analytic situation could later be studied also in the direct observation of psychotics, in so-called applied psychoanalysis, or in the direct observation of children. What I want to emphasize in this context is that the comparative study of reconstructive data and data of direct observation of children leads, on the one hand, to the confirmation of analytical propositions; on the other hand it leads to the formulation of more specific hypotheses.

The essential importance of constructs for the coherence of the psychoanalytic system (or whatever we choose to call it) can be gathered already from the brief outline I have given in the first part of this discussion. Theories, or hypotheses of a different order, connect them with observational data. That these constructs, which are introduced because of their explanatory value, cannot be directly defined in terms of observational data, but that inferences from the constructs can be tested by observation, has long been known in psychoanalysis (Hartmann, 14). Still, some of these constructs seem particularly suspect to many critics of analysis. An occasional lack of caution in the formulation of its propositions, or Freud's liking for occasional striking metaphors, has led to the accusation against analysis of an anthropomorphization of its concepts. But in all those cases a more careful formulation can be substituted which will dispel this impression.

There is, then, the question whether and in what sense such constructs are considered "real"; and, more specifically, the question has often been asked whether and in what sense Freud considered constructs like libido, the "system unconscious," and the substructures of personality in the sense of structural psychology, as real. He said that the basic concepts of science form rather the roof than the foundation of science and ought to be changed when they no longer seem able to account for experience; also that they have the character of conventions. But he certainly thought that what he meant to cover by these basic concepts had effects which could be observed. He was in no danger of confusing concepts with realities; he was a "realist" in a different sense. He does not seem to have thought that "real" means just "the simplest theoretical presentation of our experiences," but rather that those basic concepts pointed to something real in the ordinary sense of the word.

It is quite possible that Freud, as Frenkel-Brunswik (10) has remarked on "scientists of great ingenuity," sometimes proceeded "from observation directly to hypothetical constructs and . . . derived the intervening variables later." But it is also evident from Freud's work that he by no means always spelled out the ways in which he had arrived at the formulation of his constructs. It is hard to say in a general way under what conditions a direct transition from data to constructs would seem legitimate or fruitful. It has been suggested by Ellis (9) that "where intervening variables are of a limited usefulness in scientific theorizing, hypothetical constructs take in the widest range of relevant phenomena, lead to a maximum success in the prediction and explanation of behavior."

It is obvious that among the intervening variables "dispositional concepts" play a significant role in analysis. The term "mental disposition" has actually been used in analysis, but the same kind of concept is often also covered by different terms. It has been pointed out (Hartmann, 14) that the concept of "latent attitudes" used by Koffka and others comes rather close to psychoanalytic thinking. The term mental tendency is ubiquitous in psychoanalysis, and many of these tendencies, as mentioned before, are understood to be not manifest but in the nature of a disposition.

Speaking now of the series independent–intervening–dependent variable, I want to quote to you a passage from Rapaport (30) about a significant aspect of intervening variables in analysis, which states clearly the point I have in mind: "Let us assume that an aggressive drive is our independent variable and overt behavior towards an (actual or thought) object our dependent variable. It will be noted that in a certain subject at certain intensities of the drive we will observe aggressive behavior (in deed or thought) toward the object, at other intensities we will observe no overtly aggressive behavior but rather excessive kindness (reaction formation). In other subjects at certain intensities the aggressive behavior will be diverted from the object to other objects (displacement) or upon their own self (turning round upon the subject), or will be replaced by ideas and feelings of being aggressed by the other (projection). In these observations the defense of reaction-formation, displacement, turning round upon the subject, projection, etc., will be conceptualized as intervening variables." Here let me remind you of what I said before, that the explanation of manifest behavior presupposes in every single case the consideration of a great number of variables. The statement, current in analysis, that the same manifest action, attitude, fantasy may have different "meanings" (that is, may be the result of the interaction of different tendencies) has often been misunderstood. It has been said that it opens the door to bias or arbitrary interpretation. This argument seems to neglect the point I have just made. What the psychoanalytic approach has shown is a complex interdependence of a variety of factors, and of patterns of factors. I may mention too, in this context, that working with unilinear causal relations alone has not always proved satisfactory. The essential fact of interdependence of mental functions does not always allow a clear-cut answer to the question of which variable has to be considered as independent and which one as an intervening variable. A stimulus from the outside world will sometimes be considered an independent variable; but in another context it may be considered also an instinctual tendency or an autonomous tendency of the ego (Rapaport, 30). We came across this problem of relative independence in speaking of the secondary autonomy of the ego, but it has a much wider significance in psychoanalytic psychology.

Turning now to the validation of psychoanalytic hypotheses, I shall follow Kris (24) in distinguishing validations in analysis from validations outside of it. To begin with the former, I may repeat that the amount of time spent in the study of any single individual is vastly greater, and the wealth of data considerably richer, than in any other clinical set-up. This alone would make the use of the analytic method in the analytic situation the *via regia* to the psychology of personality. In this setting, data do appear which are not, or not easily, accessible to other methods. This asset as to fact-finding has, of course, a disadvantage in another respect: an observation an analyst makes may seem entirely credible to another analyst who possesses the necessary experience, an interpretation quite convincing, while the same observation may appear hardly credible, the same interpretation highly improbable or artificial, to one who approaches the field with a different method and in a different setting. For the analyst, one constant angle of his work is the observation of data and of sequences of data, the tentative interpretations (in search of the common elements in such sequences), and the checking of his interpretation against the subsequent (and past) material. It is safe to say that the greater part of evidence for the psychoanalytic propositions still lies with this work.

To broaden the reach of intersubjective validation beyond the relatively small group of workers in psychoanalysis, and also for teaching purposes and for comparing different techniques, the recording of interviews has been recommended by many (Kubie, 27) and practiced by some. More recently, records of analytic interviews were submitted to other analysts, who were asked to predict the developments in subsequent sessions (L. Bellak). Such studies are likely gradually to attract a greater number of research workers, but, for the present, their potential contribution to the scientific status of analysis cannot yet be estimated.

As to the genetic propositions of analysis, the direct observation of children has not only become a rich source of information, but also given us the possibility to make our hypotheses more specific and to check their validity. A great number of Freud's hypotheses on childhood could be confirmed by direct observation of children. But to validate more completely our genetic propositions, "systematic observations of life histories from birth on" are necessary. "If the longitudinal observation in our own civilization were to be systematized and the study of life histories were to be combined with that of the crucial situations in Freud's sense, many hunches might be formulated as propositions, and others might be discarded" (Hartmann and Kris, 20).

The literature on experimental research, both in animals and in man, devised for the purpose of testing propositions derived from psychoanalysis has become very extensive. It has been repeatedly reviewed (Sears, 31; Kris, 24; Benjamin, 3; Frenkel-Brunswik, 10; and others), and I do not think I should go into it in any detail here. The following remarks are, then, random remarks and do not attempt to be in any way systematic. The classical animal experiments of Hunt, Levy, Miller, Masserman are probably known to many of you. Many of the animal experiments were conducted with considerable insight and great skill. Where the experimental set-up is adequate, the frequency of "confirmation" is impressive. Or, as Hilgard (22) states, "It has been possible to parallel many psychoanalytic phenomena in the laboratory. When this is done, the correspondence between predictions according to psychoanalytic theory and what is found is on the whole very satisfactory."

Of course, we would not expect that every psychoanalytic proposition can be tested in animal experiments (Frenkel-Brunswik, 10). But there are also definite limitations to so-called "experimental psychoanalysis" in the human. It appears difficult (though it has been attempted occasionally) to study "real" conflicts with the tools that "experimental psychoanalysis" has at its disposal (Hartmann and Kris, 20; Kris, 25). And I may insert here that even experimentation that tends to remain close to "life situations," as does the work of K. Lewin, Dembo, Zeigarnik and others, is not quite free from those limitations.

A rather harsh criticism of Sears's "Survey" has been voiced by Wisdom (32). But also with others who do not share his point of view, a certain amount of dissatisfaction has become apparent (A. Freud, 11; Rapaport, 30; Kubie, 27). Sometimes in those experiments the hypotheses tested were not psychoanalytic propositions at all, though the author had meant them to be. Sometimes they were taken over literally from psychoanalytic writings, but the context in which they appear in analysis, and thus their function, being not sufficiently considered, the results had to be ambiguous. It also happened that, looked at from the vantage point of analysis, experiments could be considered as validations of certain points in analysis, though not of those the author had in mind. In evaluating the results of "experimental analysis," there is, in addition, the perspectival character of every method to be considered, highlighting certain aspects and throwing others into the shade. Every method implies a selection, and data are being centered in different ways, depending on our approach (Hartmann, 18; Rapaport, 30). That is, an analysis of the methods used, and an attempt to correlate them, becomes of prime importance.

On the whole, this field of research has not so far decisively contributed toward a clarification or systematization of psychoanalytic theory. As a rule, these studies do not go beyond what has been demonstrated in analysis before (Hilgard, 22, and Kubie, 27); they have often not achieved new insights nor stimulated research. But, at their best, they have a value as confirmatory (or nonconfirmatory) evidence. Apart from this, they have greatly contributed to bridging the gap between psychoanalysis and other psychological disciplines. Also, "experimental psychoanalysis" continues to expand, and there is the possibility that certain drawbacks of its beginnings will be overcome.

Another source of potentially fruitful contacts is the confrontation of psychoanalysis with learning theory. Thus Dollard and Miller (8) have attempted "to give a systematic analysis of neurosis and psychotherapy in terms of the psychological principles and social conditions of learning." They concentrate their study on Freudian principles, and the theorist of analysis, though often disagreeing, will profit from this and similar ventures.

This review of experimental checking of psychoanalytic hypotheses is admittedly a sketch only. But even if it were not, even if I had given the full picture, it would remain beyond doubt that the main body of evidence does not rest on these studies, but on the wealth of empirical data gathered by the analytic method in the analytic situation. The task to better define his concepts, to work toward a higher level of clarification and systematization of his hypotheses, rests, in the main, still with the analyst. This is, of course, far from saying that attempts at validation using extra-analytical methods, or criticisms originating in points of view different from those of analysis, are not to be welcomed by analysis. It is to be hoped, though, in the interest of sound interdisciplinary communication, that these criticisms, more than has often been the case in the past, will be based on a close familiarity with the methods of analysis, with the special nature of its subject matter, and with the role theorizing has played and plays in its development.

Bibliography

1. Adrian, E. D., "The Mental and the Physical Origins of Behaviour," *International Journal of Psychoanalysis,* XXVII, 1946.

2. Allport, G., *Personality.* New York: Henry Holt, 1937.

3. Benjamin, J., "Methodological Considerations in the Validation and Elaboration of Psychoanalytical Personality Theory." *American Journal of Orthopsychiatry,* 20, 1950.

4. Bernfeld, S., "Der Begriff der Deutung in der Psychoanalyse," *Zeitschrift für Angewandte Psychologie,* XLII, 1932.

5. ———, "Freud's Earliest Theories and the School of Helmholtz," *Psychoanalytic Quarterly,* XIII, 1944.

6. Bonaparte, M., "Notes on the Analytical Discovery of a Primal Scene," *Psychoanalytic Study of the Child,* I, 1945.

7. Deutsch, F., "Analytic Posturology." *Psychoanalytic Quarterly,* XXI, 1952.

8. Dollard, J. and Miller, N. E., *Personality and Psychotherapy.* New York: McGraw-Hill, 1950.

9. Ellis, A., *An Introduction to the Principles of Scientific Psychoanalysis,* Genetic Psychology Monograph, 41, 1950.

10. Frenkel-Brunswik, E., *Psychoanalysis and the Unity of Science,* Proceedings of the American Academy of Arts and Sciences, 80, 1954.

11. Freud, A., "The Contributions of Psychoanalysis to Genetic Psychology," *American Journal of Orthopsychiatry,* XXI, 1951.

12. Freud, S., *The Claim of Psychoanalysis to Scientific Interest.* London: Hogarth Press, Standard Edition, Vol. XIII.

13. ———, *Psycho-Analysis.* London: Hogarth Press, Standard Edition, Vol. XVIII.

14. HARTMANN, H., *Die Grundlagen der Psychoanalyse*. Leipzig, 1927.

15. ———, "Ichpsychologie und Anpassungsproblem," *Internationale Zeitschrift für Psychoanalyse*, XXIV, 1939. Partly translated in: D. Rapaport, *Organization and Pathology of Thought*. New York: Columbia University Press, 1951.

16. ———, "Comments on the Psychoanalytic Theory of Instinctual Drives," *Psychoanalytic Quarterly*, XVII, 1948.

17. ———, "Comments on the Psychoanalytic Theory of the Ego," *Psychoanalytic Study of the Child*, V, 1950.

18. ———, "Psychoanalysis and Developmental Psychology," *Psychoanalytic Study of the Child*, V, 1950.

19. ———, "The Development of the Ego Concept in Freud's Work," *International Journal of Psychoanalysis*, XXXVII, 1956.

20. ——— and Kris, E., "The Genetic Approach in Psychoanalysis," *Psychoanalytic Study of the Child*, I, 1945.

21. ———, Kris, E. and Loewenstein, R., "Comments on the Formation of Psychic Structure," *Psychoanalytic Study of the Child*, II, 1946.

22. HILGARD, E., "Experimental Approaches to Psychoanalysis," in: *Psychoanalysis as Science*, ed. E. Pumpian-Mindlin. Stanford University Press, 1952.

23. KLEIN, G., "Cognizant Style and Motivation," in: *Assessment of Human Motives*, ed. G. Lindzey. New York: Rinehart, 1958.

24. KRIS, E., "The Nature of Psychoanalytic Propositions and their Validation," in: *Freedom and Experience*, ed. S. Hook and M. R. Konvitz, Cornell University Press, 1947.

25. ———, "Notes on the Development and on some Current Problems of Psychoanalytic Child Psychology," *Psychoanalytic Study of the Child*, V, 1950.

26. KRIS, M., "The Use of Prediction in a Longitudinal Study," *Psychoanalytic Study of the Child*, XII, 1957.

27. KUBIE, L., "Problems and Techniques of Psychoanalytic Validation and Progress," in: *Psychoanalysis as Science*, ed. E. Pumpian-Mindlin. Stanford University Press, 1952.

28. LOEWENSTEIN, R., "Some Thoughts on Interpretation in the Theory and Practice of Psychoanalysis," *Psychoanalytic Study of the Child*, XII, 1957.

29. MISES, R. v., *Kleines Lehrbuch des Positivismus*. The Hague, 1939.

30. RAPAPORT, D., "The Structure of Psychoanalytic Theory (A Systematizing Attempt)," in: *Psychology: A Study of a Science*, ed. S. Koch. New York: McGraw-Hill, 1958, Vol. III.

31. SEARS, R., "Survey of Objective Studies of Psychoanalytic Concepts," Social Sciences Research Council *Bulletin*, 1943, 51.

32. WISDOM, J., *Philosophy and Psycho-Analysis*. New York: Philosophical Library, 1953.

2.

Methodological Issues in Psychoanalytic Theory

ERNEST NAGEL
John Dewey Professor of Philosophy
Columbia University

DR. HARTMANN'S comprehensive paper makes amply clear that psychoanalytic theory is intended to be a theory of human behavior in the same sense of "theory" that, for example, the molecular theory of gases is a set of assumptions which systematizes, explains, and predicts certain observable phenomena of gases. Accordingly, he is in effect inviting us to evaluate the merits of Freudian theory by standards of intellectual cogency similar to those we employ in judging theories in other areas of positive science. It would of course be absurdly pedantic to apply to Freudian theory the yardstick of rigor and precision current in mathematical and experimental physics. Proper allowance must certainly be made for the notorious difficulties encountered in all inquiries into distinctively human behavior, and for what is perhaps an inevitable fuzziness of all generalizations about human conduct. Nevertheless, unless I have misconstrued the burden of Dr. Hartmann's paper, no apology is required for raising substantially the same kinds of issues of fact and logic concerning Freudian theory that are pertinent to a general examination of the cognitive worth and standing of a theory in the natural or social sciences.

However, I am not a professional psychologist. I have neither been psychoanalyzed nor am I a profound scholar of psychoanalytic literature, and I am therefore not competent to discuss the detailed observational data upon which Freudian theory supposedly rests. In any event, my interest in Freudian theory is

Notes to this section begin on page 55.

primarily methodological; and my aim in this discussion is to raise two related groups of logical questions concerning which I would very much like to receive instruction. The first group deals with issues relating to the logical structure and empirical content of psychoanalytic theory, and especially of the so-called "metapsychology" to which Dr. Hartmann's paper is so largely devoted. The second group of questions is concerned with the general nature of the evidence that is used to support the theory. The two groups of issues nevertheless do not fall into watertight compartments, so that I have not found it possible in discussing questions in the first set to avoid entirely considerations belonging to the second.

I

Freudian theory maintains, and I think rightly so, that it is not possible to account for most human conduct exclusively in terms either of manifest human traits or of conscious motives and intentions. Accordingly, the theory introduces a number of assumptions containing terms that ostensibly refer to matters neither manifest nor conscious, and that are not explicitly definable by way of what is manifest and conscious. In so far as Freudian theory employs notions of this kind which do not describe anything observable (let me call such notions "theoretical" ones for the sake of brevity), the theory is quite like the molecular theory of gases or the gene theory of heredity. I do not think, therefore, that there is any substance in those criticisms of Freudian theory which object to the theory *merely* on the ground that it uses theoretical notions.

a) My first difficulty with Freudian theory nevertheless is generated by the fact that while it is unobjectionable for a theory to be couched in terms of theoretical notions, the theory does not seem to me to satisfy two requirements which any theory must satisfy if it is to be capable of empirical validation. I must state these requirements briefly. In the first place, it must be possible to deduce determinate consequences from the assumptions of theory, so that one can decide on the basis of logical considerations, and prior to the examination of any empirical data, whether or not an alleged consequence of the theory is indeed implied by the latter. For unless this requirement is fulfilled, the theory has no definite content, and questions as to what the theory asserts cannot be settled except by recourse to some privileged authority or arbitrary caprice. In the second place, even though the theoretical notions are not explicitly defined by way of overt empirical procedures and observable traits of things, nevertheless at least *some* theoretical notions must be *tied down* to *fairly definite and unambiguously specified* observable materials, by way of rules of procedure variously called "correspondence rules," "coordinating definitions," and "operational definitions." For if this condition is not satisfied, the theory can have no determinate consequences about *empirical* subject matter. An immediate corollary to these requirements is that since a consistent theory cannot imply two incompatible consequences, a credible theory must not only be *confirmed* by observational evidence, but it must also be capable of being *negated* by such evidence. In short, a theory must not be formulated in such a manner that it can always be construed and manipulated so as to explain whatever the actual facts are, no matter whether controlled observation shows one state of affairs to obtain or its opposite.

In respect to both of these requirements, however, Freudian theory in general, and the metapsychology in particular, seem to me to suffer from serious shortcomings. I lack the time to argue the matter at length, and some examples must suffice to illustrate the nature of my difficulties.

i) Dr. Hartmann has stated for us the four classes of assumptions that constitute metapsychology; and among the energic principles he mentions the following two: "The drives [in particular "sexuality" and "aggression"] are the main sources of energy in the mental apparatus"; and, secondly, "The regulation of energies in the mental apparatus follows the pleasure principle ["the tendency to immediate discharge"] the reality principle [i.e., "considerations of reality"] derived from it under the influence of ego-development, and a tendency to keep the level of excitation constant, or at a minimum." Now is it really possible to deduce from these assumptions, even when they are conjoined with the remaining ones, any *determinate* conclusions in the familiar sense of "deduce"? For example, can one conclude anything even as to the general conditions under which the sexual drive will discharge its "energy," rather than (to use Freud's own locutions) combine with the aggressive drive to form a "compromise" or have its "level of excitation" raised because of "considerations of reality"? My question is not whether, *after* the theoretical general conditions for such alternatives have been ascertained in some independent manner, it is possible to assign corresponding "degrees of strength" to the drives and the restraining influence of the ego, so that the alleged "conclusions" will then in effect be *explicitly* contained in the premises. It is, I take it, no great feat to play the role of Epimetheus. My query is whether such conclusions can be deduced from the theory *prior* to knowing just what consequences the theory must have if it is to be in agreement with assumed matters of fact.

I will not conceal my doubts about the possibility of obtaining such conclusions from the theory, although I admit that all sorts of things may be *suggested* by its assumptions. The reason for my doubts is that the theory is stated in language so vague and metaphorical that almost anything appears to be compatible with it. I am not objecting to the use of metaphors *per se,* for I am fully aware of the great heuristic values of metaphors and analogies in the construction and development of theories in all departments of science. My point is the different one that in Freudian theory metaphors are employed without even half-way definite rules for expanding them, and that in consequence admitted metaphors such as "energy" or "level of excitation" have no specific content and can be filled in to suit one's fancy. In short, Freudian formulations seem to me to have so much "open texture," to be so loose in statement, that while they are unquestionably suggestive, it is well-nigh impossible to decide whether what is thus suggested is genuinely implied by the theory or whether it is related to the latter only by the circumstance that someone *happens* to associate one with the other. I appreciate the fact that considerations of time alone would have prevented Dr. Hartmann from giving us a less opaque formulation of the principles of metapsychology. Unfortunately, I have not found that the point of my comment is blunted by comparable statements by Freud himself.[1]

ii) Dr. Hartmann is himself quite aware of the difficulty I am raising, as is evident from his references to the notion of overdetermination, as well as from his comments on the passage he quotes from Rapaport. Now I agree that if aggressive drive is taken to be the independent theoretical variable in a given case, there is no necessary incompatibility between maintaining, on the one hand, that a certain intensity of the drive in an individual is manifested by overtly aggressive behavior, and also maintaining, on the other hand, that other intensities of the drive in that individual are manifested by excessive kindness in his conduct. For the differences in overt behavior may be accounted for in terms of different intensities in the drive, perhaps in conjunction with additional stipulated differences. What is by no means clear, however, is that the allegedly different intensities of the drive are not postulated *ad hoc* and *ex post facto,* and that without *antecedent* knowledge of just how a given individual will behave, relatively unambiguous statements about his overt behavior can nevertheless be deduced from the hypotheses of the theory when appropriate initial conditions are supplied.

In any event, there is an uncomfortable ambiguity in the way the theoretical notion of aggressive drive appears to be associated with observable behavior. This ambiguity is equally present in the rules of correspondence for the notion of sexual drive, which is sometimes coordinated with almost any form of *sensuality.* A similar lack of even moderate precision can be noted in the correspondence rules Freud seems to have proposed for the theoretical notions of the id, the ego and the superego. I do not have the time to discuss the vague way in which these theoretical notions are themselves formulated, nor the amazingly loose way in which their postulated interrelations are specified. But it will be instructive to consider briefly the coordinating definitions

Freud appears to have had in mind for them. According to him, the id represents the influence of heredity, the superego corresponds to the moral standards of society, and the ego represents the accidental and current events of an individual's own experience.[2] I construe this account as an attempt to provide "operational definitions" for these theoretical notions. If I am right in this assumption, one cannot help being impressed by the extraordinary vagueness of the correspondence rules. Just how is one to distinguish in the gross behavior of an individual those features which are responses, for example, to the impact of current events, from those features which are the outcome of social pressures? It seems to me that in general the distinctions are enormously vague, and that the line between them can be drawn only in an arbitrary manner. Even if one overlooks the imprecise way in which the theoretical notions are themselves specified, it is difficult to see how conclusions about manifest behavior—ostensibly deduced from metapsychology on the basis of such rules of correspondence—can be anything but the products of a large measure of arbitrary decision.

iii) My final example is also drawn from Freud. Freud claimed that the analysis of dreams reveals "ideational contents" in the dreamer's unconscious that could not have been acquired in either the dreamer's adult or childhood experiences. Freud therefore maintained that "we are obliged to regard it as part of the *archaic heritage* which a child brings with him into the world, before any experiences of his own, as a result of the experiences of his ancestors." [3] He also declared that "this state of affairs is made more difficult, it is true, by the present attitude of biological science, which rejects the idea of acquired qualities being transmitted to descendents. I admit, in all modesty, that in spite of this I cannot picture biological development proceeding without taking this factor into account." [4] Well, in all modesty myself, I must therefore ask whether the statement that some acquired characteristics are biologically inherited follows from Freudian theory when the latter is conjoined with a number of initial conditions. If it does, and apparently Freud believed it does, and since the biological evidence indicates that the statement is false, why does not this fact constitute a refutation of the premises of the argument? It may indeed be impossible to say which of those premises are thus shown to be false, since Freud piled hypothesis upon hypothesis, for each of which the available independent evidence, if any, seems to be equally precarious. But in any event, Freud did not think that his conclusion, though regarded by all competent biologists as false, refuted *any* of his premises. It is therefore pertinent to ask what could refute those premises and whether they are at all refutable.

On the other hand, if that conclusion does not really follow from Freud's premises, and some of Freud's disciples do not think it does, why could this fact not have been clearly demonstrated to Freud? My own opinion is that the premises are far too loosely formulated to permit a clear decision of such questions. One is therefore led to inquire further whether there are any statements which, unlike the above example, are unmistakable instances of deduction from Freudian theory, or whether the theory has the remarkable feature that a statement can be shown to be a theorem only if it is first accepted as a postulate. Do any of the familiar Freudian theses, such as those about infantile sexuality and sexual development, frustration and aggression, or totemism and social taboos, follow logically from the theory, when suitable assumptions not identical with those theses are added to the theory? More generally, what is the logical relation of Freudian metapsychology to any of the more specific Freudian contentions? I do not believe straightforward replies to such questions can be given, for the reason already stated. But if this is so, there is surely good ground for the suspicion that Freudian theory can always be so manipulated that it escapes refutation no matter what the well-established facts may be.

b) I must now turn to a second difficulty I find in the declared content of Freudian theory. The theory is intended to explain human behavior on the cardinal assumption that all conduct is *motivated* or *wish-fulfilling*. But since most of our conduct is not in fact *consciously* motivated, the theory postulates the complex "mental apparatus" summarized by Dr. Hartmann, which includes under various names what are in some sense *unconscious* motives or wishes. As I understand Freudian theory, and as I think Dr. Hartmann's paper also makes quite plain, these unconscious motives, wishes, drives, urges and intentions must be regarded as "psychic" or "mental processes," as "purposive ideas" which are directed toward definite "aims" or "objects," and not simply as latent somatic dispositions possessing no *specific goals.* Indeed, if these unconscious drives were not strongly analogous to conscious motives and wishes, the claim that psychoanalytic theory explains human conduct in motivational terms would be difficult to make out and would perhaps collapse. On the other hand, these unconscious motives have an enduring character and tenacious attachment to specific objectives that conscious wishes do not exhibit. Indeed, on Freudian theory a thwarted wish of early childhood, directed toward some person, may not completely vanish, but may enjoy a repressed existence in the unconscious, and continue to operate in identical form into the present even though that person has long since died.[5] In consequence, there is an important failure of analogy between conscious motives and unconscious mental processes, so that it is only by a radical shift in the customary meanings of such words as "motive" and "wish" that Freudian theory can be said to offer an explanation of human conduct in terms of motivations and wish-fulfillments.

This comment would perhaps be calling attention only to a relatively verbal matter, were it not for the fact that the unconscious mechanism postulated to account for human conduct is emphatically said to be a *psychical* or *mental* apparatus which is endowed with all the customary attributes of substantiality and causal agency. As is well known, Freud hoped that this mental apparatus would eventually be identified with physiological processes in the body; and he himself observed that the question whether the unconscious processes he postulated are to be conceived as mental or as physical can easily become a war of words.[6] Nevertheless, he not only insisted that the apparatus of metapsychology is *mental,* but also described its parts as if they were things struggling with one another or with the external world. He admitted that the assumption of unconscious mental activity was in a sense an extension of that primitive animism which attributes a consciousness to the things around us, even though he noted that the mental, like the physical, may "in reality" not be what "it appears to us to be." [7] And he repeatedly talked of the id, the ego and the superego as inhabited by drives charged with energies, acting like forces, and in some cases immutably directed toward quite specific objects. *"Psychic reality,"* he once vigorously asserted, "is a special form of existence which must not be confounded with *material* reality." [8] Dr. Hartmann's language is similarly equivocal. He sometimes describes the main theoretical components of the mental apparatus as "units of functions," and suggests that unconscious drives are something like dispositions. But he also declares that these components possess energies and conflict with one another—though without explaining in what sense functions can be charged with energies or dispositions can be engaged in conflicts.

It is certainly tempting to read all this as just metaphorical language, a convenient and dramatically suggestive way of talking about some of the complex but still unknown detailed mechanisms of the body. On this reading of Freudian theory, its assumptions would be formulations of the relations between, and the teleological organization of, various latent capacities and dispositions of the human organism. Accordingly, its "motivational" explanations of human conduct would then not differ in kind, though they would differ in not specifying the detailed mechanisms involved, from teleological explanations of the behavior of such teleologically organized (or "feed-back") systems as an engine provided with a governor or the human body as a self-regulative structure for the maintenance of its internal temperature.

However, such a reading is difficult to carry through if one is to make consistent sense of the theory, in part because of the characterization the theory gives of many drives as immutably fixed to specific objectives, but in larger measure because of the causal powers the theory ascribes to its theoretical entities. If these causal ascriptions are themselves construed figuratively, I cannot make ends meet in understanding the theory as a supposedly "dynamic" account of human personality and conduct. On the other hand, if those ascriptions are taken seriously (i.e., more or less literally), then on the suggested reading of the rest of the theory the latter would in effect be asserting what is to me the unintelligible doctrine that various *modes of organization* of human activities are the *causes* of those activities.

In point of fact, Dr. Hartmann adds to the difficulties of construing the theory in the proposed manner. For he represents Freud as having believed that the theoretical psychic entities have "effects which can be observed" and that the mental apparatus is "real in the ordinary sense of the word." Limitations of time and space prevent me from examining what various things might be meant by the word "real" in this context; and in any event, the whole issue this word of protean meanings raises may not be worth pursuing. But I do want to conclude this part of my discussion with two confessions, even at the risk of being thereby convicted of a failure to understand the actual intent of Freudian theory. The theoretical "mental apparatus" as he apparently conceived it seems to me to reduplicate on an ostensibly "psychic" level the admittedly unknown detailed somatic mechanisms and capacities of the human organism. Accordingly, though psychoanalysis explicitly proclaims the view that human behavior has its roots in the biophysical and biochemical organization of the body, it actually postulates a veritable "ghost in the machine" that does work which a biologically oriented psychology might be expected to assign to the body. Dr. Hartmann denies that the mechanism of metapsychology is anthropomorphic; but I must confess that the theoretical literature of psychoanalysis with which I am acquainted does not seem to me to confirm this denial. And as for the notions of unconscious psychic processes possessing causal efficacies—of unconscious, causally operative motives and wishes that are not somatic dispositions and activities—I will not venture to say that such locutions are inherently nonsense, since a great many people claim to make good sense out of them. But in all candor I must admit that such locutions are just nonsense to me.

II

I come to the second group of questions, those dealing with the nature of the evidence for Freudian theory. There appear to be three major types of such evidence: clinical data, obtained from patients in psychoanalytic interviews; experimental findings in psychological laboratories; and anthropological information gathered by studies of primitive and advanced societies. Since the clinical evidence is regarded by psychoanalysts as by far the most important type, as well as because of limitations of space, I shall devote the remainder of my comments to it. For the sake of the record I think I ought nevertheless to state my conviction, although without supporting reasons, that even when the best face is put on the experimental and anthropological evidence the available data do not uniformly support Freudian theory. Some of this evidence can certainly be construed as being favorable to, or at any rate compatible with, the theory; but some of the evidence is decidedly negative.

The psychoanalytic interview (or method) is the distinctive procedure used by analysts for arriving at psychoanalytic hypotheses, for obtaining evidence for or against such hypotheses, and for effecting therapies. Although Dr. Hartmann has stressed the role of clinical data as the *source* of psychoanalytic hypotheses, this is not a relevant consideration to my present objective. For my concern is not with the origins of such hypotheses, but with the logic of their validation. As everyone knows, the aim of the psychoanalytic interview is to discover the causes of a patient's neurosis or psychosis, on the assumption that his present condition is the manifestation of internal conflicts produced by an unfulfilled but repressed "wish" of early childhood, which is still operative in the unconscious and which is usually sexual in character. Briefly stated, the method of ascertaining such alleged causes consists in having the subject engage in "free association" narration of his conscious thoughts, until the "latent meaning" of his fragmentary recollections of childhood experiences—i.e., the frustrated but suppressed wish that is the source of his present difficulties—is uncovered by the "interpretations" which the analyst places upon what is told him. Accordingly, the crucial issue is how such interpretations are established as valid.

Judging by what analysts themselves say on this question, the grounds for regarding an interpretation as sound are its coherence (or compatibility) with all the things disclosed by the patient in the interview, its acceptance by the patient, and (at least in some cases) the improvement in the condition of the patient when he accepts the interpretation and so recognizes the alleged source of his troubles. Now although the probative worth of such evidence has been frequently challenged, and some of its defects have been acknowledged even by psychoanalysts, I have never come across adequate answers to what seem to me grave criticisms. In the hope of eliciting better answers, permit me therefore to enumerate the difficulties, however familiar they may be, that I regard as important.

a) Only passing mention need be made of the circumstance that although in the interview the analyst is supposedly a "passive" auditor of the "free association" narration by the subject, in point of fact the analyst does direct the course of the narrative. This by itself does not necessarily impair the evidential worth of the outcome, for even in the most meticulously conducted laboratory experiment the experimenter intervenes to obtain the data he is after. There is nevertheless the difficulty that in the nature of the case the full extent of the analyst's intervention is not a matter that is open to public scrutiny, so that by and large one has only his own testimony as to what transpires in the consulting room. It is perhaps unnecessary to say that this is not a question about the personal integrity of psychoanalytic practitioners. The point is the fundamental one that no matter how firmly we may resolve to make explicit our biases, no human being is aware of all of them, and that objectivity in science is achieved through the criticism of publicly accessible material by a community of independent inquirers. It is well to remind ourselves, in this connection, of Stekel's observation that "patients dream in the dialect of whatever physician happens to be treating them. . . . Sadger's patients will dream about urinary eroticism; mine perhaps of the symbolism of death and religion; Adler's of 'top-dogs' and 'underdogs' and of the masculine protest." [9]

Moreover, unless data are obtained under carefully standardized circumstances, or under different circumstances whose dependence on known variables is nevertheless established, even an extensive collection of data is an unreliable basis for inference. To be sure, analysts apparently do attempt to institute standard conditions for the conduct of interviews. But there is not much information available on the extent to which the standardization is actually enforced, or whether it relates to more than what may be superficial matters.

b) The mere coherence of an interpretation with the data supplied by a subject seems to me to carry little weight as evidence for its truth, especially if more than one such coherent interpretation can be given, whether within the general framework of Freudian metapsychology or on the basis of quite different assumptions. I have read enough of the analytic literature to have been impressed by the ingenuity with which the reported data of various cases are made to dovetail into psychoanalytic interpretations. Nevertheless, I am also familiar with the fact that analysts themselves sometimes differ in their diagnoses of the same case; and I have little doubt myself that for every ingenious interpretation of a case, another one no less superficially plausible can be invented.[10] Accordingly, even if we waive the important point to which Dr. Hartmann himself calls attention, that the analyst may base his interpretation not on *all* the information given by the patient, but on an unwittingly biased selection of the data, the question remains whether there is any objective way of deciding between alternative interpretations.

Dr. Hartmann suggests two such ways. One of them is the making of successful predictions, the other is the use of established laws based on experience with various types of patients. I want to consider each of these briefly.

c) What sorts of predictions can be made by an analyst? Dr. Hartmann is not very informative on this point. But apart from therapeutic prognoses, which for the moment I will ignore, the only kinds of predictions I have found mentioned in the relevant literature refer to the reactions of the patient. Thus, Ernst Kris cites as examples of such predictable reactions "the reactions of acknowledgment to any interpretation given, for instance, that of sudden insight combined with the production of confirmatory details or substitute reactions of a variety of kinds," such as the recall by the subject of past experiences which he was previously unable to remember.[11] However, neither the *acceptance* of a given interpretation by a subject, nor his *claim* to a sudden insight into the alleged source of his difficulties, seems to me to constitute, by itself, a critical confirmation of the interpretation. For the interpretation does not, as such, predict either its own acceptance by the subject or the insight claimed by him; and in any event it is pertinent to ask how often an interpretation of a certain kind when proposed to comparable subjects is neither accepted by the subjects nor accompanied by a sense of illumination about themselves. Nor is it clear why the mere say-so of a patient that he now understands the source of his difficulties is competent evidence for the assumption that the alleged source is indeed the actual source. There have been countless numbers of people throughout human history who have believed quite sincerely that their successes or failures could be attributed to various things they did or did not do or that were done to them; nevertheless, most of such beliefs have subsequently been shown to be baseless. Why is not this lesson of human experience relevant for assessing the analogous claims of psychoanalytic subjects?

Moreover, as Kris himself notes, the improvement in recall which sometimes follows the presentation of an interpretation must not be assumed to "produce" the recall: the interpretation can be viewed only as a *help* to better recall. Even with this reservation, however, one is begging the question in supposing that it is the *specific content* of an interpretation, as distinct from the over-all directed prodding of the subject's memory that takes place during the interview, that accounts for the improved recall. More generally, the changes in various symptoms which the patient exhibits as the interview progresses do not constitute critical evidence for an *interpretation,* unless it can be shown that such changes are not produced by some combination of factors for which the interview as a whole is responsible. There is at any rate some ground for the suspicion that the interpretations are frequently imposed on data which are themselves manufactured by the psychoanalytic method. Can an adult who is recalling childhood experiences remember them as he actually experienced them, or does he report them in terms of ideas which carry the burden of much of his later experience, including the experience of a psychoanalytic interview? Is an adult "regressing" to a childish attitude who, in order to recapture a childhood experience, may find it necessary to put himself into a childish frame of mind? I do not pretend to know the answers to such questions. But neither am I convinced that adequate attention has been paid to them by most analysts.

d) Dr. Hartmann is not very explicit about his second suggested way of supplying an objective support for an interpretation, namely, by the use of established laws in developmental psychology. If I understand him correctly, he is saying that different types of neurotic personality can be distinguished, and that each type is in fact associated with a fairly distinctive kind of childhood traumatic experience. Accordingly, once the analyst has determined by way of the interview to which type his patient belongs, his interpretation is supported by an appeal to the corresponding law. Now I agree that such a procedure would make an interpretation prima facie credible, if indeed there are well-established regularities of the kind indicated. Nevertheless, though I am not in the position to question the claim that there are such regularities, I would like to be clearer about their nature. In the first place, do the regularities hold between manifest neurotic symptoms and the *allegations* patients belonging to a certain type make concerning their childhood experiences, or between neurotic symptoms and *actual childhood experiences* whose occurrence has been ascertained independently of the subjects' memories of them? If it is the former, the evidential value of such a regularity for a given interpretation is dubious, for reasons too obvious to need explicit mention.

But in the second place, and on either alternative, the fact that some event or attribute B occurs with a certain relative frequency p when some other event or attribute A occurs, is not sufficient to show that A and B are significantly related—unless there is further evidence that the relative frequency of B in the absence of A, or the relative frequency of the nonoccurrence of B in the presence of A, is markedly different from p. Thus, the fact that many men who have certain kinds of traumatic experiences in childhood develop into neurotic adults does not establish a causal relation between the two, if there is about the same proportion of men who undergo similar childhood experiences but develop into reasonably normal adults. In short, data must be analyzed so as to make possible comparisons on the basis of some *control* group, if they are to constitute cogent evidence for a causal inference. The introduction of such controls is the *minimum* requirement for the reliable interpretation and use of empirical data. I am therefore not impressed by Dr. Hartmann's assertion that psychoanalytic interpretations are based on a great wealth of observations, for it is not the sheer *quantity* of data that is of moment but their probative strength. I am not aware, however, that analysts have in fact subjected their clinical data to systematic and critical statistical scrutiny. I have not read everything that Freud wrote, and I may be doing him an injustice in supposing that he cannot be rightly accused of having made such a scrutiny. But at any rate I have not found in the books of his I have read, in some of which he announced what he regarded as important changes in his theoretical views because of fresh clinical evidence, that these changes were controlled by the elementary logical principle to which I have just been calling attention.

e) This is a convenient place to say a few words about the evidence supplied for Freudian theory by psychoanalytic therapy. I agree with Dr. Hartmann that the adequacy of the theory should not be *equated* with the success of its therapy.

Nevertheless, the evidence from the latter is surely not irrelevant to the former. Unfortunately, information about the effectiveness of Freudian therapy is notoriously difficult to obtain, and I am in any case not sufficiently familiar with whatever material is available to have a reasoned opinion about it. However, I would like to mention Dr. P. G. Denker's study of 500 cases of psychoneuroses treated, without psychoanalytic intervention, by general medical practitioners.[12] The study finds that the percentage of improvements was as high as the ratio of improvements sometimes claimed for psychoanalytic therapy. It would certainly be rash to claim that the findings of his study are conclusive on the point at issue. But I think the study does indicate that therapeutic success as supporting evidence for Freudian theory cannot be taken at face value.

f) There is one final point I wish to make. Psychoanalytic interpretations frequently assert that the present difficulties of a patient have their source in an unfulfilled wish of early childhood, which persists in self-identical manner and produces discord in the unconscious stratum of mentality.[13] It is pertinent to ask, therefore, what is the evidence for the tacit assumption that none of the events that have transpired since that early traumatic experience need be considered in accounting for the patient's present neurosis. For even if one grants that such a childhood experience is an indispensable condition for an adult neurosis, the assumption that the repressed wish has continued to operate essentially unmodified in the subject's unconscious, despite the countless number of more proximate happenings in the subject's life, cannot be accepted as a matter of course. If I understand correctly the import of investigations such as those on the impact of thirst on cognition, to which Dr. Hartmann refers, they are not only irrelevant for establishing this assumption, but point in the opposite direction. Indeed, the available evidence on the influence of education and cultural conditioning upon the development of human personality casts serious doubt on that assumption. Without this assumption, however, the clinical data obtained in psychoanalytic interviews do not confirm the typical interpretations that, were they sound, would support Freudian theory.

A possible rejoinder to the difficulties I have been raising is that despite the dubious character of the evidence for Freudian theory, it is the only theory we do possess that explains in a systematic way an extensive domain of important phenomena. To such a comment I can only reply that this is indeed most unfortunate if true, but that nonetheless the imaginative sweep of a set of ideas does not confer factual validity upon them. I do not minimize the importance of having *some* theory, even a dubious one, if it helps to open up fresh areas of investigation and if it is a source of fruitful ideas for the conduct of controlled inquiry. I certainly acknowledge the great service Freud and his school have rendered in directing attention to neglected aspects of human behavior, and in contributing a large number of suggestive notions which have leavened and broadened the scope of psychological, medical and anthropological inquiry. But on the Freudian theory itself, as a body of doctrine for which factual validity can be reasonably claimed, I can only echo the Scottish verdict: Not proven.

Notes

1. Dr. Hartmann's account of Freudian theory is in fact only a condensed paraphrase of Freud. Cf. S. Freud, *An Outline of Psychoanalysis* (New York: 1949), pp. 108–10; also "The Unconscious" in *Collected Papers* (London: 1956), Vol. IV.

2. S. Freud, *An Outline of Psychoanalysis,* p. 17.

3. *Ibid.,* pp. 49–50.

4. S. Freud, *Moses and Monotheism* (New York: Vintage Book, 1955), pp. 127–28.

5. Cf. "The Unconscious," *loc. cit.*, pp. 118–19.

6. *Ibid.*, p. 100.

7. *Ibid.*, p. 104.

8. S. Freud, *The Interpretation of Dreams*, in *The Basic Writings of Sigmund Freud*, ed. A. A. Brill (New York: Modern Library, 1938), p. 548.

9. W. Stekel, *The Interpretation of Dreams* (New York: Liveright), I, 14.

10. Freud maintained that absence of agreement among psychoanalysts is sometimes the consequence of insufficient training. He thus declared, for example, that "We shall not be so very greatly surprised if a woman analyst who has not been sufficiently convinced of the intensity of her own desire for a penis also fails to assign an adequate importance to that factor in her patients."—*An Outline of Psychoanalysis*, p. 107.

11. Ernst Kris, "The Nature of Psychoanalytic Propositions and Their Validation," *Freedom and Experience, Essays Presented to Horace M. Kallen*, ed. S. Hook and M. R. Konvitz (Ithaca, N. Y.), p. 246.

12. P. G. Denker, "Results of Treatment of Psychoneuroses by the General Practitioner," *New York State Journal of Medicine*, Vol. XLVI (1946).

13. "In the id there is nothing corresponding to the idea of time, no recognition of the passage of time, and (a thing which is very remarkable and awaits adequate attention in philosophic thought) no alteration of mental processes by the passage of time. Conative impulses which have never got beyond the id, and even impressions which have been pushed down into the id by repression, are virtually immortal and are preserved for whole decades as though they had only recently occurred."—S. Freud, *New Introductory Lectures on Psycho-Analysis* (New York: 1933), p. 104. Cf. also a similar statement in "The Unconscious," *loc. cit.*, p. 119.

3.

Psychoanalysis and Scientific Method

LAWRENCE S. KUBIE, M.D.
Clinical Professor of Psychiatry
Yale University School of Medicine

PSYCHOANALYSIS is one of the controversial frontiers of psychiatry and of science in general. To assay the right of psychoanalysis to a place among the sciences will require that we recognize its virtues, its present limitations and its scientific future (i.e., its future research potential).

I am going to confine my discussion to a consideration of psychoanalysis as a process. I am not going to discuss the superstructure of psychoanalytic theory, the many phases and stages of its evolution, its deviations, or its various currently accepted forms. Dr. Hartmann has presented certain aspects of this. Nor is it my purpose to indicate the areas where I agree with Dr. Hartmann or where I disagree, beyond pointing out that although we represent the same general "school" of analysis, there are areas of disagreement as well as agreement between us, which is an indication of health in psychoanalysis as in any scientific discipline. Nor am I going to try to answer Professor Nagel's brilliant, incisive, blunt, challenging, hard-hitting and illuminating paper. In it there are almost as many points with which I agree as I find in Dr. Hartmann's paper. But there are also premises and implications from which I dissent. To go through it point by point would take some time and would fail to put forth any additional concrete data for consideration. Finally, I want to state emphatically and explicitly that I am not going to

Note: *The text of this contribution was submitted after the Institute was concluded as a statement of "What I was trying to say."*—EDITOR

References in this section are to the bibliography, which begins on page 75.

discuss the evaluation of psychoanalysis as a therapeutic instrument. For this there are several quite specific reasons, which again would take me too much time to discuss in detail. These have been presented fully and repeatedly in the literature on several occasions, in studies to which I would refer the interested reader.*

I mention this literature to underscore a fact that is often overlooked: namely, that ever since 1930 (when the Berlin Institute published its honest yet naive report on the therapeutic results obtained during the first ten years of its existence), psychoanalysts have devoted an enormous amount of time and thought and attention to the problems of evaluation of therapy.

I cite these publications also because there is so much continuing naiveté about this problem current among psychologists with inadequate clinical experience, who because of their inexperience fail to appreciate the complex difficulties of such an evaluation, and the even greater difficulty of comparative evaluation. The problem of maturity for psychiatric research has been analyzed in another study (1 and 5h).

Also at this point I want to state unequivocally my regret that from the very outset psychoanalysis became a therapeutic instrument, instead of having had the benefit of starting out as an instrument for and as an object of basic research in the technique

* (a) A Symposium on the Evaluation of Psychoanalytic Results held in Boston in the late forties and published in the *International Journal of Psychoanalysis* in 1948 (7); (b) a discussion of the Objective Evaluation of Psychotherapy (2) published in the *American Journal of Orthopsychiatry* in 1949; (c) a statistical study on Variations of Psychoanalytic Practice (5c) which was published in *Psychiatry* in 1950; (d) a consideration of the special difficulties of setting up control groups in all psychotherapies, as discussed in the Hixon Fund Lectures (5e), delivered at California Institute of Technology and published by Stanford University Press in 1952; (e) a consideration of various other factors which make the comparative study of psychotherapeutic results premature at this time, and also the special conditions which must be met if such a study is to have any value, in "Some Unsolved Problems of Psychoanalytic Psychotherapy" (5j), in the volume entitled *Progress in Psychotherapy*, edited by Frieda Fromm-Reichmann and published by Grune and Stratton in 1956; (f) a description of the necessary structure of a multidisciplinary Institute for Basic Research in Psychiatry (5l) published in the *Bulletin* of the Menninger Clinic in 1956; (g) a still unpublished paper on The Neurotic Process as the Focus of Physiological and Psychoanalytic Research, delivered in London last September and to appear this year in the British *Journal of Medical Psychology* (5o).

of microscopic psychological investigation, unbiased by therapeutic needs, demands, and urgencies. This of course is not the first time that new scientific instruments have been introduced into medicine only to be misunderstood and misinterpreted and in some measure misused even by their discoverers and proponents, because they were used prematurely for therapeutic purposes. It has been true of many drugs, of many biological agents such as sera and antibiotics, of many physical agents such as heat, electrical stimulation, the X-ray and other forms of radiant energy. In the end such errors are corrected. It is misleading to assume that mercenary reasons alone account for this. The basic reason for the headlong rush into therapeutic application is that the heartbreaking urgency of sick people stimulates the therapeutic optimism of the physician. Freud repeatedly predicted that in the retrospective view of history psychoanalysis will be regarded as more important as a method of psychological investigation and as a theory of human psychology than as a therapy. Moreover, Freud repeatedly warned against the biases, both subtle and gross, that are introduced into analysis by an overemphasis on therapeutic demands and needs. Yet these efforts at self-correction, however honest, cannot eliminate all of the distortions that attend premature therapeutic applications.

Nevertheless we are justified in being in some measure philosophical about the unfortunate fact that analysis was tossed into the therapeutic arena prematurely, simply because it was unavoidable. Without a therapeutic drive people would not then have subjected themselves to analysis. This would not be as true today. Men and women now go into analysis for training purposes, as part of research projects, and even out of philosophical and intellectual curiosity. The very fact that they will do this is one of the important indices of the change that has occurred in the temper of our culture, i.e., a lessened defensiveness, a humbler willingness to accept the complexity and the motley color of human personality, a greater humility about the role of conscious processes in personality. Yet this very change is a product of analysis, and has occurred in spite of its many scientific deficiencies.

Sixty years ago human beings would not have subjected themselves to analysis, unless driven to it by the failure of other forms of therapy, and by their awareness that somehow in the course of analysis a certain number seemed to achieve a resolution of difficulties. Lest this be misunderstood, I will quickly add that I am not prejudging even those cases in which there seem to be therapeutic results, or the question of what role the analytic experience plays in this change. I am merely stating that the fact that improvement occurred during the course of analysis encouraged others to go on. Consequently, as we look back historically, the fact that analysis began as a therapeutic instrument is seen to have been inevitable and unavoidable, even if it clouded many scientific issues. Now, however, we have reached a point at which we must turn back to use analysis for pure research, and to subject it to pure research. In fact, this is already starting in many centers, gropingly, fumblingly but with dedicated purpose. I do not doubt that the outcome will be many important changes in technique and in the superstructure of concept, terminology and theory.

I want next to list what I consider to be some of our basic limitations and gaps. I will then describe what I consider to be the essence of psychoanalysis as a process, and how this process fits into the framework of scientific methodology. Then I will add a few words about what we might call the philosophy of the basic concept of psychodynamics.

Limitations

The limitations that I will describe will not constitute an exhaustive or all-inclusive list, nor will they be organized systematically. They are rather a fairly representative sample of the limits within which we have operated in the past, and from which we are now trying to escape.

(1) Psychoanalysis and psychiatry in general have been unique among all scientific disciplines and methodologies in that they have been dependent almost exclusively upon auditory data. This has never been absolutely true, but because of the over-

whelming importance of the spoken word as a means of communication, and because of the slowness of written communications, the ear is the major source of our observational data. Yet auditory data are transitory. Even more than visual data they are limited by temporal restriction. Furthermore, they are vulnerable to distortions even at the moment of perception. Here I would remind you of Professor Abraham Kaplan's brilliant comment on how the advance of a science is dependent upon the abandonment of the doctrine of immaculate perception (5m).

Anyone who has followed the work on subliminal and preconscious perceptions (most of which unfortunately has been restricted to the tachistoscope and visual inflow) must be aware that the bombardment of the individual by an incessant assault of preconscious auditory afferents must play a more important role than has been appreciated in the past by Freud or anyone else. Indeed, evidence from daily experience has been with us for years that it plays an enormous role in the auditory, olfactory, tactile and kinesthetic spheres; yet its implications have been overlooked. Therefore, although our dependence upon auditory inflow has certain limitations and certain unique fallibilities, it also has unique potentialities. Ultimately, when this has been subjected to future critical studies, it will become a source of strength to psychiatric and psychoanalytic technique instead of a source of weakness, as at present. Indeed, future analytic research will include the investigation of processes of preconscious perception in every sensory modality.

When I say that auditory data are susceptible to distortion even during the process of perception, I mean quite specifically that, as we listen to words, we alter what we hear. We do this automatically, without being aware of it, as an essential part of the technique of communication. If anyone doubts this, record an interview or even a reading; have the best available secretary transcribe the record; then sit down and listen to the recording while reading the transcript. You will note that as the secretary listened to the machine, she corrected even what the tape said. Moreover, the better the secretary, the greater are the corrective distortions that she will have imposed upon the record. The conclusion is inescapable that, until quite recently, when it became possible to introduce techniques of precise recording and reproducing, our raw observational material rested on insecure grounds. Yet it is equally clear that the introduction of mechanical contrivances, especially into highly-charged human relationships, brings in new distortions. This, however, is equally true in all science. The microscope introduces distortions, as does the stethoscope. Blood drawn from the vein and put into a test tube for chemical analysis has been changed. Science advances by learning how to recognize the changes introduced in the process of observation and measurement, to limit them, to allow for them and to correct them as it interprets data and builds its theories. Here analysis stands on the frontier of new developments, based on a precise study of the raw material of analytic communications. But we cannot say that, except for a few isolated instances, we have had the benefit of this type of study in the past.

(2) Auditory data are peculiarly susceptible to retrospective distortions of memory; and unfortunately it was quite impossible to correct these distortions, so long as we had no way of recording and reproducing the auditory material of the psychiatric or analytic interview so that it could be re-examined, reheard, and rethought, not by one observer alone but by many.

(3) The third limitation has been in the sphere of controls. This is a complex subject which has been discussed in several publications to which I have already referred the reader (5e, 5g). Here I will say only that the use of paired groups is so full of fallacies as to make them not absolutely but relatively meaningless. Therefore one is forced to make use of individuals studied down to the most minute detail, which in turn introduces other new sources of error. My personal belief is that the answer is ultimately going to be found through the development of techniques of pooling experience of many observers on many patients, each of whom is studied meticulously. (A timid start towards this has been made by the Central Fact-Gathering Agency of the American Psychoanalytic Association.) That the

superficial study of large numbers has value is undoubtedly true; but it loses much of its value unless out of the larger groups representative individuals can then be subjected to undivided microscopic scrutiny. (Such a combination of techniques was urged on Kinsey repeatedly and would have made of the Kinsey studies something of infinitely greater value than was achieved.)

(4) There are gross defects in our techniques of validation. It has been pointed out on many occasions that it is not difficult to prove that certain interpretations of the meanings of behavior are *possible*. This is easy. It is not too difficult to take a step beyond that and to prove in many instances that an interpretation is *probable*. What is difficult is the critical final step. This involves the proof that an interpretation (i.e., an hypothesis) is *adequate, unique, and necessary*. Analysis has rarely been able to present data that meet this ultimate criterion of validity.

This degree of evidence is of utmost importance for the validation of our procedures and of our techniques. Yet it is only rarely that we achieve conclusive validation for a specific interpretation in a specific situation. This has been possible chiefly with the material from uninformed children, naive psychotics, and subjects under hypnosis. In the literature there are many examples from these three sources where the patient sounds as though he had written the textbooks. These data carry the validity of precise experimentation.

(5) The criteria by which we have approximated validation in the past, namely, the effect of an interpretation on a patient's emotions, on his subsequent material, on the freeing of memories, on free associations, and on our ability to *predict* future behavior, all lead to approximate and not precise validations. They have been useful; and they are not to be despised. But we have no right to pretend that they are conclusive.

(6) A great deal has been written and said about the importance of *prediction* for validation. There is no question but that in the daily practice of analysis, and particularly in the supervision of students, important predictions can be made as to what is going to occur in the life of a patient, the kind of material that he is going to produce, the kind of dream that he is going to

have, the kind of feelings that he is going to generate. Moreover these predictions are not infrequently correct. However, no study has been made as yet of the frequency with which such predictions are incorrect. Nor has anyone studied how frequently *no* predictions are made; which is vital to any statistical survey, because the withholding of a prediction must be included. The confidence to venture any prediction may depend upon a special constellation of circumstances, and may therefore not be representative of the process as a whole. Thus we may fail to make predictions out of a preconscious fear of making an incorrect prediction. This would weight our samples of correct predictions in our favor. Nor has anyone tested the effects of any change in technique or of any interpretation on the ratio of correct to incorrect predictions. Therefore although we cannot dismiss the occurrences of correct predictions as meaningless, we should be cautious in any claims that we base on such predictions. This points up the importance of research on analytic methodology and analytic validation, which remains to be done.

(7) There are limitations to our right even to make assumptions as to quantitative differences, much less to attempt to make measurements. Here I would refer to a paper published in 1947 on the Fallacious Use of Quantitative Concepts in Dynamic Psychology (5b), as well as to many recent elaborations of this topic. The point that must be borne in mind is that it is almost impossible to talk of processes of any kind without speaking of "more" and "less." Yet the assumption that quantitative changes are the only changes that can account for differences in activity, in personality, and in illness is an unwarranted assumption. This whole area is being subjected to critical scrutiny today by a number of analysts, who are concerned with the changes in thinking that the development of cybernetics, of communication engineering, of electronic computers, etc., are forcing upon us (cf. Pumpian-Mindlin, 9; Warren McCullough, 6, and 5f, p. 27; and Colby, 3).

(8) Two other grave deficiencies in our current conceptual equipment are closely related to the problem of quantitative differences. These are the inadequacy of our criteria of change

(5j), together with a tendency in all systems of psychology toward an illusion that a new description (which is sometimes just a new nomenclature and sometimes a new and more precise description) has greater explanatory value than the old. The distinction between description and explanation is one of vital importance, yet it has not been solved.

(9) This leads finally to certain instrumental lacks, i.e., to deficiencies in our instruments of precision. I have already mentioned one, namely, that which derives from the fact that we depend so exclusively upon the ear. This is a lack which is being overcome. The use of infrared photography will make it possible to compare night activity with day activity and will take us another step. But we still lack techniques by which to validate any assumptions with respect to quantitative changes in general. We lack precise criteria of change. We lack instruments with which to assay the relative roles played concurrently by conscious, preconscious and unconscious processes. Strangely enough, it is easier for us to study the impact of unconscious processes on conscious activity than the impact of conscious communications on what goes on behind the iron curtain in the level of unconscious processes. Here again we need new instruments.

(10) As a result of these procedural limitations we find ourselves with certain conceptual limitations. We cannot yet be certain what constitute the internally cohesive clinical syndromes or conglomerates of behavior that operate as units in the personality. These have been formulated and reformulated in many ways; and there have been brief times when analysts have agreed about them. Then dissatisfaction with the formulation starts and disagreement leads to fresh formulations. This is not unnatural; but it means that we have not yet settled one of the most critical steps in our development. Moreover we are not sure what are the sources of energetic processes, or the forms that energetic processes take, or the role that hypothetical differences in energy may play in psychological affairs. We have not been able to eliminate from our thinking the figurative language of physics, of mechanics, of hydraulic engineering and of the electricity of

the 1890's, which still dominate our speech and our theoretical constructions. The process of conceptual clarification is just starting. But it is being given serious and earnest attention.

Now, having listed our faults, let me turn to what I consider the essential virtues of psychoanalysis as a process and why I consider analysis to be of such basic importance to science in general.

Psychoanalysis as a Process

It is possible to divide psychoanalysis into components in many ways. I can claim no ultimate virtue for those that I will use here, except that I find them helpful in the consideration of our problem.

The goal of analytic exploration is to illuminate the concurrent roles of conscious, preconscious and unconscious processes in human thought, feeling, purpose, behavior, and relationships. As a therapy, psychoanalysis attempts to redistribute these roles; but this is outside of the range of this paper. For exploratory purposes, therefore, I will consider only the following elements of psychoanalysis as a process:

- The constancy of the setting
- The constancy of attitudes
- The analytic incognito
- The role of interpretations in general as working hypotheses
- The role of transference interpretations
- The crucial significance of free association

In the struggle to explore the inner space of human psychology and human personality, the basic challenge is the clarification of the interplay among and the respective roles of three "levels" or systems of concurrent processes. I will say at once that there is abundant evidence, largely overlooked, that among them the most important is neither conscious nor unconscious, but what we call *preconscious*. This constitutes a continuous, turbulent and rapid stream of afferent, integrative, creative and efferent human mentation. Of this continuous preconscious stream our conscious symbolic processes provide at best a relatively slow, limited and weighted sample; and our unconscious symbolic processes constitute in turn an even smaller and distorted sample, sometimes of the conscious samples, and perhaps sometimes of the underlying preconscious stream. No matter how we structure the personality or organize it, no matter how we use such concepts as id, ego and superego, concepts of repressions, of defenses, of identification, of incorporation, etc., since each of these operates on all three of these levels concurrently, the critical problem remains the same: how do we determine their relative roles and their interplay? To determine this will require the development of techniques by which we can study all human activity on all three levels. At present psychoanalysis, faulty though it is, is the only instrument that even approximates this achievement. That out of it more precise instruments must and will evolve I do not question. But these will be rooted in the pioneer work of Freud.

Let me be quite explicit that I characterize the goal of the analytic process as an attempt to clarify the continuous interplay of concurrent conscious, preconscious and unconscious processes in every moment of life and in every aspect of human personality and behavior. Moreover this is the core of the understanding of all human psychology, sick or well; since their interaction enters into every creative act in science, art, music or literature, and into the neurotic process as well.

Implicit in this is a concept of the relationship between neurosis and health which involves the essential nature of the neurotic process, its genesis, and the role of conflicts on all three levels. It is not my purpose here, however, to discuss this. Instead I will refer you to two studies of the issue (5f, 5i). But with this premise in mind I will discuss in what analysis *as a process* consists.

It designs a situation sufficiently standardized to enable us to make comparable observations on one person at different times, and also on different people. This framework maintains a relative constancy of all external variables, making it possible to repeat observations day after day in relatively unchanged situational circumstances. It minimizes, although it cannot eliminate, changes introduced by the fluctuating state of the *observer*—to wit, the analyst. It also minimizes the distortions introduced by the analyst's unconscious processes, turning him as far as possible into a relatively passive and inert recorder of his own "preconscious perceptions of the patient's productions." Of these he makes his own conscious samples and conscious summaries; and from time to time he shares these with the patient in the form of "interpretations," which is what the analyst calls his working hypotheses.

This creates a situation in which the major variables introduced into the stream of observations arise in the subject who is under analysis, so that a situation can be approximated in which it is possible to study someone else's mind without too much distortion and interference from the observer's.

I must explain this further. By remaining as ill-defined as is humanly possible, by masking his own emotional reactions, his esthetic tastes, his political and religious views, the details of his personal life, his feelings about the patient and the patient's communications, the analyst attempts to remain a blank about whom the patient can imagine anything he feels, and feel anything he must. As long as the analyst is not a real person to the patient, whatever the patient thinks, feels, and imagines about the analyst is not anchored to reality. Instead, the patient's fantasies and feelings are a product of his own imaginative and creative psychological potentials. The unknown analyst remains a sample of humanity drawn from a grab bag; and on this image of the analyst the patient can drape his fantasies as one might drape a costume on a dummy in a store window (5d, ch. VIII). The study of this process gives the patient insight into the subtle ways in which similar processes distort all of his daily human relationships; with the stranger he passes on the street, the man who greets him, a boss, an associate, a child. Gradually it becomes clear to him that none of these is a simon-pure reality; but that all are mixtures of reality plus projections of his own unconscious needs and conflicts and fantasies. In short, the patient uses the unknown analyst in the same way that someone who is being given a Rorschach or a thematic apperception test uses a stimulus card, i.e., as an object on which to project his feelings and fantasies. The study of the distortions of reality that these projections produce illuminates for him the distortions that can enter into all interpersonal relationships. With a virtually unknown analyst the patient can explore the nature of these distortions. This is what is meant by the study and clarification of transference processes. To the extent to which the analyst becomes active, he will anchor the patient to reality, thus obscuring the role of unconscious needs and feelings. Transference processes operate in all relationships; but the more real the analyst becomes to the patient, the less helpful for the exploration of unconscious components in the patient's psychology are his transplanted feelings about the analyst.

Note that I have not said that this eliminates countertransference processes. But I can say that the careful protection of the analytic incognito lessens the activity of countertransference processes on all three levels, and reduces to a minimum the distortions that they otherwise introduce. All of this has been carefully explained in readily available studies and in nontechnical terms (5d, ch. VIII; 5g).

Please note that I am not talking about therapeutic leverage, but about the scientific and exploratory values of what is called the analytic incognito and the analysis of transference. These devices are essential for protecting the material observed from contamination by the observer.

Free Association

These considerations bring us to another essential element in the analytic process, i.e., the way in which the "analytic incognito" and the clarification of transference processes enable the patient to use the essential analytical technique, namely the technique of free association.

It is strange that the scientific significance of free association has been so little appreciated. It has not been adequately studied even by analysts. Indeed I consider it one of the major deficiencies of our development as a science that we have not studied the process of free association more objectively and precisely. I should add, however, that it has been only since we have had recording methods that this has become possible. I have already indicated that it is impossible to participate in any conversation without distorting it. Obviously, then, it is even more impossible to listen to a string of free associations without distorting them. This is true no matter how phonographic the mind. We can remember a sentence as a whole; but if we break up that sentence into syllables and scramble them it becomes impossible to remember the same number of "nonsense" syllables. Yet free associations, if they are truly free in the technical analytic sense, approximate strings of unrelated topics, ideas, words and thoughts. Consequently the task of recording and reproducing becomes so difficult that only a recording device can do the job. Until recent years this has limited the dependability of our raw data.

Why, however, is the production and study of free associations important? It happens, and not by chance, that free association is the mirror image of the conditioned reflex. This was first pointed out in 1934 (5a). Even this, however, is not its major importance in the framework of all psychology, and of psychoanalytic psychology in particular. The deeper importance of free association arises from the fact that it is our only approximation of a technique by which to secure relatively unweighted representative samples of *all* that is going on in the mind. Any conversation that is goal-directed, any effort to talk on a topic, involves an automatic, preconscious process of selection and rejection. If I talk about baseball, I do not talk about football; and if I talk about football I do not talk about science or philosophy. The result of talking "about" anything is a preconscious screening, selecting, and rejecting which goes on all the time at enormous speeds. Under such circumstances, what is spoken is a selected and weighted fragment of *all* that is going on in the speaker's head at that time; and it is this which makes up human conversation. If we seek a representative cross-section of another's mental processes, if we want to conduct an approximation to a Gallup poll of them, we can do so only if the speaker talks without any chosen topic. This is precisely what free associations provide. First, through the agreement not to exclude or select anything deliberately, free associations are free of *conscious* choice, selection, or rejection. Secondly, because there is no goal or topic, the automatic selection and rejection by *preconscious* processes are minimized. What is unmasked thereby is the influence of *unconscious* processes on the linkages among feelings, ideas, actions, and purposes (5d, ch. VII, 5g). The technique of free association thus has a unique significance as a method for unmasking the concurrent influence of conscious, preconscious and unconscious processes in mental activity. In fact, as Glover said long ago, as long as you are securing free associations, the analysis is moving. Although this sounds like an oversimplification, it is the core of the matter. If one can set up a situation in which one eliminates all of the factors that distort free association, one is polling the human thinking machine.

Up to the present we have no other comparable device. And also up to the present time we have designed no other experimental or observational situation which for this specific purpose is comparable to the analytic situation. Every element in the formal analytic situation, i.e., the analytic incognito, the constancy of external variables, the noninterference by the analyst, the calculated interpretation, the watchful eye on countertransference pressures and the tracing of transference attitudes to their sources, is essential to the facilitation of free association. Do not misunderstand this. They do not facilitate the easier gratifications of conversational interchange. Quite specifically and rigorously they facilitate free associations.

We should challenge ourselves next with the question: How do we know that associations are free? If we are honest, we answer that we do not *know;* that we have only approximate knowledge; and that we will not have conclusive indications of how truly free free associations are until through the application of recording methods and their meticulous quantitative and qualitative study (including timing) we secure more precise data on the nature and production of free material than have yet been available to us. When this type of research is carried out we will achieve a wholly new phase in the scientific development of psychoanalytic methodology.

The Philosophic Position

I have said above that I would end with a brief philosophic discussion of the concept that dynamic interactions can occur among psychological events. This issue has been spelled out in considerable detail in a paper which was written several years ago, but which has appeared just recently (5n), entitled "The Psychodynamic Position on Etiology." With a few essential changes to make it more precise and accurate, what was said there stands up fairly well:

> Any consideration of dynamic interactions on the level of psychological experience stirs a venerable philosophical conundrum out of its Rip Van Winkle slumbers. Fortunately, although the problem is ancient, I have the temerity to believe that it can be resolved simply. . . .
>
> The idea that sequences of psychological events can exert dynamic influences on one another seems at first thought to do violence to all scientific concepts of the world, and to the laws governing the conservation of mass and energy. Yet this need not worry us. There is no difficulty in understanding in physical terms how perceptual stimuli which arise from *immediate* occurrences initiate chain reactions in the central nervous system, and thereby influence the psychological expressions of central activity; because such perceptual units initiate the immediate discharge and transmission of energetic [(?) or signalling] processes. . . .
>
> Furthermore, once these processes are launched in the nervous system, they can continue in transmutable forms even for years, and in this sense can be "stored." Thereafter, any symbol which represents past, or spatially distant, or even future perceptual events acts on the nervous apparatus as a coded signal which can trigger off or redirect or redistribute these . . . processes. Therefore, it is merely using a legitimate verbal shorthand to talk of cause and effect on a psychological level. This is semantic economy, and does no violence to our basic concepts of the physical world.
>
> From this we may generalize and say that it is the coded signal (or its symbolic representative) which enables one group of psy-

chological states to cause alterations in other psychological states. It may seem strange that we even stop to explain this, since its occurrence is an elementary fact of human experience. If it did not happen, our past could never influence our present or future, nor could there be any communication on any level of psychological interaction. If this were not true, no mere event could have a lasting influence on anyone. Yet we know that the thoughts and feelings of today are integral with those of tomorrow; and that words, expressions, gestures, and events communicate with one another, in a manner of speaking. We also know that my symbolic activities, acting as perceivable signals, are incorporated into the psychological processes and ultimately into the personalities of other human beings, whose symbolic responses in turn and in the same way become incorporated into mine. Thereby comparable sequences are initiated within each of us. Moreover, once my own symbolic events have occurred, they become events to me quite as potent as are the symbolic attitudes, expressions, gestures, and acts of a friend or stranger. In short, the symbolic process, which is that which stamps the human race with its uniqueness, and the extraordinary development of which distinguishes man from even the highest primate, is also the mechanism by which all psychological interactions and interrelatings occur both within and between individuals. It is the mechanism by means of which internal psychological events are capable of having psychological and also psychosomatic consequences. The symbolic process is not only the instrument for communicating signals, information, and interactions; it is also the instrument by which experience on the psychological level can be translated into somatic changes, and, conversely, somatic experience into psychological change. It is the source of our greatest creative power, but also the source of our greatest vulnerability [5f, 5i].

Evidently, then, the symbol is the psychophysiological implement an understanding of which is essential for an explanation both of normal and of pathological human psychological function. It is the key concept in psychodynamics and psychogenesis, whether of normal or sick activity. That from earliest childhood the symbolic process can go off its rails is perhaps the greatest challenge that medicine faces today; because if this did not happen, there could be neither the neurosis nor the psychosis as we know it in the human being.

At the same time the symbolic representation of remote events binds widely separated times and far places into one immediate interacting psychological continuum. This is one of its several essential functions; and whereas on conscious levels, and to an uncertain degree on preconscious levels, we can sharply distinguish the past from the present, and the near from the far, on the more obscure levels of dynamic unconscious processes, near and far, past, present, and future all fuse into a continuum so complete that differentiation among them is lost. This was first described clinically by Freud [4]. More recently it was demonstrated experimentally by Penfield [8].

We can summarize this salute to an ancient philosophical dilemma by stating that, in the study of dynamic interrelations on the level of psychological experience, no assumptions which violate basic scientific concepts of the world are needed, since by means of symbols, acting as coded signals, effective and sustained interactions can occur among sequences of psychological experiences, with a binding of time and space and with effective "storing" of continuing processes.

If I were formulating this discussion today, I would elaborate on the distinction between the coded signals that mediate preconscious processing and the symbolic process that mediates symbolic sampling, as well as the distorted symbolic processes of unconscious sampling. However, these issues would take us far afield. Here I would add only that the symbolic process has vital implications for the whole concept of the human apparatus as a machine. It is through the interposition of the symbol that the human system anticipates any thrusting impulse from within or any thrusting impulse from without and corrects *before* the responsive deviation occurs. This indeed is the essential distinction between instinctual processes in the human animal and in all other animal forms so far as they have been studied (5k). As a matter of fact, even exteroceptive receptors can anticipate external thrusts, through the intervention of symbolic processes. All of this must be studied by analysts with a reformulation of the instinct theory in mind. Analysts must also turn their attention to the role of the subsymbolic type of signalling which occurs within the machine—something which is close to the coded signal of the communications engineer, implementing all preconscious processes, and which in the human apparatus responds to an incessant bombardment of subliminal stimuli in many sensory modalities which have not been studied sufficiently.

This leads directly to another area for basic research which derives from the newer knowledge of feed-back and cybernetics and their relationship to psychological functions in general and to psychoanalysis in particular. The tendency inherent in all feed-back mechanisms to minimize the stimulus–response deviation is recognizable in all central nervous activity, from the reciprocal innervation of Sherrington to the Freudian concept that pleasure is characterized by a reduction of tension. Without going into this question, I would venture to say that in the long run the application of principles based on models derived from modern electronic engineering, communications engineering, mathematical machinery, digital and analogic computers, and electronic devices in general, will clarify much that at present is confused and muddy in psychoanalytic theory, concepts and terminology, and eventually will furnish us with further techniques for critical self-examination.

Bibliography

1. Brenman, Margaret et al, "Research in Psychotherapy," Round Table, 1947; *American Journal of Orthopsychiatry,* Vol. XVIII, No. 1 (January 1948), pp. 92–118.

2. Bronner, Augusta F. et al, "The Objective Evaluation of Psychotherapy," Round Table, 1948; *American Journal of Orthopsychiatry,* Vol. XIX, No. 3 (July, 1949), pp. 463–91.

3. Colby, Kenneth M., *Energy and Structure in Psychoanalysis* (New York: Ronald Press, 1955), p. 154.

4. Freud, Sigmund, *The Unconscious* (1915), Standard Edition (London: Hogarth Press, 1957), Vol. 14, pp. 159–209.

5 (a). Kubie, Lawrence S., "Relation of the Conditioned Reflex to Psychoanalytic Technique," *Archives of Neurology and Psychiatry,* Vol. 32 (December, 1934), pp. 1137–42.

(b). ———, "The Fallacious Use of Quantitative Concepts in Dynamic Psychology," *Psychiatric Quarterly,* Vol. 16, No. 4 (October 1947), pp. 507–18.

(c). ———, "A Pilot Study of Psychoanalytic Practice in the United States: With Suggestions for Future Studies," *Psychiatry,* Vol. 13, No. 2 (1950), pp. 227–45; abstracted in *Annual Survey of Psychoanalysis,* ed. J. Frosch (New York: Josiah Macy, Jr. Foundation, 1950), Vol. I, p. 251.

(d). ———, *Practical and Theoretical Aspects of Psychoanalysis* (New York: International Universities Press, 1950), p. 252; also especially ch. VII on free association and ch. VIII on transference, the analytic incognito, etc.

(e). ———, "Problems and Techniques of Psychoanalytic Validation and Progress," in *Psychoanalysis as Science,* ed. E. Pumpian-Mindlin (from the Hixon Fund Lectures of the California Institute of Technology, 1952). Stanford: Stanford University Press, 1952, pp. 46–124.

(f). ———, "Some Implications for Psychoanalysis of Modern Concepts of the Organization of the Brain," *Psychoanalytic Quarterly,* Vol. XXII (1953), pp. 21–68.

(g). ———, "Psychoanalysis as a Basic Science," in *Twenty Years of Psychoanalysis,* ed. F. Alexander and H. Ross (New York: W. W. Norton, 1953), pp. 120–45.

(h). ———, "The Problem of Maturity in Psychiatric Research," *Journal of Medical Education,* Vol. 28, No. 10 (October, 1953), pp. 11–27.

(i). ———, "The Fundamental Nature of the Distinction Between Normality and Neurosis," *Psychoanalytic Quarterly,* Vol. 23, No. 2 (1954), pp. 167–204.

(j). ———, "Some Unsolved Problems of Psychoanalytic Psychotherapy," in *Progress in Psychotherapy,* ed. F. Fromm-Reichmann and J. L. Moreno (New York: Grune & Stratton, 1956), pp. 87–102.

(k). ———, "Influence of Symbolic Processes on the Role of Instincts in Human Behavior," *Psychosomatic Medicine,* Vol. XVIII, No. 3 (June, 1956), pp. 189–208.

(l). ———, "An Institute for Basic Research in Psychiatry," *Bulletin of the Menninger Clinic,* Vol. 20, No. 6 (November, 1956), pp. 281–87.

(m). ———, *The Use of Psychoanalysis as a Research Tool* (No. 6 of "Psychiatric Research Reports"), American Psychiatric Association, October, 1956, pp. 112–36.

(n). ———, "The Psychodynamic Position on Etiology," in *Integrating the Approaches to Mental Disease,* ed. H. D. Kruse (New York: Hoeber-Harper, 1957), pp. 14–33.

(o). ———, "The Neurotic Process as the Focus of Physiological and Psychoanalytic Research." Read before the Royal Society of Medicine, London, September, 1957. In press.

6. McCullough, Warren, Personal communication (cf. Kubie No. 5f above, p. 27).

7. Oberndorf, C. P. et al, "Symposium on the Evaluation of Therapeutic Results," *International Journal of Psychoanalysis,* Vol. XXIX (1948), Part I, pp. 7–20. Reprinted in *Yearbook of Psychoanalysis,* ed. S. Lorand (New York: International Universities Press, 1950), Vol. 5, pp. 9–34.

8. Penfield, W., "Memory Mechanisms," *Archives of Neurology and Psychiatry,* Vol. 67 (February, 1952), pp. 178–98.

9. Pumpian-Mindlin, E., "Propositions Concerning Energetic-Economic Aspects of the Libido Theory." Read before the Conference of Conceptual and Methodological Problems in Psychoanalysis, New York Academy of Science, March 4–5, 1958 In press.

PART II

PSYCHOANALYSIS AND SOCIETY

4.

Social and Cultural Implications of Psychoanalysis

ABRAM KARDINER
Clinical Professor of Psychiatry
Columbia University

I HAVE been asked to discuss the social and cultural implications of psychoanalysis. This ambiguous title permits me to address myself to any aspect of psychoanalysis in so far as it has any bearing on the social sciences. The limitations of time necessitate selectivity. I have, therefore, chosen to discuss with you a certain impasse that has been reached both by psychoanalysis and correspondingly by the anthropologists or students of culture. Small and simple cultures give us an opportunity to get certain holistic impressions that larger and more complex cultures do not. And such cultures provide an ample testing ground for the uses of psychodynamics in elucidating some aspects of the social processes.

Such an undertaking runs across the natural opposition of interests vested in academic departments and in their traditions. We have taken these risks, and so far I can report to you that psychoanalysis came and saw but did not conquer. We must try to see why it failed, because I know that psychoanalysis is a powerful implement with the aid of which man may learn to understand and to direct himself.

Let me begin with a thumbnail sketch of the methods and frames of reference that evolved in anthropology for 100 years. Shipwrecked sailors and missionaries had no frame of reference. Their purpose was to amuse and to astonish. The first systematic frame of reference was supplied by the evolutionary thinkers—Herbert Spencer, Tylor and Sir James Frazer. Perhaps Spencer really set the pattern for this whole style of thinking. He was an evolutionist—a plausible position. But this evolution was conceived of as unilinear, uniform in all humanity, and apparently driven by the same force that makes an acorn into an oak. The evolutionists were also pervaded by a Lamarkian conception of institutions as survivals of more primitive types of organization. This unilinear assumption gave all of these thinkers the license to leap from one culture to another, pulling out of each what they needed for a consistent theory. It is sad to relate that this line of thinking persisted for some 50 years, until it was finally put aside by Boas and Goldenweiser.

In the meanwhile there appeared another line of approach, which has since developed into what came to be known as the functionalist school. Its first protagonist was Emile Durkheim, in his book, *The Elementary Forms of Religion.* Here the emphasis shifted from institutions as survivals to the relation of institutions with each other. Institutions, said Durkheim, must be treated as "things," and the process he was observing was some form of *interaction.* This process he saw, by analogy with physics, as things interacting with and upon one another.

This had been, ever since, the guiding idea of all functionalists. The unit they used was the institution, and institutions related to each other; they meshed like gears, or they failed to mesh. Under the aegis of this guiding idea some brilliant work was done. It was Boas who introduced new standards of accuracy in description, and the necessity of studying individual cultures exhaustively. Malinowski and Ruth Benedict introduced some variations in the functionalist point of view. Both were impressed with the necessity of defining institutions through some recognizable relation to human beings. Malinowski proposed that institutions existed for man and were purposely created by man for specific needs. But he lacked the technical knowledge to follow through. Ruth Benedict used an inspiration of Nietzsche much popularized by Oswald Spengler—the culture pattern. This contribution consisted of an elaboration of the functionalist point of view. Institutions were indeed related to each other; not, however, like a system of gears, but on an analogy with human characterological types. Thus there were Dionysian, Apollonian,

Faustian, etc., cultures. Today the value of this kind of analogy is dubious. It is hard to believe now that people took this seriously.

The crowning achievement of functionalism is to be found in the work of Alfred Kroeber and Leslie White. According to these two, institutions interact with one another to create the superorganic. Kroeber studied cultures over long time-spans and observed that different gifted individuals in the same culture catch a something that is in the air. The creator of this something is superorganic; that is, the something is created by the impact of institutions on each other, without human intervention, and also without regard for human affairs. I submit that this position of functionalism is tantamount to the anthropomorphization of institutions. By placing the control of culture in the hands of the superorganic, it takes it out of the hands of man. Any doctrine that takes the government of human affairs out of the hands of man increases his helplessness and his hopelessness.

What we see here is the *reductio ad absurdum* of an operational frame of reference that completely excludes man. Dr. Kroeber knows this, for he claims that he wishes he knew of a way of including the human unit in his studies. But he is completely dissatisfied with what psychology can yield. Dr. Kroeber was Freud's first reviewer in 1919. In 1939 he reconsidered his first review and reaffirmed his first conclusions.

Let us, therefore, cast a glance over the kind of information that Kroeber rejects.

Freud, who was the greatest psychological influence of our time, set to work on the social sciences in 1911. This task had been originally assigned by him to Carl Jung; but instead of following Freud's suggestions he came out with a book called *Symbole und Wandlungen der Libido*. This was Jung's final break with Freud, who thereupon set to work on this job himself. The result was *Totem and Taboo,* the book that Kroeber reviewed and found wanting. Let us see the cultural background of this book. In 1910 Frazer had published his large work, *Totemism and Exogamy*. It is not commonly appreciated how many of Freud's assumptions, and how much of his whole style of thinking, were influenced by the evolutionary anthropologists. His whole conception of "stages of development" was borrowed from Herbert Spencer. All other assumptions and patterns of arranging ideas he took from Darwin, Robertson Smith, Atkinson, Marett. Throughout his life he preferred the assumptions of Lamark to those of Darwin. In addition to all of these, there was Haeckel's law of biogenesis, which stated that ontogeny repeats phylogeny.

When Freud wrote *Totem and Taboo* in 1912, he was not aware that this style of anthropological thinking had gone completely out of fashion and was thoroughly discredited as a method of investigation. Naturally Kroeber, who was much under the influence of Boas, could not accept such ideas as the theory of primal parricide as the *origin* of culture or of the Oedipus complex; nor could he tolerate the idea of an infantile recurrence of totemism—that is, the theory that animal phobias in children represent a recurrence (recapitulatory) of totemism. Similarly, the latency period was looked upon as a recapitulation of the ice age. Nowadays one does not regard underwriting Lamark as an excusable and amusing foible.

In his subsequent writings Freud took up different slants of the problems in the social sciences. Two of the books were of a polemical nature: *Group Psychology and the Analysis of the Ego* and *The Future of an Illusion.* In the first he went out to attack the Adlerian point of view and to demonstrate that the libido theory, which by that time he regarded as his greatest achievement, could explain the data of sociology. He attempted to show that relations between people could be accounted for by this theory. For his social prototypes he took the army and the church—both nonfamilial hierarchies. This book contains some exceedingly valuable ideas concerning the process called "identification" and the formation of the ego ideal. *The Future of an Illusion* is important in that he here crystallized his ideas concerning the origins of religion as projections of constellations formed within the family setting—an extremely useful idea, of which more presently.

His most exciting sociological work, *Civilization and Its Dis-*

contents, was the result of his reflections about society and its control of instincts. But Freud was now using his revised instinct theory. Originally he used the sexual vs. the ego instincts. By a series of reflections he came to the conclusion that there were two new classes of instincts: life instincts vs. death instincts. He then recast many of his old ideas in terms of the new classification of instincts.

His book has many exceedingly wise reflections about the vicissitudes of culture. But it, like all the others that preceded it, contains no methodical approach to culture, and attempts to solve no concrete problems. Some people prefer to see in Freud's view of the fate of man, as depending on the outcome of the eternal battle between life and death instincts, great profundity and wisdom. As an empiricist, I cannot share this enthusiasm. I cannot wager man's fate on the capricious outcome of a battle between life and death instincts, to which man cannot address himself and which he cannot in any way control.

II

I now come to the heart of the matter of which I am inviting your consideration. Here are two disciplines, both in possession of vast stores of information, both landing themselves in the frustrating situation where the knowledge they have in abundance cannot be used in the service of man. They are both suffering from the same disease—*frame of reference trouble.* Kroeber goes about mourning over the circumstance that he does not know how to include the human unit; the Freudians go about complacently with the conviction that they do not need to concern themselves with the cultural environment, or settling for the lip service that, of course, the environment must be taken into account, when the fact is that there is no technique for so doing. Since both are engaged in the appropriate mourning processes, Kroeber anthropomorphizes institutions, and Freud anthropomorphizes instincts.

We could spend much time discussing how this strange impasse came about. Both came to it honestly. The anthropologists came to their difficulty through a faulty conception of what an "institution" (the unit of study) really is. Because it was identified largely by its morphology and not by its function (what it did), anthropologists who were concerned with institutions of a bizarre nature forgot that they were conceived by man and served man, even when the institution's original function was forgotten or distorted. Institutions pattern human relations or the relations of man to his natural environment. They have no existence outside of man and no meaning without him. We cannot, in the name of common sense, take the position that an abstract construct, which is the name of a pattern of a specific form of relationship (like family or ritual), does anything or acts by itself on anything, much less on another abstraction.

There is a way of introducing the human unit into anthropology. But it cannot be done by protecting a vested interest in a tradition and defending oneself against the necessity of learning a new technique. On the other hand, I cannot blame Kroeber for refusing to utilize what Freud has bequeathed to us in *Totem and Taboo* or in *Moses and Monotheism*. I feel like saying here that I am led to the belief that Freud was not a very good judge of the best things he had done. I surely cannot blame Kroeber for rejecting the mixture of fine ideas and gobbledegook one finds in the writings of Geza Roheim.

It is worth taking a moment to tell you how Freud got into his particular frame of reference trouble. From 1890 to 1900 (up to and including his *Interpretation of Dreams*) Freud used a frame of reference in which he recognized the governing control apparatus of the organism—the ego. This ego initiated certain identifiable adaptive maneuvers, such as repression, and a large number of others described in the *Interpretation of Dreams*. It was largely in connection with repression that Freud had difficulty in reconstructing dynamic reasons. He first thought that repression, i.e., sexual repression, was initiated by traumatic experience, an idea he later had to abandon. He then discovered that the sexual instinct had a varied history, and that arrests of development could take place anywhere along the line. The idea of arrest of development was an exceedingly useful one;

but just as it was the libido that developed, it was the libido that was arrested.

This was a shift that cost Freud heavily in clarity and precision. While he was occupied with the ego, he was occupied with means–end devices, the end being homeostasis. Thus repression, condensation, projection were means to the end of altering cognition and meaning; but when he became occupied with the libido, he was occupied with what now looks gratuitous, the principle of the conservation of energy. The means that were used to this end were energy transformations by means of charges or cathexes. His reasoning consisted of proof by assumption. At first he identified these changes by alterations in morphology; later he explained them as alterations in energic charges. The first were demonstrable. The second were not. This aspect of the theory created an illusion of knowledge but was really a series of tautologies that added no new information.

The real stumbling block to the theory of transformation of libido from zone to zone, from repressed libido into character traits or into sublimations, came with the necessity to recognize a nonerotic aggression. This necessity finally led to the purely verbal reconciliation of life and death instincts.

It was the work of Otto Rank, who himself embarked on a psychological wild goose chase in defining adaptation in terms of the overcoming of the birth trauma, that woke Freud up to the fact that something was wrong with his original conception of neurotic anxiety as a transformation of repressed libido. He therefore went back to his original frame of reference of the 90's, reinstated the ego as the central agency, and restored the position of common sense that anxiety was a response to a real or expected danger situation. Following this, his daughter Anna rediscovered the adaptive devices described by her father in 1900, but which since that time had enjoyed a position that was extraterritorial to the theory. They were now called mechanisms of defense.

However, there persisted in the literature a hangover of the old theory, in the sense that there now existed a libido psychology and an ego psychology. The ego used a neutralized energy for its ends, just as the sexual instinct used the libido. The energic concepts, tautological as they are, are retained, but in addition are used to invent concepts that make no semantic sense at all—such as desexualized libido and deaggressivised aggression. Concepts like these are misleading chiefly because they create the illusion of knowledge.

Now please do not misunderstand me. I well know that all these manipulations are in the interest of solving clinical problems. This effort must be respected. It is not a form of idle speculation. It is just a technical matter. But unfortunately technical matters ultimately decide meaning. For example, oral erotism has a very different meaning from dependency; yet the same symbols can be used to express both. This libido theory that I am criticising from a methodological point of view has, notwithstanding its handicaps, trapped a vast store of useful information. The information remains useful; the frame of reference needs revision.

In short, both frames of reference went awry, one because it did not know how to include the environment, the other because it did not know how to include the human unit. I must make mention of one valiant effort to include the environment in the frame of reference. That was by Alfred Adler. But unfortunately he included only the social directive and excluded the organismic response. This was the equivalent of throwing the baby out with the bath. Freud's success lay basically in the fact that he taught us how to follow the reactions of the organism. Without this, there is no psychodynamics. Freud grappled with this problem—bequeathed to him by Adler—for many years and did not succeed. He came closest to it in 1926 in *The Problem of Anxiety*. But he could not tear himself away from the triumphs of libido theory. He therefore left a libido psychology and an ego psychology. This is an incredibly confusing situation.

Perhaps we can learn something about how to resolve this impasse from the quandary in which both disciplines have landed. The anthropologists have developed a tradition and a frame of reference that deal only with certain identification tags of patterned relationships to other humans or to the outer world.

These are called institutions. Preoccupation with these left no room to consider either the impact of these institutions on those exposed to them, or how to undertake the study of that impact. Freud invented a technique but did not use it because he imputed the responses of the organism, which he correctly observed, not to an interaction but to the autonomous action of an instinct. That the instinct was in itself a kind of adaptation that was handed down ready-to-use with the organism did not matter. However the case may be with lower forms of life, adaptation in man is not predominantly governed by inborn and ready-to-use devices. Freud was therefore trapped by his earliest assumptions; and when it came to including the environmental factor in the frame of reference, he found there was just no room for it. He therefore ascribed to the environmental factor a coincidental role. He thus recognized that rage and defiance had something to do with the so-called anal-sadistic stage of development. But in the final formulation this was a recapitulatory and developmental stage, and the character traits associated with it were transformations of an anal libido. You see that Freud had not only all the relevant data but also the causal sequences quite correct. The fault lay in the assumptions on which the frame of reference was based. Instead of using this rather abstruse and wholly undemonstrable and gratuitous conception of the transformation of energies, why not just pit the organism, with all its inborn equipment, against identifiable conditions outside itself? You then have a series of interactions. The greatness of Freud's discoveries lies precisely in the fact that he taught us how to identify two vital factors in the whole process of adaptation: (1) the adaptive maneuvers of the organism in response to both internal and external disturbances in homeostasis, and (2) the end products of these adaptive maneuvers; and how to evaluate their success or failure.

Now when the psychologist tries to work with an incomplete inventory of what the organism is reacting to, he must perforce attribute its reactions to something he already knows or thinks he knows. The same fate overtook the anthropologists who tried to work without benefit of organismic response. Not knowing anything about this, they had to attribute what they also correctly observed to something they could identify, namely, institutions. When I therefore propose to you that the psychologist cannot work without the student of the human environment and the student of the internal environment (the biologist and physiologist) and vice versa, I am not proposing either a horse trade, a mutual back-scratching agreement, or a marriage of convenience. I am merely calling your attention to the sad fact that the autonomy of academic departments can be respected only at the peril of insuring our ignorance.

III

Now to complain that Freud did not use the tools he himself invented to the greatest advantage is like complaining that Galileo did not invent calculus. That does not belittle his accomplishment.

Let us have a look at what kind of information is yielded by a new adaptational technique.

The data of anthropology provide a vast source of information concerning the effectiveness or ineffectiveness of different types of social patterning. We can judge of this because the contact with these institutions leaves an indelible imprint on the human personality. This is available knowledge without guesswork. Years ago when I first propounded this idea and the evidence for it, it was greeted with some enthusiasm. Then the question became: "So what!" ("Years ago we were told some people do one thing and some do another. Now you tell us that some people have one type of personality and some another. So what!") This cavalier attitude is not warranted. Knowledge of the impact on the human personality is exceedingly valuable information if you want to know whether your social patterning is having a good or pernicious effect. Moreover it gives you much more specific information than that; it tells you just what particular institutions are at fault. We now know enough about adaptive patterns and integrative processes to be able to identify those miscarried integrations. This is, therefore, an important facet of the whole social process. It is not true that anything goes in social patterning; some patterns are more effectual than others; some lead to great discomfort, and others to mutual destruction.

Let us take a specific instance. The Alorese have a very capricious division of labor. The female does most of the gardening. She therefore leaves the house at sunrise and returns at sundown. The children shift for themselves in the meanwhile. Maternal neglect is not institutionalized; the division of labor is. The former is only an accidental by-product. It could be remedied by a papoose arrangement. This neglect has identifiable consequences in the character of the children—all or most of them. Man is an integrative animal. What maternal neglect does is that it increases the burden of adaptation for the young child, for which it has no resources. The resulting integrative processes bear the imprint of this adaptive struggle from that time forward.

Now suppose all people in a society are constituted in this way. They will have common fears, common suspicions, common aspirations, and common needs for which they will invent appropriate adaptive devices. We can expect that they will have a religion that is consistent with their character. And so it is. We find a religion based on the family cult—in common with hundreds of other societies. But there is something in this community's religion that is very like the relation of children to their parents. They call on the deity only in dire emergencies, sacrifice reluctantly, do not store up merit. They have no permanent representations of the deity or temples; they improvise the effigies for the occasion, then throw them away.

Their folk tales have a distinctive character. The motif of parent hatred is quite prominent. (Grandparents get a better break.)

They have a distinctive set of values. They have no conception of truth, only of expediency. They cannot plan in advance—no consistent life goals. They just live from day to day. They have no conception of honesty or value. They have no conception of sin or forgiveness. (This is where the missionaries would be up against an impenetrable wall. They could not form any idea of original sin or grace, etc.) They tolerate dilapidation and decay, and let things go to rack and ruin. They have no artistic sense; do not seek to idealize nature. They cannot do this since the world is a constantly traumatic place.

Now what we have here is a record of an adaptive process by a whole group of people in a specific environment, who have worked out during the course of their history certain ways of cooperating in order to make the outer world submit to their needs. They are not social engineers, and do not therefore know what the effects of their institutions are. In fact they are the last to know. This is a marginal society in the sense that the gratifications they get seem to us to be rather minimal. Yet they survive—largely because no one has bothered to conquer them. They submit to the Dutch, having no alternative. If anyone were to point out the failure of their social patterning, they would probably be astonished and deny it. "We're getting on fine!" would probably be their answer.

Here is also evidence of the kind of personality that emerges from this institutional set-up. This information is important, because society depends on the capacity for cooperation. That capacity must be built into the human unit; it cannot be preached at him. The knowledge of how the human personality of a given society is integrated gives you the best information about where the homeostats of the society are. They are in the human unit. There is no other locus, because society, not being an organism, has no built-in homeostats. They lie in the human unit. Furthermore the needs of the constituents of a society are conditioned by their character. Hence the folklore of a people is always distinctive; it comes from a common base of experience.

IV

We now come to a consideration of a further application of this new type of knowledge, and that is to history. History is culture in motion. Not many historians have this conception; but some of them do, and it will soon show itself in the histories yet to be written. This is the most complex of all social processes to follow—culture in motion. Students like Kahler, Barzun, Hauser, and others are in revolt against the king-and-battle historians as well as against the Toynbees who seek to use history as a platform for preaching a return to a universal religion—whatever that may mean.

Like the anthropologists and sociologists, the historians refuse to have any traffic with psychology. But don't believe them. They behave like children who don't like grammar but who talk in sentences. They can no more avoid the implication of motivation than they can avoid words. All things considered, some of them do a very good job without benefit of psychology. They would do much better with it. Barzun, Hauser and Kahler would all profit by it.

Let us take a good illustration of history written in the new view; Barzun's *Romanticism and the Modern Ego*. Here the so-called history is draped around the central core of the human personality. He studies the transition from the classical culture of the age of Louis XIV to the Romantic movement. He there describes the *ethos* of two epochs, each with a different social organization, social directives, social machinery, and social opportunities.

Bertrand Russell in his *History of Modern Philosophy* starts his book with the assumption that philosophy is the product of the problems of adaptation at a given time, just as Harold Laski once observed that Newton was occupied with those problems that were defined for him by the businessmen of his time. There was another historian who had a glimmer of this—Oswald Spengler. But he had no technique for investigation. Instead he used a series of postulates concerning society as an organism and echoing Nietzsche's culture pattern inspiration on the basis of characterological prototypes, Apollonian, Dionysian, Faustian.

Of course, one can write long books with such a master plan; but I fear there is nothing here but entertainment. Its value is largely esthetic. Its morale value is zero because it contains the assumption that man can do nothing for himself.

We do not need inspirational efforts. We need methods of

investigation in order to arrive at reliable knowledge. We also need the hope requisite to work with them.

The technique for studying cultural change has hardly begun. It is the most difficult of all psycho-cultural undertakings. But it is easier to try a bit of the past than the complex present, without an established technique for a guide.

When we study the contrast between the ethos of classicism and that of romanticism, we are presumably studying an alteration in the style of human expression. I think it is much more than that; we are studying the impact of a vast social change on the emotional expressions of man.

In other words the social change was responsible for the emotional attitude. This in turn was a reaction to the creation of new opportunities for self-expression. One cannot understand this as an autochthonous outburst led by one inspired man—J. J. Rousseau. A new social machinery was well on the way to being created, and the feudal order, which had long since lost its real power, was about to be publicly proclaimed bankrupt. Liquidating the old political gadgets was in some places a bloody formality. But the essence of the whole matter lay in the circumstance that opportunities for enterprise and contractual service were now open to a vast number of people. The social machinery for manufacture, commerce, travel, credit, etc. were the institutions that defined the ambit of individuality.

One of the reasons that the study of cultural change is of such great importance is that there is in contemporary literature an endless confusion about the concepts of individuality and the origin of values or value systems. The novelists, the philosophers, the ministers (among whom we must put Fromm), and the historians are engaged in a jeremiad against the fragmentation of man, the collapse of individuality, and the devaluation of values. The confusion comes not from a belief that there is not much truth in the allegations they make. There is. But we do not know what the individuality is they are mourning about; nor the source of the values whose disintegration they are bemoaning. There is much danger in spreading these alarms. And although each has a different conception of individuality and of values, if we followed all of them, except as onlookers at an academic debate, we would come away with a great headache.

I think the trouble is that none of these thinkers, Fromm, Kahler, Camus, etc., have taken the pains to define their terms or come to grips with the sequences in the culture process. They all tend to think of values as something one can take on or put off; or of the assumption of values as a voluntary process. They scold people for having the wrong values and exhort them to take on new ones. Most of all they bemoan loss of individuality, which is not defined. I think they are mourning the loss of Renaissance man, or, as T. S. Eliot more explicitly puts it, the English gentleman who had wealth, leisure, and accomplishment. In any case the badge of individuality is a claim to distinction, if not privilege. If it is not this, then there is no power on earth that can rob anyone of "individuality" and uniqueness. For there are no two human beings who are alike—nor two dogs either.

Let us take a few contrasts. In the mediaeval way of life, what was the equivalent of individuality was not character but status, into which you were born. Of course there was character too; but that did not count. The status housed the character, not the other way around. In the 18th and 19th centuries, individuality became important as character, because in the new social order character became the implement of social interaction, and hence the implement of success or failure. With the new social opportunities created by the liberal way of life, it also became obligatory to be successful. One might not choose the way of the merchant, i.e., the accumulation of wealth or increase in standard of living. One could choose the reverse—contempt for it. But one could not renounce the claim to distinction of one kind or another.

Let us turn to another facet of the same problem. Let us examine the values promulgated by St. Benedict and St. Francis of Assisi. These men preached the only socially relevant message of the time—namely, tolerance for hard and unrewarding work, and tolerance for suffering. In its most extreme form, suffering became the claim for distinction. Was this just perversity? I don't think so. It was a device to make suffering, which was almost everyone's lot, bearable and to promise reward. It was therefore not a gratuitous credo, a faith; it was a powerful social control, because it channeled hope, contained aggression, and made postponement of gratification acceptable. This is what made the church powerful and the lay orders so successful. Moreover the source for these values was not perversity, but the particular opportunities that existed in the social order of the day. Mutual hatred and aggression ran high, and rebellion and protest took specific forms like heresy and abandon. The remedy for this was to go after the heresy, with the institution of a special police to deal with it—the Inquisition. This made everyone a partner in the universal cruelty that was about. If you want to have an idea of what it is like to live in a society where there is universal ill will of everyone toward everyone, or where everyone is looked upon by everyone else as a means to an end, think of what it is like (to take an extreme instance) to live in a community where there is mutual cannibalism. It is not very pleasant.

Values are most likely expressions of the structure of the personality as it is integrated in a given social patterning. When we study the alteration of our society under the impact of a new social order, as we did in the transition from the classic to the Romantic mode, we witness an alteration of values. Let me give you an illustration of the first order: the value systems of the Alorese. The chief feature of the integrative pattern is that the child has more adaptive burdens thrust upon it than it can manage. That is the consequence of maternal neglect. Let us see some of the consequences of this:

1. Esthetic sense is completely absent. There is no idealization of nature, for it is constantly painful and traumatic.

2. They have no concept of virtue. There is no consistent punishment–reward system.

3. There is no concept of heroism. There are culture heroes, but they are not heroes at all noteworthy for their achievements. On the contrary, it is the sneaky vengeance on parents that is often the deed of the "hero."

4. Systematization and order have no value. Hence the Alorese tolerate dilapidation and decay.

5. They have no conception of honesty, only of expediency.

We could go on to give more illustrations of the origins of value systems. But we can at least localize their source: (1) in the integrations of personality formation; (2) in the alterations of culture that permit the personality new forms of expression: e.g., the feudal system had one set of values; middle class liberation initiated a new set. Values cannot therefore be preached at people if the makings for the reception are not there. You cannot preach the concept of grace to people who in their life experience have had no opportunity to learn about love, punishment and reinstatement after punishment.

I believe that those who set themselves up as critics of one society (like Fromm and Kahler) ought to stop confusing the people who take them seriously by telling them that the world is falling apart because man's persona (meaning his various social roles) is ruining man the individual—a compact and integrated whole (Kahler). This is Kahler's thesis of the disintegration of modern man. According to Fromm, the persona is the market personality of modern man, stemming from capitalism. In short, these two and other observers detect a certain collapse in the kind of personality integration we accepted as the norm in 1900. This is quite true, and I share some of the views of Fromm and Kahler. Neither of them gives us any of the evidence for this disastrous state of affairs. Kahler has no answer to this terrible situation, for the simple reason that he does not know where the trouble comes from. Nor does he know whether the symptoms are transient or permanent and leading to ultimate mutual annihilation. He does not examine the only source for this information—himself, but he goes to the poets, the novelists, and the philosophers. This is evidence of a certain kind, but not the best.

Let me present to you a different kind of evidence: the kind of disorders one finds in clinical practice today.

1. A considerable increase in schizotypal disorders. This is a pandemic disease but increases at certain times of stress.

2. An increase in male homosexuality (not statistically measurable).

3. A marked change in the character of the family—a distinct increase in the egocentric tendencies of each member.

4. A marked increase in juvenile delinquency—enough to make headlines in America, just as the increase in male homosexuality has reached cabinet consideration in England.

These are all signals of social distress. Above all, there is a great deal of free-floating anxiety and mutual hostility all around. The individuality Kahler is talking about has reached an anarchic stage; it is showing its true color—the claim for privilege at everyone else's expense. In science it shows itself in the fact that communication (except for students) is at a complete standstill. In the exact sciences there is still some left. In the disciplines of opinion, there is almost no communication or exchange of ideas. The general attitude seems to be "Everyone is a fool but me."

This is the very bankruptcy of a way of life much acclaimed one and a half centuries ago.

What is wrong? Is it capitalism? Is it the loss of the wholeness of the personality and its fragmentation into different social roles? I do not think so. Something has eroded the capacity of man for cooperative and affectionate relationships. Either disturbances have occurred in the integrative pattern, or the society has suffered an alteration that makes it difficult or impossible for man to use these potentials even after they have been effectively integrated.

It is one of the most elementary lessons in psychiatry that problems of self-preservation tend to erode the capacity for affectionate and cooperative relationships.

There are many doubtful facets of psychiatry. But we may never permit ourselves to doubt the truth of what we have learned about how man's adaptive tools are shaped during development or how development can be interfered with. If you doubt this, then you may discard the rest. That will leave you with the academic psychologies and their quantifying criteria. Nor can you ignore the evidence that the emotions of man are inborn and function through life only as far as fear and rage are concerned; the tender emotions have to be fostered and nurtured. They may remain permanent equipment of the personality, but under certain social conditions they tend to vanish—in self-preservative crises of drastic proportions. This is what was learned in concentration, D.P., and detention camps. This is the great danger to humanity—the disintegration of the patterns of cooperative living, the atrophy of the emotions that sustain them, and the increase in egocentric tendencies. This unleashes the flood tides of fear and rage. Fear sometimes and in small doses acts as a stimulant and incentive to problem-solving; in large doses it paralyzes the intelligence. Rage on a social scale is always destructive.

I should now like to sketch for you some of the factors of the social scene that are responsible for the clinical phenomena we have described. Do they localize the sources of the breakdown? No, not altogether. But if we study the problems of adaptation of the individuals of today we can piece together the total picture.

We are witnessing the *reductio ad absurdum* of the promises of the liberal way of life in which one is responsible for one's own fate, granted the assumption that the social machinery for implementing these approved goals exists. To make use of this machinery requires planning and the requisite capital, neither of which is available to any but a few. Most people live unplanned lives and improvise as they go along, even if the rate of those who get college education has increased 200 per cent in fifty years. Most people do not reach middle classdom, but have to engage in the fringe activities and drudgery. At the same time they are stimulated to need and want things, for they have now become the "consumers." They have learned to live by the religion of things and gadgets, each of which simplifies, adds a small increment of pleasure or triumph. Henry Ford made every man a Columbus and a conqueror. The higher the social stratum, the greater the pressure for accomplishment and the greater the risks to self-esteem. A great many give up the fight; it is not, however, a resignation, but a resentful defeat. Life has become harder because there is no ceiling on aspiration, and in the past two generations, from 1914 on, the external barriers to fulfilling life goals have been seriously increased by two world wars and a depression.

During this very time, 1914–1950, we have seen the fruition of two powerful influences that have altered the character of life in the western world: the influence of feminism and the influence of psychology (especially psychoanalysis).

Of the two, the first is the more important because it has led to institutional changes—the alteration of the position of the female in society and in the family, which has influenced the generic patterns in the family. Confusion is created in the mind of the growing child as to the differences in role between male and female. The hard and fast, though perhaps inequitable, Victorian role differentiations have disappeared. The egocentric tendencies of both partners in a marriage have disrupted the unity of the family and augmented the child's insecurity. The "education" in character and morality has been taken out of the hands of the parents, school, and books and been transferred to the mass media, which preach the purely instrumental use of human beings as the standard morality. If we add together all these familial influences, and the external influences that keep insisting that you should need and want things, and that you use other human beings as means to these ends, or regard them as obstacles to be removed, you have the formula for the collapse of public morality.

The influence of these factors on sexual development can be appraised only in the light of the knowledge that homosexuality is a symptom of failure of development. Inequalities in self-assertion always exist; but most forms of homosexuality are due not merely to the special conditioning of the arousal and expectation patterns, but to the wish to ingratiate oneself with the powerful father and to incorporate his magical implement orally or anally. I could, for this occasion, invoke the evidence from primates and birds who, in danger situations of defeat in combat, assume what looks like the feminine sexual posture. However, the same monkey in a victorious situation has the defeated monkey make the same gesture. We do know that this situation is self-preservative; we do not know for certain that it is sexual in intent. Judging from the behavior of man, it is. But it is not a certainty in animals.

The increase in male homosexuality is therefore like the increase in schizophrenia: it arises from (1) an increase in the general hardship of adaptation and (2) confusing or inconsistent cultural directives and restrictions. The schizotypal failure is irrespective of intelligence, and great intellects have been harnessed to schizotypal assumptions and modes of thinking. A considerable proportion of our "art" is today being created by schizotypical characters. The plight of the male who is ground between the compulsory public ideal of achievement of the higher living standard and the dread of a collapsed self-esteem is severe. He either flees from the female altogether into the delusion of homosexuality, or he exploits the female's sexual availability and makes her pay for her new freedom. Under these conditions he is hard to trap into a marriage, or demands a "dutch" arrangement with his wife, or demands support from her. He is willing to surrender his Victorian prerogatives for security. The upkeep on masculine ideals has gotten too high.

In certain urban centers, the influence of psychiatry has not been an unmitigated blessing. Oddities of character heretofore pridefully displayed as badges of individuality have been ground down to the lesser proportions and stigmatization of pathology. As the influence spread in the early part of the century, the new deity called Normality was in for its quota of worship and sacrifice. If you were impotent or frigid you not only failed to live up to a new specification for happiness, you were also a failure and a victim of your own past. Skeletons were now rattling not as they formerly had and should, in closets, but down the labyrinthine ways of your own mind. This called for new deceptions, remedies, and new ways for establishing claims for individuality. The public had to refrain from criticism, because they were taught that everyone is by nature bisexual anyway. Confusion replaced the simplicity of the Victorian parental education, and we bred in the twenties a group of the most terrified and intimidated parents the world has ever seen. Parents must now be encouraged not to be afraid of their children.

This is another way of saying that psychoanalysis issued confused and inconsistent directives to a public that respected its authority. In many instances the public did what it wanted with these directives—as it did in the twenties, when it made sexual freedom a necessity for mental health. This was the public's doing, not Freud's. He never said that sexual promiscuity was a cure or prophylactic of neurosis. But for the greater part psychoanalysis made parents self-conscious and terrified of inflicting neurosis on children. They acquired a phobia for discipline and direction and subscribed to the now exposed fallacy that an undirected child knows best what is good for it. Some of these parents, so eager to prevent neurosis in their children, exposed them to promiscuity. Among these cases there has been no lessening of sexual neurosis. Psychoanalysis is responsible for the fiction, promulgated largely by Freud, that culture is predominantly restrictive; the reverse is true. It is predominantly directive. And the child should not be asked by itself to discover those truths about social expediency that are incorporated in the general directives of sex morality. We can mitigate its extravagances and correct its errors; but we cannot dispense with it entirely.

In my brief discussion on the study of history as culture, I began by showing you what the social sciences, anthropology, and history did without the ability to keep track of what is happening to man in the culture process when it is static and when it is in motion. We cannot afford to ignore the contribution of psychiatry in diagnosing the effects of institutions on man. You may ignore this at your peril, because these are the only homeostats in society. Man does not know in advance the effects of his social improvisations. Very often he wakes up to the effects of institutions when it is too late, and they have to run their course to ruin. An instance of this is the effect of the break-up of the family in the Israeli kibbutzim; a second is the effect of feminism 150 years after it started—all for good and sufficient reasons. The human unit lets you know long before disaster that a given institutional set-up is creating trouble. The evidence is there for those who can see and they must convince the rest of us of the urgency of the observations.

Finally, let me urge again the value of undertaking a large series of empirical studies to aid us in gathering data. We do not need rhapsodists or those who, in the interests of psychology, have assumed the role of prophets, if not messiahs. We need hard workers and empiricism, not inspiration. We, in all the social sciences, must wake up to the fact that we do not enjoy any authority. Perhaps we do not deserve it. There is a vast storehouse of data in those primitive societies, or what is left of them, to teach us about those social patterns that have viability. (We cannot visit the unmarked cemeteries of dead cultures that have failed because of faulty patterning of human relations.) Secondly, we have the vast storehouse of recorded history that needs restating. Finally, we have the vast and intricate laboratory of our own troubled cultures, which we ought to study for the long pull rather than have our methods appropriated by big business. Let us hope that if we do this we may establish an authority we do not yet have, to awaken the self-preservative instincts of man and to give him some intelligent guidance about where the dangers lie in his otherwise astonishing performance that makes his brief sojourn on this planet the greatest success story of all time.

5.

Psychoanalysis and Its Discontents

ERNEST VAN DEN HAAG
Adjunct Associate Professor of Sociology
New York University

I BELIEVE Professor Kardiner's viewpoints play an important enough role among contemporary students to warrant critical analysis. I hope, however, that he will excuse me if some of my comments should turn out to be based on misunderstandings. The boldness of his speculations, the profusion of intriguing points, and the imaginative leaps that make his paper so interesting also left me somewhat disoriented, as though I had been taken on a long and rapid journey and my vision had become blurred.

I

Professor Kardiner stresses certain severe limitations of anthropologists and social scientists and, on the other hand, of psychoanalysts; these limitations, he feels, prevent both from fully understanding the subjects they are studying: both therefore should change their faulty "frames of reference" and thus avoid their mistakes. Although no doubt many errors are committed on all sides, I have been unable to identify and find those mentioned by Professor Kardiner.

I do not know any social scientists that hold the "superorganic" theory of culture in the form ascribed to Kroeber by Professor Kardiner. If some do, they are hardly representative. Social scientists do not—as Kardiner thinks—"exclude man

Notes to this section begin on page 115.

from the operational frame of reference" or "anthropomorphize institutions," or find "no room to consider the impact of institutions on those exposed to them and do not know how to undertake such a study." For example, the text used to teach freshmen at City College defines an institution as "a regular way of doing something—an established procedure." [1] I define institutions in *The Fabric of Society* [2] as "permanent group behavior patterns." In short, social scientists define institutions as the behavior of people. Hence, people are not "excluded from the operational frame of reference" in any intelligible sense.

Anthropological literature abounds precisely with studies of the impact of institutions on people. Anthropologists know that culture is created and borne by men. When they define culture as "superorganic" they wish to stress (1) that culture, including institutions, exists before and after the lifespan of the *individual organism* and molds him more than vice versa; (2) that culture is not reducible to individual organisms or simple aggregates but involves socially patterned and transmitted relationships which are best explained in terms of the functions they serve in the society in which they occur—although at times they become dysfunctional. It is to the study of these relationships that sociology and anthropology are dedicated. They do not reflect intrapsychic phenomena but abstract from them so as to artificially isolate their subject. This procedure is followed in all sciences. None, therefore, aspires to answer all questions. Unlike Professor Kardiner, I see no inconsistency between this view and any of Freud's views.[3] Indeed, unlike Professor Kardiner, I think that many anthropological studies explain the interdependence of institutions and personality types almost too well: so well that one finds it hard to see how this relationship came into being, how it developed and how it might change from within. And yet there is such a thing as history, although it is discreetly ignored in most anthropological studies—a neglect so easily accepted with regard to primitive peoples because usually little is known about their history.

Having chided social scientists for some views that would be foolish, but are not held by them, Professor Kardiner goes on to attribute some rather odd views to Freud; Freud is said to have invented "a technique [of studying the individual in his environment] which he could not use" because he imputed the responses of the organism which he correctly observed not to interaction but to the autonomous action of an instinct."

I find this baffling. What is psychoanalysis concerned with if not the relationships among people? Did Freud think of the Oedipus complex as an intrauterine relationship? Psychoanalysis is *centrally* concerned with "interaction." The vicissitudes of the drives which Freud described are largely due to the impact of culture—by means of persons other than the subject—on these drives. The whole ego is, as Freud observed, a creation of the relationship between the inborn needs—e.g., hunger—and outer reality, including, pre-eminently, society. The superego is almost exclusively a social creation via the primary group. And, according to Freud, these two parts of the personality—these results of the interaction of society with the individual which are internalized by him—determine how and to what extent the individual can acknowledge and satisfy instinctual demands. To say that Freud "found there was just no room for including the environmental factor in his frame of reference" is, in my opinion, a profound misunderstanding. In Freud's theory, the environmental factor transmitted through the primary group is internalized quite early. It is *part* of the "frame of reference"—wherefore it need not be added later.

In short, I do not believe that either the anthropologists or Freud hold the views or are limited in their method in the way Dr. Kardiner thinks they are. The conflict that Dr. Kardiner sees never existed in the form he perceives it; and his attempt to repair frames of reference is, to my mind, irrelevant to any of the many actual and serious problems that anthropology and psychoanalysis seek to solve.[4]

II

I must find fault even with some of Dr. Kardiner's minor criticisms of Freud. Not that Freud's theories do not leave much still to be explained. Even when they provide an explanation, it is often ambiguous. And very seldom do we have more than hypotheses, so formulated that they will be hard to prove or disprove with the degree of exactness that is desirable and exists elsewhere. One difficulty—which I can do no more than mention—is that methods of observation often must include the scheme of interpretation that the observations should validate. (But I am confident that this difficulty—which is not confined to psychoanalysis—can be overcome.) Admirable and immensely fruitful as is Freud's achievement, it is in this sense largely heuristic: it has not led us into the promised land, though it may well have shown us the way. We will know about that only after having arrived.

But with all this, I cannot agree with Dr. Kardiner that "Freud anthropomorphizes instincts." Freud's speculations on drives may be true or false. His metaphors may or may not be well chosen. But no literate person takes them literally. Drives are not anthropomorphized by Freud beyond considering them a part of our human heritage that is not wholly controlled by our consciousness. Similarly, I find Dr. Kardiner's objection against "desexualized libido" (which he thinks is oxymoronic) unsubstantiated. The expression is far from graceful, but the meaning quite clear: energy that is supposed to have an original sexual source and aim but which losing the marks of source and aim continues to serve as energy. There are legitimate questions about this: (a) Can the sexual source and the originally sexual aim be proved? (b) If not, is the hypothesis of such original source and aim fruitful? I would be doubtful on the proof, affirmative on the fruitfulness of the hypothesis. But this is not Dr. Kardiner's question. He objects to the whole concept for reasons not stated in his paper. (Incidentally, with this reasoning, one could also object to the idea of libidinized functions—which is rather basic to some syndromes.)

III

Let me now return to a major point. I share Professor Kardiner's view—and Freud's—that personality structure is strongly influenced by the treatment the infant receives. But, summarizing his very interesting work on the Alorese, Professor Kardiner suggests that social values in turn can be traced to the same source, and therefore "cannot be preached at people if the makings for the reception are not there." This may be a tautology, and as true as it is trivial. But if it is more than that, if Professor Kardiner really means by "the assumption of values [is not] a voluntary process" that the normative system of a society depends decisively on how the cradle is rocked, I think he raises many more questions than he answers. What about the success of Christian missions or, generally, people's ability to change values? What about infants brought up in primitive cultures and making adjustments to the Western world? I certainly believe there is a relationship between disposition to accept values and personality structure, and between personality structure and upbringing. But how important this relationship is—how many other relationships are involved and how—I don't think we know. Are we really to suppose that Germany changed from Imperial Germany to the Weimar Republic to Hitler's Germany and now in the West to Adenauer's democracy, in the East to Moscow's dictatorship—and surely there are different value systems involved—because of changes in the treatment of infants? Are both Max Weber and R. H. Tawney quite totally wrong in their different views about the origin of the capitalist system? Would it not be more reasonable to say that these and many other value systems can be accepted by adults with nearly any kind of infantile conditioning? In short, infantile conditioning does not stand, as Professor Kardiner seems to think, in a one-to-one relationship to value systems but permits a broad range. And we know little about the focus and limits of each range.

I have commented earlier about the absence of historical dimension in many anthropological studies. Professor Kardiner's remarks about St. Benedict, St. Francis, and the Inquisition indicate that this fault is not confined to anthropologists. The message of the two saints, Professor Kardiner explains, is "a device to make suffering . . . bearable and to promise rewards." But St. Benedict and St. Francis (who lived 700 years after him) had very different messages. Surely St. Francis preached *ora et ama;* he did not stress "tolerance for hard and unrewarding work." The whole idea of the value of "hard and unrewarding work" smacks more of Jansenism, of Calvinism and of the nineteenth century than of the earlier ages which, according to Professor Kardiner, should have preached these values, but didn't. On the other hand, St. Benedict preached *ora et labora.* If the Benedictines ever went in much for suffering, it's news to me. Moreover, suffering had not just been invented. Nor has it ceased since. Professor Kardiner's "explanation" then, at most, suggests why the phenomena were possible, not why they occurred, nor why quite different reactions to suffering did not occur. And I might comment similarly on Professor Kardiner's remarks on the Inquisition—which, compared to Nazism and Communism, seems a rather benign institution, even though it occurred in times which, according to him, should have produced a more ferocious one.

When Professor Kardiner goes on to explain that "it is one of the most elementary lessons of psychiatry that problems of self-preservation tend to erode the capacity for affectionate and cooperative relations," he seems to undermine his own point. We should find the Middle Ages and many primitives bereft of the capacity for affectionate and cooperative relationship. Moreover, this capacity should be at a maximum now, for, as I see it, the problems of self-preservation are at a minimum. Yet I am sure that Professor Kardiner does not think that people are more affectionate and cooperative than ever. This suggests at best that he defines "problems of self-preservation" not as an external reality matter but an internal psychological matter, in effect as that which makes people uncooperative, etc. This seems circular reasoning. It might be added that concentration camps showed the effect of sudden changes as much as the effect of the intensity of the struggle for self-preservation. Finally, note that the guards did not have the inmates' problems of self-preservation; did they have more capacity for "affectionate and cooperative relationships"? In reality, that capacity seems to depend on the intensity, the quantity and the type of the problems of self-preservation

—*and* on conditioning. Often problems of self-preservation strengthen tendencies toward cooperation more than the absence of such problems does. Moreover, "self-preservation" depends on one's concept of self, which seems largely a function of one's reference group. "Self-preservation" for the slave owner means keeping his slaves; for the slave it means being fed; and for Dr. Kardiner it includes keeping his patients, his professorship and, in general, his status.

IV

In the last part of his paper, Professor Kardiner offers a fascinating theory to explain phenomena which no one has shown to exist. These phenomena are increases in male homosexuality, schizophrenia,[5] juvenile delinquency, and egocentric tendencies of family members.

Take juvenile delinquency. According to Lecky's *History of European Morals:*

> In 1712 a club of young men of the higher classes, who assumed the name of Mohocks, were accustomed nightly to sally out drunk into the streets to hunt the passers-by and to subject them in mere wantonness to the most atrocious outrages. One of their favorite amusements, called "tipping the lion," was to squeeze the nose of their victim flat upon his face and to bore out his eyes with their fingers. Among them were the "sweaters" who formed a circle round their prisoner and pricked him with their swords till he sank exhausted to the ground, the "dancing masters" so-called from their skill in making men caper by thrusting swords into their legs, the "tumblers" whose favorite amusement was to set women on their heads and commit various indecencies and barbarities on the limbs that were exposed. Maid servants, as they opened their masters' doors, were waylaid, beaten and their faces cut. Matrons enclosed in barrels were rolled down the steep and stony incline of Snow Hill. Watchmen were beaten unmercifully and their noses slit. Country gentlemen went to the theatre as if in time of war, accompanied by their armed retainers. A bishop's son was said to be one of the gang and a baronet was among those who were arrested.

Is it in comparison to the Age of Enlightenment that juvenile delinquency has increased? Or, to what period? As Professor Kardiner agrees, there is no actual evidence for an increase in homosexuality. I submit there is evidence only for some increase in awareness. Nor is there any reason at all—and Professor Kardiner gives none—to consider increased homosexuality, delinquency or schizophrenia singly or together as "signals of social distress." Indeed, as far as we know, some of the most brilliant periods of cultural development have been marked by at least some of these phenomena. Possibly they are part of the price we pay. They may be signals, not of distress but possibly of a stress which might be incidental to beneficial developments. Possibly also of relaxation. I don't know, and I wonder how Professor Kardiner does.[6]

I do agree with Professor Kardiner's low estimate of the psychological climate of our time. In fact, I have tried to explain it myself elsewhere.[7] But I do not believe that the symptoms named by Professor Kardiner would show what they are meant to show if they did exist. And there is no evidence that they do. Nor is there evidence to show a worsening of social health. In short, the theories offered seem to me, if not entirely clear, entirely unsupported. The major difficulties lie in two premises implicit in Professor Kardiner's paper: that psychological health is related to moral goodness; and secondly, that society can be diagnosed almost as an individual patient can.

V

Although scornful of the views of such moralizers as Erich Fromm—and here I do not dissent—Professor Kardiner competes with them. His own views on "the *reductio ad absurdum* of the promises of the liberal way of life," on "the egocentric tendencies of both partners in marriage," on "signals of social distress," on "a considerable proportion of modern 'art' being created by schizotypical characters," [8] rest on a relationship or identification of the morally or esthetically "good" with the psychologically "healthy," which as a minimum suggests that *only* what is psychologically healthy can be good—i.e., psychological health is a necessary condition for goodness; or, as a maximum, Professor Kardiner might say that whatever is psychologically healthy is good, i.e., psychological health is a sufficient condition for goodness. I do not believe that either of these propositions is correct: i.e., the unhealthy—e.g., Durkheim's altruistic suicide—can be morally good; and the healthy—e.g., some murders or running away with your neighbor's wife—may not be. It is because psychological health and goodness are not identical that psychoanalytic therapy is not connected with transmission or acceptance of the analyst's moral views. Psychoanalysis may help restore the possibility of moral choice to a patient. But it does not make that choice for him.[9]

Further, if one wishes to derive a prescription for action from a diagnosis of a society as unhealthy—and Professor Kardiner does—one must have a value system from which one can infer that the advantages possibly procured by the conditions producing unhealthiness are not worth it, and that the disadvantages of the proposed therapy are. I doubt that the implied value system would be acceptable to many people if made explicit. And, of course, I know no way of justifying it. Perhaps optimal mental health requires an egalitarian homogeneous society or a Huxleyan "brave new world." Perhaps Hitler and Stalin helped the mental health of more people than they injured. Would we—if that were true—have to support their systems? Or, perhaps optimal mental health is achieved in a Jeffersonian rural system with low living standards. Would we favor such a social optimum should it be inconsistent with the economic one?

To avoid such difficulties, sometimes morality is defined as nearly coextensive with mental health. This is increasingly done. (I suspect it is implicit in the last part of Professor Kardiner's paper.) But I can see no warrant for it. Moral preferences remain no more (for that matter, no less) than moral preferences, however much disguised as pseudoscientific judgments on "maturity," "stability," "normality," and other unspecified or irrelevant qualities.[10] The disadvantage of the change in terminology is that it makes serious moral discourse impossible. (In the end, it will impair scientific discourse, too.) You may object to your views being called wicked, and try to justify them. But the person who instead calls them "neurotic" makes it easy for himself not to take them seriously, just as a Communist might by calling them "Fascist." He has simply ousted your views from the realm of discussion. Yet nothing would be proved about the wrongness of your views, even if your motive for proclaiming them could be shown to be neurotic.[11]

The second major premise implicit in Professor Kardiner's paper is that psychoanalytic theory can diagnose a society as though it were an individual patient. However, I do not believe that group behavior can be interpreted psychoanalytically the way individual behavior can be. Psychoanalytic theory becomes the less reliable the less it is applied to live patients. The less the object of study is able to respond—if we apply the theory to remote historical figures or to groups—the less reliable the theory. As various symptoms appear, and as the patient reacts to therapeutic behavior, an analyst with a live patient before him will be guided in his theoretical formulation. Almost each segment of patient behavior permits a considerable range of interpretations from which the analyst chooses. His choice is shown to be appropriate or inappropriate by the patient's reaction. The trouble in interpreting the behavior of groups or absent persons is that they do not respond with reactions that can be utilized to narrow the interpretative range. As a result, that range remains insufficiently restricted to be meaningful; there are quite a number of interpretations compatible with general psychoanalytic principles that could "explain" the behavior of absent patients, or of groups. Hence, the explanation chosen tends to reflect predilection which is not fully justified. I think that Freud here allowed himself to be seduced by his own speculations. But we need not follow him. Moreover, we seldom will even approximate knowledge of the relevant facts as well with groups, as absent patients, as we do with live individual patients. This leads me to conclude that we should leave absent patients alone (or be aware that we are playing a parlor game) [12] and that psychoanalysis can only *contribute* to the explanation of group behavior—and we do not know yet how much.

One additional point needs to be made about groups, including the behavior of individuals as group members. Tempting as it may be to conceive of sociology as macropsychology, it is no more correct than it would be to reduce psychology to microsociology (though this seems to be the major point of Harry Stack Sullivan and of his school). There are needs of the human personality that are inborn, however socially transmuted; and an explanation of behavior that disregards intrapsychic relations cannot account for it completely and economically. On the other hand, the behavior of groups cannot be accounted for by studying individuals. The group as such and its history must be studied. If this be true, then psychoanalysis can contribute to the study of group behavior, but it cannot by itself account for it. Nor can it account for the behavior of individuals acting as group members. To illustrate, some people are criminals despite a "normal" social environment. Some are law-abiding despite a criminal milieu. In both these cases, we would do well to concentrate on psychological factors for an explanation. But some people are law-abiding in a law-abiding environment, and some violate the law in accordance with the norms of a criminal milieu. Here we do best in concentrating on social factors for an explanation, particularly if we are interested in finding out what creates and changes the social milieu.

Psychoanalysis offers a reservoir of hypotheses connecting individual personality with social milieu; these hypotheses—in many cases the only ones available—are worth exploring. However, they offer no more than hints contributing to the understanding of the diversity of human culture. To behave as though they already offered the explanation to which some day they might contribute is, in my opinion, a disservice to both psychoanalysis and social science.

Notes

1. Robert Bierstedt, *The Social Order* (New York: McGraw-Hill, 1957).

2. Written with Ralph Ross (New York: Harcourt, Brace & Co., 1957).

3. I am similarly astounded by Professor Kardiner's incidental remarks about historians such as Kahler, Hauser and Barzun being "in revolt against the king-and-battle historians as well as the Toynbees." It seems odd to reassert the well established importance of cultural history by denying the need for political and military history or for philosophical studies of history.

4. Among recent instances of fruitful collaboration, let me mention August B. Hollingshead and Frederick C. Redlich, *Social Class and Mental Illness* (New York: John Wiley & Sons, 1958). Note that it is a psychiatrist and a *sociologist* that collaborate. I think that this is the more relevant collaboration with respect to *our* society. Of course, I need hardly remind you of Dr. Kardiner's own most interesting work on the Alorese in *Psychological Frontiers of Society*, ed. A. Kardiner, R. Linton, C. Dubois, J. West (New York: Columbia University, 1945).

5. I am aware that more schizophrenics and schizoids seem to turn up in private practice than before. Perhaps more than a third of all diagnoses in private practice now refer to schizoids or schizophrenics. But this may be due to increased awareness, different diagnosis, better prognosis, different age and family structure, etc., rather than to more schizophrenia. (Note that the supposed general increase in psychosis has been shown to be very unlikely by Herbert Goldhamer and Andrew Marshall in *Psychosis and Civilization* (Chicago: Free Press, 1953).

6. Note that I am discussing, as did Professor Kardiner, the social meaning of these phenomena—not their meaning for the individuals afflicted, although I suspect that Professor Kardiner's conclusion owes something to confusing the individual and the social.

7. See Chapter 15 of *The Fabric of Society.*

8. I wonder on what research this proposition rests? And on what criteria of discrimination? And in what way the health of the artist is to be relevant to the work of art?

9. There are some exceptions that occur in the treatment of schizophrenia. But psychotics are legally deemed unable to make moral choices.

10. I do not wish to give the impression that psychoanalysts are alone in such confusions. Note, e.g., my criticism of Professor Kenneth Clark's "scientific proof" of the injurious effects of prejudice in *The Fabric of Society,* pp. 165–66.

11. Moreover, there is no workable definition of mental health in general. Fortunately, there is no need for such definition so long as workable definitions of particular diseases are available. Note, however, that I do not wish to deny wholly the possibility of a philosophical anthropology, which, if it could not decide what values men ought to have, could help establish the range of actual and possible value systems as it relates to the range of human possibility.

12. The matter is illustrated admirably by Meyer Schapiro's "Leonardo and Freud," *Journal of the History of Ideas,* April, 1956.

6.

Psychoanalysis and Sociology

ALEX INKELES
Professor of Sociology
Harvard University

In his discussion of psychoanalysis and social science, Dr. Kardiner tells us that at the "heart of the matter" is the "frame-of-reference disease." He means by this that anthropologists—and presumably other social scientists—have not effectively incorporated the human unit into their design, and in their turn "the Freudians go about complacently with the conviction that they do not need to concern themselves with the cultural environment." I hope to extend Dr. Kardiner's analysis by consideration of yet another discipline, namely sociology.

Modern sociology may conveniently be regarded as having begun with the publication of Durkheim's *Rules of Sociological Method,* and his *Suicide* may be taken as the first distinctively sociological empirical research of the modern variety. Durkheim noted the great variation in suicide rates between the nations of Europe and within particular subgroups in any nation, and sought for a principle that would explain this variation. He found it in the differences in the extent to which nations or groups were characterized by a high degree of social integration or solidarity. Durkheim conceived of the sociological mode of analysis as explicitly nonpsychological, that is, he *insisted on leaving out* the human personality as an element in the chain of his analysis. Thus, he set as his goal "disregarding the individual as such, his motives and his ideas," in favor of seeking "directly the states of the various social environments . . . , in terms of

Notes to this section begin on page 129.

which the variations in suicide occur."[1] And later in his book, after reviewing the inadequacy of psychological explanations, he announced triumphantly:

> Wholly different are the results we obtained when we forgot the individual and sought the causes of the suicidal aptitude in the nature of the societies themselves. . . . The suicide rate can be explained only sociologically . . .[2]

Durkheim performed a great service and led us to vastly increased knowledge by his devotion to the idea that there are distinctive sociological forces that influence man's behavior. So great was the force of his argument and so impressive were the results he obtained by his method that his position became the standard for most of the sociologists who followed him. But in so far as Durkheim gave sociologists a clear-cut identity, it was unfortunate that it was not based mainly on the distinctive and autonomous sociological framework of their analysis. Instead, their sense of identity rested in large measure on their *counter*identification vis-à-vis psychologists. The result was that sociology, despite Cooley, Mead, and Thomas, developed and remained as a self-consciously nonpsychological and often aggressively antipsychological discipline.

Even in Durkheim, of course, the individual and his psychology crept back into sociological explanation. After locating the uniform presence of low states of social integration in groups with high suicide rates, Durkheim still had to face the questions of why and how such states of the social environment produce the different suicide rates. And this question could not be answered without considering the nature of the human being who intervened between the "suicidogenic" currents that Durkheim located in societies and the suicide rates that the currents produced. Incidentally, one of the theories Durkheim developed has many attributes akin to Freud's death instinct, and would surely have met his approval, even if to Durkheim's distress. On the whole, however, Durkheim's psychological theory was quite inadequate to the task. Yet for our purposes that is much less important than the fact that in Durkheim's analysis the psychology of personality retained an illicit quality, something not only secondary but slightly bootleg.

Sociological research in the period after World War II reveals a marked change in this pattern. There is now widespread evidence that sociologists recognize the importance of simultaneously considering the psychological and social-structural variables, and numerous studies have been completed or are under way which rest on the central premise that behavior can be understood only if due account is taken not only of the situation of action but of the actor's perception of it and his particular needs and dispositions. More and more, sociological research has come to accept the central role of general personality theory, and of measures of particular personalities, in the interpretation and prediction of social behavior. To illustrate this trend I must limit myself here to three brief references.

Perhaps most heartening is the fact that on the very topic on which Durkheim so effectively made his mark, we now have one of the most outstanding examples of the integration of psychological and sociological analysis. I have in mind the brief but impressive work of Andrew Henry and James Short, Jr., on *Homicide and Suicide*. I stress the word *integration* of psychological and sociological analysis because in this effort sociology is not replaced by or reduced to psychology. Henry and Short begin with an explicitly psychodynamic assumption—that suicide and homicide are both aggressive acts. The aggression is assumed to arise from frustration and, in common with all aggressive impulses, initially seeks an "outside" object. At this point a Durkheimian concept, the strength of the relational system, is introduced to assess the actor's situation. Where he is subject to greater external restraint it will be easier to perceive those who impose the restraint as legitimate objects of aggression, and homicide will be the more likely outcome. Where the degree of external restraint is slight, as for example in the higher and more autonomous occupational groups, it will be difficult to locate an easily legitimated external target, and the aggressive impulse will therefore most likely be directed at the self, leading to suicide.

Within the framework of this set of assumptions, Henry and Short reassess Durkheim's findings and introduce a series of new and fascinating materials on the relative variations in suicide and homicide rates which seem to follow the pattern they predict. Many problems of course remain. And alternative explanations of their very findings certainly can be entertained. Psychologists may well argue as to how adequate it is to regard homicide and suicide as aggressive acts differing only in object. Sociologists may question whether it is really meaningful to describe those higher in the status system as simply less subject to "external restraint" than laborers. But my purpose here is not to assess the adequacy of Henry and Short's analysis. I wish, rather, to call attention to the fact that their study gives equal standing to psychological and sociological theory, and that they predict behavior only after assessing the effect of psychological and sociological factors interacting simultaneously.

A very similar development may, incidentally, be found in another classical and traditional area of sociological research, namely in the study of juvenile delinquency. The standard explanation for delinquency developed by Clifford Shaw in his classic study stressed that certain areas of the city in which *social disorganization* was marked developed a delinquent subculture. The analogy with Durkheim's social integration and his suicidogenic current is evident. But as with Durkheim there remained the mystery of how a state of the society became converted into the individual's delinquent act; why some exposed to delinquent culture learned and practiced it and others not. It was only when we posited an explicit psychological mechanism in the delinquent and explored the conditions of its development that we were able to establish the link between the state of social disorganization and the thousands of individual acts that yielded the delinquency rate. I have in mind, of course, the work of the Gluecks in *Unravelling Juvenile Delinquency,* and especially their exploration of the differences in superego strength in delinquent and nondelinquent boys drawn from equally delinquent environments.

A second major realm in which psychological theory has

been applied to traditional sociological problems is the study of recruitment to and performance in occupational and other social roles. The distinctive nature of the advance here lies not in the grubbing search to discover whether by some happy chance some personality type or trait will emerge as more common and perhaps typical in a given occupational group. Much of the work being done in this area has reached a quite different level of interest and sophistication. In the best work careful analysis is made in advance of the special qualities of the job, on the basis of which the researcher specifies the distinctive personality characteristics that should influence recruitment and/or performance in the particular occupation. An outstanding example may be found in G. Swanson's study of the differences between the job of the editorial and the sports writer. Basing himself on theory earlier developed by Lasswell and Rosten, Swanson predicted that as against the sports writers, the editorialists would be markedly more phallic–aspiring, anal–expulsive and oral–passive in character. Not only were these main predictions strikingly supported by psychological test, but a large number of subsidiary predictions were also confirmed.[3] This study is but one of a series which suggest that we have begun to break ground in a great unexploited field of study of the relation of character types to different aspects of social structure and the functioning of social systems.

A third realm of sociological concern in which we have recently witnessed interesting advances in the coordinate use of psychodynamic and sociological theory is the study of child socialization. In many ways the socialization process is crucial in facilitating the continuity or in inducing the change of social systems. The study of the results or effects of particular child-rearing practices, while in itself predominantly a focus study for the psychologist, is nevertheless a subject of great significance for the sociologist. But as our horizons expand in this realm we have come increasingly to recognize that what the significant socializing agents, and pre-eminently the parents, do to the infant and child is not independent of forces in the larger society. On the contrary, the social context of the father's occupation may be strongly associated with the way in which he raises his children. For example, the degree to which his work environment approximates the model of the small, informal, personal business or the large, bureaucratic mass work setting may exert important influence on the type of discipline a man applies to his children. It is just such a problem that has been made one of the central issues in an important study by Professors Miller and Swanson at the University of Michigan, where they are exploring the types of ego defense that characterize youths whose parents have used differing disciplinary methods. The disciplinary methods used by the parents are themselves regarded not as random but as systematically related to the work environment of the parent. If we were further to extend the analysis, it is evident how we would move ahead to explore the consequences of this sequence of events in the later life performance and adjustment of the children, and in how they would in turn rear their own young.

There is, then, reason to be encouraged, even gratified. Progress is being made on a number of fronts in bringing about a coordinated, perhaps even integrated, utilization of the theory and method of personality psychology and sociology in dealing with problems of great scientific and practical interest. But you will have noticed that I speak of personality psychology rather than of psychoanalysis. There are, of course, many evidences of the direct application of psychoanalytic theory, if not method, to sociological problems. Indeed, the research I cited above was selected to illustrate this influence. In the study of the journalists the author relied directly on character typology developed by Freud, and the study of child-rearing stressed the ego defenses, perhaps somewhat neglected by Freud but later given special attention by Anna Freud. These instances are far, however, from the full-scale application of psychoanalysis to the understanding of social problems which I imagine Dr. Kardiner would like to see. Yet they represent the more outstanding applications of psychoanalytic theory in more or less traditional sociological research. The vast majority of sociological studies that make use of psychological theory and data are quite eclectic in their choice of psychological theory. An explicitly psychoanalytic frame of reference is *not* likely to be the first choice. Indeed, its explicit use is likely to be quite rare.

The failure of psychoanalysis to win a firm foothold in sociology is probably best understood in historical perspective. As I have noted, Durkheim fought a vigorous and impressive struggle against the psychological reductionism of his time, hoping to establish sociological variables as independent and important in their own right. But no sooner had this been accomplished than a new onslaught befell Durkheim's followers in what seemed to them the new psychological reductionism of Freud and many of his disciples. This challenge was, on the whole, met by rather global rejection of Freudianism as a camp hostile to sociology. Freudianism was typically classed by sociologists with other theories which sought to explain social phenomena in defiance of the sociologists' assumption that they arise only from "the complex interplay of various and diverse conditions." In the case of Freudianism, its particular monism took the form of a simple appeal to "presumptive origins . . . conceived of as organic impulses." Robert MacIver, for example, thus classifies Freud's approach to social causation. He speaks of Freud's *Totem and Taboo* as "one work in which [Freud] went so far as to designate a supposititious primal parricide," and quotes Freud as specifying this to be the "inexorable criminal act with which so many things began, social organization, moral restriction, and religion."[4] This quotation is meant to indicate to all sociologists the utter unacceptability of the Freudian explanation of social phenomena. It is reproduced with barely a line of comment. No comment is needed. All loyal sociologists would indeed spontaneously draw back in annoyance, shock, or horror.

Yet the seemingly simplistic psychological reductionism that sometimes crept into Freud's work cannot in itself explain the failure of Freudian psychology to secure a firmer place in sociological thinking. Even among those who are not frightened off by this reductionism, and indeed among those who are in general quite sympathetic to psychoanalysis, there are major obstacles to its ready incorporation into sociological research on a systematic basis.

There is one very general difficulty, of a methodological sort, which perhaps cuts across many of the more specific complaints. The Freudian method of analysis is above all "clinical"; this is of its essence. By contrast, the professional training of the sociologist stresses objective "external" and quantifiable method. Exact definition of one's variables, explicit indication of the operations to be performed, definite indication of the indices of association to be relied on, reproducibility, i.e., the possibility of replication and verification by others, are essential elements of his whole philosophy of research. Not only does he find the psychoanalytic practitioners clinical in their approach—something he himself often practices and generally accepts—but he finds them strangely resistant, suspicious, and even hostile to efforts to go beyond the clinical method in the application of tests of reliability and validity which have become the stock in trade of the sociological discipline. There is, of course, now evident a change in the willingness of psychoanalysis to permit and collaborate in such efforts. The change is coming about, as is only proper, concurrently with an insistence that the sociologist become familiar with psychoanalysis, its practice and its clinical method, through firsthand experience. But at the present time severe limits continue to be placed on the potential influence of psychoanalysis in sociology by what seems to the sociologist to be an inability on the part of the psychoanalytic school to comprehend the fundamental importance of the simple rules of the scientific method as it is generally practiced in the behavioral sciences.

While this difference about method may explain why a psychoanalytic interpretation of social phenomena may be less than acceptable to sociologists, it does not suffice to explain why more influence has not been felt in sociology from psychoanalytic thinking. Here we may point to a number of quite specific aspects of the psychoanalytic movement which have affected this outcome and continue to do so. The difficulty was well summarized by Dr. Kardiner when he diagnosed it as "frame-of-reference trouble," and traced this more particularly to the fact that

> the Freudians go about complacently with the conviction that they do not need to concern themselves with the cultural environment, or settling for the lip service that, of course, the environment must be taken into account, when the fact is that there is no technique for so doing.

In general, I agree with Dr. Kardiner's estimate of the situation, but perhaps I can make some contribution to furthering the discussion by trying to locate the difficulty more concretely and precisely.

I believe the sociologists' coldness comes first and foremost from the basic assumption underlying psychoanalysis, that man's behavior is to be understood primarily as the manifestation of incompletely socialized instinctual drives which are always seeking to break out in action. These two ideas of the prime importance of instinctual behavior and their incomplete socialization were stated by Freud, perhaps more succinctly than anywhere else in his letter to Dr. Van Eeden:

> Psychoanalysis has concluded . . . that the primitive, savage, and evil impulses of mankind have not vanished in any individual, but continue their existence, although in a repressed state, in the unconscious . . . and that they wait for opportunities to display their activity. It has furthermore taught us that our intellect is a feeble and dependent thing, a plaything and tool of our impulses and emotions; that all of us are forced to behave cleverly or stupidly according as our attitudes and inner resistances ordain.[5]

If you take this position of course it follows that all men can be understood in pretty much the same terms, that the important thing with any man is to get behind the intervening experiences to the universal, instinctual man underneath, and that the intervening experiences of men as they develop are to be understood mainly as idiosyncratic, the accidents of individual life history.

The model of man that most sociologists find congenial is

profoundly different. Although it stresses the psychic unity of man, it gives prime emphasis not to man's instincts but to his social conditioning. It assumes that the intervening learning experiences which come between natural and socialized man are the most important source for predicting behavior, and it assumes those experiences to be sufficiently orderly, uniform, and regular so that one can seek to understand the behavior of groups of men in socio-cultural terms rather than by leaping over them to the underlying instinctual man. Man is taken as first and foremost a social, not an instinctual, being, his behavior a reflection not predominantly of his instincts but of his orientation to others and to cultural and social goals. Although man's impulses are acknowledged to be a great force, his intellect is hardly written off as a "feeble and dependent thing." On the contrary, his rational strivings and purposeful behavior to achieve social goals are taken to be the chief key to an understanding of social behavior.

Beyond this difference in the general model of man and in assumptions about the sources or origins of behavior, there are a number of further differences in emphasis which deserve mention. Freudianism is primarily concerned with the *adjustment* of the individual, sociology with the *behavior* of the incumbent of a social role. The psychoanalytic interest is not so much in what a man does as why he does and how he feels about having done or not done it. The sociologist is more concerned with *what* he does, especially whether or not he does what he must to meet his role obligations. Nothing can better illustrate the difference of approach than Ruth Monroe's comment that a musician who recovers from an hysterical paralysis of the arm may look convincingly cured, but is not if he develops blinding headaches or is thoroughly exasperating to his manager and family. The sociologist might agree that the musician is not cured of whatever ultimately ails him. He would, however, give greatest weight to the fact that the musician can now play, and can therefore give pleasure to audiences, support to his wife and profit to his manager, even if he is a source of thorough exasperation to them. Performance, not adjustment, is his criterion.

Indeed, this example suggests still another difference in emphasis, which creates a gap between sociology and psychoanalysis. Although Freud did attempt to redress the balance late in life, especially in papers like "Analysis Terminable and Interminable," it is nevertheless the case that he relatively neglected to measure the difference in the current situation faced by different people. Ruth Monroe has described this attitude as stressing the dynamic or topographic aspects rather than the *quantitative* state of the psychic economy. To put it in stronger language, Freudian psychology seems very often to neglect, sometimes even to deny, the importance of the immediate situation in influencing action. If you assume, as the sociologist does, that such situational pressures are of utmost importance in determining behavior, then you must have considerable reservations about any explanation of individual or group differences in behavior which do not take these situational factors into account. Concern for the delineation of such situational variables and responsibility for measuring them where possible and assessing their significance in influencing action, are of course at the very heart of sociology.

There is another sense of the economic that is also relatively neglected in psychoanalytic thought. Whenever Freud turned his keen analytic interest to social problems they were almost always problems arising in what are sometimes called the projective subsystems of society—religion, myth, humor or wit, and art. He said almost nothing about economics and very little about politics, and he only lightly touched on most social institutions other than the family. This hiatus may be an historical accident, or it may be that the psychoanalytic theory is indeed powerless to account for nonprojective institutions. Whatever its cause, this situation makes a grasp of psychoanalysis seem far from compelling to most sociologists.

Finally, I should mention that even those sociologists who turn with interest and appreciation to psychoanalysis as an adjunct to their traditional sociological analysis, often find themselves disappointed in the categories it offers for the description of those qualities of personality in which sociologists are bound to be most interested. The Freudian vocabulary is rich in terms to describe what the sociologist calls deviance. But it is neither rich nor systematic in the vocabulary it offers for the description of the range of normal behavior, traits and types. The start that Freud made in his few essays on different character types met in the course of analysis is rich and most suggestive, but it has hardly been carried forward to yield the complex battery of categories and types for describing personality that the social scientist needs. And even for the types delineated by psychoanalysis there is the problem of measurement already alluded to. The sociologist obviously cannot psychoanalyze those he studies. He is not competent to do so, nor could he find the time if he were. The solution does not lie, however, in securing the services of psychoanalysts on sociological studies. However valuable their collaboration may be, it is generally difficult to get more than a small part of their time. And more critical, they too can reach only a small number of individuals. For most purposes sociologists need personality materials on large numbers. To insist on the clinical method, then, becomes for them a counsel of despair.

The challenge thus is clear. Whether it interests psychoanalysis is another matter. But if psychoanalysis is to become the general psychology, the "metapsychology" of which Freud so often spoke, it must accept the challenge. Implicit in accepting it are certain suggestions for the further development of psychoanalysis, for movement and growth out of the rather narrow position in which it seems at the moment fixed. It means more concern for the economic or situational aspects of man's psychological functioning, more attention to normal functioning, more interest in socially important behavior, more effort to extend and develop the descriptive or typological language of the science, more adventuresomeness in going outside the clinical situation, more support for those who seek to develop objective tests and measures of personality traits and individual functioning, and less defensive behavior about the intentions of those who seek to apply the same criteria to testing the effects of psychoanalysis and its predictive powers as are applied to other scientific theories and methods. If the challenge is met I personally have no doubt that psychoanalysis can continue to hold its position as the most complete, most adequate, and intellectually most commanding of the theories of man's psychological nature and functioning.

Notes

1. Emile Durkheim, *Suicide,* tr. John Spaulding and George Simpson (Glencoe, Ill.: The Free Press, 1951), p. 151.

2. *Ibid.*, p. 299.

3. G. E. Swanson, "Agitation Through the Press," *Public Opinion Quarterly,* 1956, XX, 441–56.

4. R. M. MacIver, *Social Causation* (Boston: Ginn & Co., 1942), pp. 108–09.

5. Quoted in Ernest Jones, *The Life and Work of Sigmund Freud* (New York: Basic Books, 1957), II, 368.

PART III

PSYCHOANALYSIS AND PHILOSOPHY

7.

The Relevance of Psychoanalysis to Philosophy

MORRIS LAZEROWITZ
Professor of Philosophy
Smith College

FREUD has described the artist in words which, there is some reason for thinking, apply also to the philosopher. About the true artist Freud wrote that

> he understands how to elaborate his daydreams, so that they lose that personal note which grates upon strange ears and become enjoyable to others; he knows too how to modify them sufficiently so that their origin in prohibited sources is not easily detected. Further, he possesses the mysterious ability to mould his particular material until it expresses the ideas of his phantasy faithfully; and then he knows how to attach to this reflection of his phantasy-life so strong a stream of pleasure that, for a time at least, the repressions are out-balanced and dispelled by it. When he can do all this, he opens out to others the way back to the comfort and consolation of their own unconscious sources of pleasure, and so reaps their gratitude and admiration . . .[1]

It can come as a surprise nowadays only to very few people to learn that a painting, like a dream, has its origin in forbidden sources in the unconscious and is valued primarily for the thoughts it conceals, its latent content. The artist will not, in all probability, be gratified to be told that his work is an externalized form of dreaming and that the taste, imagination, and skill which enter into it, though admirable on their own account, derive their major importance from the fact that their role is

Notes to this section begin on page 154.

to effect "secondary elaboration" for the purpose of concealment. Nevertheless, it is no small thing to be able to open out to others "the way back to the comfort and consolation of their own unconscious sources of pleasure."

The philosopher is even less likely than the artist to be gratified by being told that his work, like that of the artist, is to give hidden expression to fantasies in a form which makes them a source of pleasure to others; for he fancies himself to be a kind of scientist, a seeker after basic knowledge whose way is "through speculation upon ultimate truths." [2] Philosophers sometimes give the impression of thinking differently about the real nature of their theorizing. Bradley, for example, speaks of philosophy as "a satisfaction of what may be called the mystical side of our nature," [3] or remarks that ". . . when the sense of mystery and enchantment no longer draws the mind to wander aimlessly and to love it knows not what; when, in short, twilight has no charm—then metaphysics will be worthless." [4] But understandably the idea that philosophical theories are nothing more than subtle, highly intellectualized ways of expressing and satisfying needs of the "twilight" (and darker) parts of our minds does not emerge into the clear light of consciousness and probably would not be pursued if it did. The medium in which the philosopher works *seems* to be propositions about the world, propositions the truth-values of which he wishes by his special methods to determine and the consequences of which he wishes to elucidate. And if this were the case, then although the utterances of the philosopher had unconscious import in addition to their scientific sense, the latter would, so to speak, stand on its own. Science is not a plastic art, and scientific propositions do not lend themselves to moulding. There is evidence, however, for supposing that the philosopher, despite all appearances, does not use language to express scientific propositions but instead uses it in such a way as to create the illusion of doing so, while in fact he gives expression *only* to his unconscious fantasies. His plastic medium is language, and, like the artist, he has "the mysterious ability to mould his particular material until it expresses the ideas of his phantasy faithfully"; he has the remarkable ability to mould language until it expresses his secret ideas in a form which makes it possible for other intellectuals, particularly those with a highly developed gift for abstract reasoning, to participate in and enjoy them.

So far as I am aware, no psychoanalyst, including Freud, has been led by his investigations to the notion, or even to a suspicion of the notion, that the metaphysician is not the seeker after truth he seems to himself as well as to others to be.[5] Thus a distinguished psychoanalyst, in a recent paper in which he discusses two different pictures of the world built up by two types of people, states that the question as to "which of the two pictures is the correct one, belongs to metaphysics. . . ."[6] In this connection it is worth noting that J. O. Wisdom, a philosopher who is practiced in the technique of psychoanalysis, states in an analytical work on Berkeley that he was led to "the idea of psychoanalyzing the writings of a philosopher" by a theory he had formed about "the nature of metaphysics";[7] and it might be imagined that he had discovered something unusual about the subject. But apart from such unelaborated remarks as that philosophy is "perhaps the strangest of all the creations of the human mind"[7] and that "philosophy is the last refuge open to myth (though not necessarily every kind of philosophy is impregnated with it),"[8] I have been unable to discover in his work any notion other than the classical one about the nature of philosophy: namely, that the theories found in it are, in their own right and without regard to unconscious associations, what they seem on the surface to be, truth-value claims about the existence and nature of phenomena.

Elsewhere I have argued at length[9] that a philosopher plays a deceptive game with language and that his theories are theories only in appearance, or, better, that with his utterances he produces the false impression that he is pronouncing theories. With exquisite skill, which rests on the mysterious ability to perceive the innermost workings of language, he does invisible, magical things with terminology: with it he produces at one level the vivid intellectual illusion of expressing a theory about the nature of time or the unity of the world or causation, and at the same time he uses it to give voice, at another, subterranean level of our minds, to thoughts which cannot be openly stated but which have the greatest psychical value. He uses language to bring about simultaneously a double dramatic effect, the convincing semblance of deep science and the expression of a cluster of inner fantasies. This account of the work of the philosopher's utterances is certain to arouse skepticism (from which, even as *advocatus diaboli,* I must confess myself to be by no means entirely free), and I wish to make it clear that it is not part of my purpose in this essay to try to defend psychoanalysis against its critics nor to try to explain any of its fundamental concepts. I shall take it for granted that the unconscious is ubiquitous in our thought and behavior, that it surrounds us everywhere, and I shall assume as substantially correct the basic psychoanalytical tenets as to its constitution and modes of operation. My object here is to show, as well as I can in the brief compass of a few pages, that the philosopher instead of using language, as he seems, to make factual claims about the world and its various real or only apparent aspects, uses it to create the false impression of stating such claims. And I bring in psychoanalytical theory as an explanatory hypothesis, i.e., as a hypothesis which provides an explanation of the astonishing durability, the long unmasked existence, of the substanceless intellectual mirage which the philosopher's words foist upon us. In a figure of speech, we are prevented from tasting the golden fruit in the Garden of the Hesperides by a sleepless dragon which guards it. The need of the unconscious to safeguard the vehicles for its expression is the barrier which prevents us from getting close enough to the philosopher's theories to see them for the mirages they are. As a further gain, psychoanalysis *completes* for us the account of a philosophical pronouncement, gives us the whole picture of the several jobs it is made to perform.

I propose to illustrate the hypothesis that a philosophical view is a three-layer structure composed of the illusion of science,[10] an unconscious group of ideas, and an altered piece of language which creates the first and expresses the second, by analyzing several familiar views. One is taken from F. H. Bradley and the other from Spinoza, the theories, namely, that whatever is finite is a self-contradictory adjective of the Absolute, and that every event has a cause. Before proceeding to these theories, it will be useful to look at one or two philosophical disputes which can be dealt with briefly. These will serve as compact illustrations of the kind of manipulation with language which produces the idea of a philosophical utterance's being something other than it is.

One philosopher has asserted that inductive logic is not logic, and it is hardly necessary to tell professional philosophers that although he won agreement from some people he failed to win agreement from others, who instead contested his claim. As is usual, the disagreement has remained an unresolved stalemate. It is typical for metaphysical controversies, no matter how long continued, to fail to come to resolution. A doctrine may lose its popularity and, by and large, be abandoned, but there is no guarantee that it will not be revived and accepted again by thinkers with recognized competence who know the objections to the doctrine. This disconcerting feature of philosophical views puts the thought into our minds that a philosopher need not, without being irrational, give up his position if he does not *wish* to do so, and that it is the nature of the subject, the fabric from which the theories of metaphysics are woven, that makes this possible. Consider the question "Is inductive logic logic?" when asked and debated by philosophers. The question seems to be a request for truth-value information with regard to a proposition about inductive logic, one claimed answer being that the proposition is true, that inductive logic is logic, and the other claimed answer being that the proposition is false, that inductive logic is not logic. This is what, superficially, seems to be the case; but it requires little reflection to realize that the question cannot be a request for this sort of information and that the disagreement cannot be one with regard to the truth-value of the proposition. For it can easily be seen that under this construction, however naturally it may come to us, the answer to it is not disputable and no disagreement could arise. The philosophers who answer the question differently and disagree amongst themselves know what inductive logic is, know that it is logic if it is logic, or that it is not logic if it is not logic. There could be no more disagreement about this among them than there could be a disagreement between mathematicians over whether π is a number. It is not to call attention to anything not perfectly familiar to everyone to point out that no philosopher on either side of the question can produce *any* piece of evidence to which the other could not reply, "Yes, that is so, but just the same . . ."

If we do not slide over the fact that there could be no disagreement over the question, construed as a request for truth-value information about what inductive logic is, it becomes too much for us to believe that the statement that inductive logic is not logic is the obviously false factual statement it seems to be. The counterstatement that inductive logic is logic cannot, in the context of the disagreement, be given its natural interpretation either. We may be puzzled to know how rightly to read the statements; but we cannot rest content with the first readings, providing, of course, we are not tempted to give up the idea that a disagreement of *some sort* actually exists between the contending philosophers. When, however, we begin to see our way through one semantic fog another comes up to obscure our vision and lead us astray. With the dispelling of the first notion about the problem and its claimed solutions, the linguistic reality behind the appearance becomes dimly discernible. The strong temptation then is to conclude that the question asks for information about proper usage, and that the two rival answers are truth-value statements about correct terminology. But this conclusion is a mistake also, as is made clear by the fact that it leaves us with an inadmissible paradox. If we construe the question as being about accepted usage, as asking, in the nonverbal mode of speech, whether the word "logic" correctly or properly applies to what the designation "inductive logic" covers, the two statements made in answer to it also have to be viewed as making truth-value claims with regard to matters of usage; and we are faced with the paradox of people disputing over the truth-value of a proposition while in possession of its truth-value. For it cannot in all intellectual sobriety be said that one or the other philosopher has a mistaken idea about the actual use of the word "logic" and cannot be straightened out. Nevertheless, the second construction, which so many find the irresistible stopping place, shows us the way to an interpretation of the question and answers which has the merit at least of being free from paradox.

It must be plain that *any* interpretation which makes the question out to be one over which the disagreement is about the truth-value of a proposition will involve a *wild* consequence, to the general effect that the known truth-value of a proposition is being disputed. The existence of the disagreement cannot, in any way which makes intelligible what is happening, be squared with such an interpretation of the question. Hence, since the existence of the dispute is not to be denied, we are compelled to revise in a radical way our notion of what it is that the question asks and what it is that is the subject of claim and counterclaim. The direction of the required revision is not difficult to discern, although it is a way that we may be loath to take. If the division over the question whether inductive logic is logic is not about the proper application of the word "logic," it is not unreasonable and it is certainly enlightening to conclude that it is a contest over a *change of usage:* a philosopher who states that inductive logic is not logic has decided to *contract* the application of the word, and a philosopher who states the opposite resists this contraction. The question can, without straining the language in which it is couched, be construed as a request for a reconsideration of the current use of the word "logic," raised by a person who, for whatever reason, finds himself being impressed by the *difference* between inductive logic and deductive logic. The statements made in answer to it, then, represent terminological decisions. The statement "Inductive logic is not logic" represents the decision to curtail the application of the word "logic" so that it is no longer applicable to what is at present called "inductive logic," and the statement "Inductive logic is logic" gives expression to the decision to preserve its present application. On this account we can understand how the dispute can have an indefinitely long life, and we can also see how the illusion is generated that a theory is being stated about the nature of inductive logic. The dispute can be continued indefinitely in the way in which disagreements over matters of taste can and do go on with undiminished vigor, because no sort of fact is in question. The appearance of a theory's being pronounced and disputed is brought about by the manner in which the terminological contraction is introduced and contested, i.e., by being expressed in language which masks what it is used to convey.

Let us consider another view, again in the context of philosophical disputation: the view, namely, that physical objects are attributes. This view usually occurs as part of a larger metaphysical system which is charged with strong feelings, but taken by itself and treated as a "logical" theory it can be dealt with compactly. F. P. Ramsey has remarked that ". . . when, for instance, Dr. Whitehead says that a table is an adjective, and Mr. Johnson that it is a substantive" they are arguing about "its logical nature." [10a] As in the case of the preceding philosophical disagreement, it looks as if a question about the truth-value of a proposition is being argued. The question "What is the logical nature of tables?" has the air of asking about what tables are, and the two statements "A table is an attribute" and "A table is not an attribute, it is a thing or a substance" appear to be truth-value utterances about what their nature is. But again, if appearance is taken for fact we are left with the bewildering paradox that people are disputing about what they all know. A person who knows what chairs, books, and the like are will be ignorant of many physical facts about their composition, etc., but he cannot fail to know whether or not they are attributes. There is no theoretical process of examining any physical object to see what its "logical nature" is, whether it is an attribute or is not an attribute but a substance; and there is no pointing out a feature F of a physical object, like a table, such that overlooking F leads to a mistaken notion about the nature of the table, while as a result of seeing F a correct notion is formed. This means that the disagreement is not open to theoretical resolution by any sort of examination of things and that it is not, therefore, about their nature. Seeing this brings us to the second appearance that the question and answers present. They begin to emerge in the guise of statements about the *grammar* of such words as "table" and "book": their seeming to be about the nature of things changes into their seeming to be about the grammar of a whole class of words. But the second appearance is also easily seen now to be delusive. For turning the question "What is the logical nature of tables?" into the grammatical question "Is the word 'table' a substantive or an adjective?" leaves no room for disagreement. For all parties to the disagreement know perfectly well the grammar of words like "table" and "book." It is, in fact, knowledge of the actual grammatical classification and function of such words that makes those who seem to be mistaken so stubbornly uncorrectible; what these philosophers do not themselves count as going against their position they can hardly be expected to accept from others as counting against it.

The disagreement becomes comprehensible if, as in the preceding illustration, it is understood as a divergence over some sort of language innovation, in the present case over a grammatical reclassification of general nouns with adjectives. The question "What is the logical nature of tables?" is then seen to be a logician's request to reconsider revising part of standard grammar. The statement "A table is an adjective" represents one logician's decision to change accepted grammar in such a way as to permit general substantives to function only adjectivally in sentences, while the statement "A table is a substantive" represents another logician's decision to preserve that part of grammar. When a philosophical logician like Russell complains that "Metaphysical errors arose through supposing that 'all men' is the subject of 'all men are mortal' in the same sense as that in which 'Socrates' is the subject of 'Socrates is mortal,' " [11] and (elsewhere) says, "Parts of speech, as they appear in grammar, have no very intimate relation to logical syntax," [12] he is concerned to justify the fact that the special notation that some logicians have constructed departs in certain respects from the grammar of ordinary language. One such departure is of special interest in the present connection. In the theory of monadic functions as developed in *Principia Mathematica,* ordinary subject-predicate grammar is modified by the stipulation that in the sentence-form "ϕx," "x" is to count as an *individual* variable, which cannot be replaced by general substantives, and "ϕ" as a predicate variable which can be replaced by general nouns as well as adjectives. The new grammar may achieve notational uniformity, but it is not a truer or a more correct syntax, nor does it reflect more accurately the "structure of fact."

The syntactical reclassification of general substantives with adjectives can be presented in the form of a theory about the "logical nature" of things, or it can be presented as part of an imposing metaphysical theory about the ultimate nature of reality. Russell, who adopted the reclassification in logic but not in metaphysics, makes the second possibility discernible when he describes Spinoza and Bradley as philosophers "who have asserted that there is only one thing, God or the Absolute, and only one type of proposition, namely that ascribing predicates to the Absolute." [13] Another philosopher also describes Bradley's view in words which tend to reveal the same underlying fact: "Reality is the ultimate subject of judgment." [14] Bradley's metaphysical system is well known, and it will be realized that my discussion is confined to only one of its aspects. The following two statements from *Appearance and Reality* present an undistorted summary of this aspect. One statement is: "There is nothing which, to speak properly, is individual or perfect, except only the Absolute." [15] The other statement is: "Anything less than the Whole has turned out to be not self-contained . . . Everywhere the finite is self-transcendent, alienated from itself, and passing away from itself towards another existence. Hence the finite is appearance because, on the one side, it is an adjective of Reality and because, on the other side, it is an adjective which itself is not real." [16] It will be remembered that Bradley in the role of analytical "spectator of all time and all existence" surveys for us space, time, physical things, selves, and thought, in short "the bewildering mass of phenomenal diversity," [17] which he claims to show is self-contradictory and no more than appearance. What the nature of the contradictions is that he discovers everywhere, contradictions which have the mystifying property of not making it impossible for there to be self-contradictory sensible appearances while eliminating the possibility of self-contradictory realities existing, and what he does with the term "appearance" cannot be gone into here. What is of some concern in the present paper, although it cannot be dwelt on, is how he arrives at the claim that "anything that in any sense 'is,' qualifies the absolute reality." [18] It is plain that at least one path to this claim is the contention that "all appearance must belong to reality. For what appears is, and whatever is cannot fall outside the real." [19] Roughly the progression is somewhat as follows: contradictions are, somehow, generated in phenomena; these contradictions are taken to expose them as being bare appearance and as showing them to be dependent [20] on something other than themselves, i.e., as belonging to something, or as being attributes of it. Restated in terms of language, contradictions are introduced into everyday nouns and noun phrases descriptive of spatial phenomena, temporal phenomena, selves, physical things, etc., contradictions which, it is professed, show that these terms have a use only as the descriptive parts of appearance expressions of the form ". . . appearance of *x*" or of the form "*x* locks . . ." This ostensibly brings out their linguistically dependent character and reveals their status to be that of adjectives.

It is hardly necessary to point out that the nouns and noun phrases descriptive of various phenomena in ordinary language are not contradictory, that they have a use other than in the context of appearance expressions, and that they are not adjectives. Nor is it necessary to call attention to the fact that all this is perfectly well known and cannot be soberly denied by anyone who knows and uses ordinary language. What has happened, behind the profoundly impressive but delusive image of the metaphysician as a gazer into the cosmos, is that the nouns of ordinary language have, for one reason or another, been reclassified with adjectives. This, it will be immediately realized, is a grammatical maneuver that is central to monistic metaphysics, a type of view which may be described as being in essence a reconstituted subject-predicate language in which only one term plays the role of noun. Russell's characterization of Spinoza's and Bradley's views puts the thought into our minds that behind the appearance of a view about the ultimate nature of the universe and how it is related to the variety of phenomena everywhere encountered is a grammatical reformulation of ordinary language, and the results of our examination of the dispute to which Ramsey refers makes this quite certain. It is plain that if all nouns are grammatically turned into adjectives while the subject-predicate sentence structure of language is preserved, terms will have to be introduced to function as subjects in such sentences. At this point the way is open to introducing a plurality of purely grammatical subjects or a single term. The monist takes the latter course and introduces what may be called the cosmic noun. This is nothing but an *x*, a semantic *blank*, which has a syntactical function and is given different names by metaphysicians, Being, Substance, the Absolute, the Whole, Reality, etc. If we go back now to the first two statements from Bradley we shall see this clearly embedded in them; briefly paraphrased, they are that the Absolute is the only "individual" and the finite is its adjectives.

It should be pointed out that Bradley allows the existence of "limited subjects":

> All judgment (I have argued elsewhere) predicates its idea of the ultimate Reality. Certainly I do not mean by this to deny that there is a limited subject. On the contrary in all judgment the subject is in some sense limited. But notwithstanding the presence of this narrowed subject, I urge that the assertion is made of the Universe. For the judgment affirms reality, and on my view to affirm reality is to predicate of the one Real.[21]

It seems plain that what is referred to by "limited" or "narrowed" subjects are the familiar substantives of common and scientific discourse, nouns like "Socrates," "time," "star" which are the subjects of everyday subject-predicate sentences. The existence of these is acknowledged, but they are looked on as having a shadowy function in a language which serves well enough for the superficial purposes of "rude" common sense[22] and "self-contradictory" science.[23] It is in fact not too much to think that behind the admission that there are limited subjects is the wish to call attention to the unaltered subject-predicate sentences of nonmetaphysical speech in order to give contrast to the metaphysician's artificially renovated language, to make it appear profound by throwing ordinary language into a light which makes it look like a practical makeshift. Ordinary subject-predicate discourse is pluralistic. It has a plurality of subject terms, a "plurality of independent reals." [24] But behind it, the metaphysician wishes to make it appear, is a monistic language which has only one subject term and is the Language of Reality. This is plainly what is to be gleaned from a careful reading of the words:

> "Reality is one. It must be single, because plurality, taken as real, contradicts itself. Plurality implies relations, and, through its relations, it unwillingly asserts always a superior unity." [25]

By calling attention to the limited subjects of ordinary speech, he enhances the illusion that he has discovered the true nature of things and the form of language adequate to its expression. What he has done is to make up a language, not, obviously, for practical use, but for the air it creates of expressing a super-scientific theory about the structure of the universe. Concealed behind the screen of this striking intellectual illusion there must be the expression and gratification of needs buried deep in the mind. In order to be convinced of this it is not necessary to become aware of anything more than the obsessive, repetitive manner in which Bradley expresses the general parts of his doctrine. Furthermore, it is hard to think that the deception would have gone undetected without protection from deeper sources in our minds. The controversy remarked by Ramsey is relatively aseptic emotionally and consequently can be seen through with comparative ease; and the durability of Bradley's view can be accounted for only by supposing that it has become connected with ideas which are charged with powerful affect.

Anyone who is familiar with the writings of Bradley will know how very metaphorical his language is, and it seems quite plain that his choice of terminology is a sound clue to the unconscious fantasies that get worked out in his philosophizing. When he writes that "incompleteness, and unrest, and unsatisfied ideality, are the lot of the finite," [26] that "everywhere the finite is . . . alienated from itself," [27] and speaks of it as suffering from "self-estrangement," [28] we certainly shall not go far wrong if we interpret these remarks as being autobiographical. The lot of the finite is the state of Bradley's inner life, and he can give voice to his melancholy discontent only in a form which conceals his condition from himself—in the form of a metaphysical utterance. The expression of this is made possible by an artificial language in which all ordinary nouns are transformed into adjectives. Ramsey has remarked on "the peculiar incompleteness of adjectives." [29] This incompleteness, which seems to have rather mystified him, is grammatical. An adjective requires a substantive for it to function in sentences,[30] while a substantive does not require an adjective. And the fact that this incompleteness struck him as being peculiar shows that it has become connected with something in the unconscious. When Bradley speaks of the finite as "passing away from itself towards another existence" or as being "essentially related to that which is not-itself," [31] he is taking veiled cognizance of the same grammatical fact, and he uses it also to voice his inner inadequacy. Bradley has the compulsive need to give expression over and over again to his felt inner incompleteness and "unsatisfied ideality," and this he can do by modeling language to his need, that is, by changing nouns into dependent, incomplete adjectives.

It is clear that anyone who suffers from a pronounced feeling of inadequacy and self-estrangement will not be satisfied merely with expressing it, although he may take pride in the subtlety and inventiveness with which he conceals his complaining. He will also search for a resolution of his difficulty, and Bradley discovers it in the Absolute, the ultimate reality in which harmony is achieved. The term "the Absolute" is in Bradley's artificial language the name of a spurious subject, an empty, syntactical *x* which the unconscious can use for its own ends; and in his system the *x* becomes the vehicle for a great number of different unconscious ideas. One particularly intriguing, if perhaps also baffling, description of the Absolute suggests a plausible interpretation:

> "The Absolute has no seasons, but all at once bears its leaves, fruit, and blossoms. Like our globe it always, and it never, has summer and winter." [32]

This together with his talk of the finite's being "absorbed," [33] "swallowed up" [34] and "dissolved" in the harmony of the Absolute in fact makes one interpretation inescapable.

It has been said that without death there would be no philosophy,[35] and the idea of death does not fail to play a role in the metaphysics of the Absolute. "The Absolute" denotes a number of things, two of which are easily recognized. For one thing it clearly stands for the earth, "our globe," by which we are in the end "swallowed" and "absorbed." It is the Whole in which we are "fused" [36] and in which our being is "overruled." [37] In addition to standing for that which receives the dead, the earth to which we all return, the Absolute also symbolizes death itself, the *x* which is "a mere blank." [38] It is pertinent to note in this connection that in dealing with the objection that the Absolute is "a mere blank or else unintelligible," [38] Bradley considers the charge that it is unintelligible and forgets the other alternative. Death, of course, *is* a blank, and forgetting to meet the objection that the Absolute is a blank is an indirect admission that the Absolute is a symbol for the blank which is the inevitable lot of everyone. It is of interest in this connection to recall the spurious December 1901 publication of *Mind!* in which the Portrait of "Its Immanence the Absolute" is given—a blank underneath a square of tissue. In transfigured, remodelled language Bradley describes the unsatisfactoriness of life and the resolution of this condition in death. What is most dreaded (and what in fact is responsible for one of life's conflicts which is especially acute in those who suppress their sexual instinct), death, is "turned into its opposite" and becomes the highest and most desired of all things. The equivocation which is a well-known example in the logic of material fallacies comes to mind: The end of a thing is its perfection; death is the end of life; therefore death is the perfection of life. The Absolute is perfection.[39]

With his sentence, "The finite is an adjective of the Absolute," the metaphysician does an impressive and complex piece of work. He creates with it, for one thing, a double illusion, the illusion of announcing the discovery of a language more basic than that in daily use, and the illusion that with it he inducts us into the mysteries of the universe. For another thing, and we might say primarily for this, he expresses with it both an unconscious complaint and an unconscious remedy. The sentence is an invisible description of a grammatically altered language, and in giving it utterance the Metaphysician of the One skilfully makes us dupe to his semantic legerdemain, while he also voices a complaint and holds out the consolation, to himself and to those who play his language game, that all this sorrow will come to an end in death. Some people, and perhaps all, will readily see that much more of unconscious import than has been brought out here is expressed by Bradley's words. But what has been brought to light of their unconscious meaning can be seen to be charged with a sufficient quantity of affect to keep us at a distance from the conscious impression they generate and prevent our perceiving its fraudulent character. The metaphysician's theory is a subtle and remarkable work of verbal art. Its underlying mechanics are a grammatically changed language which is not meant for practical discourse but, like a work of art, is meant only for contemplation. It creates the appearance of a profound theory about the cosmos, while it actually expresses inner psychic dramas. And the appearance and dramas are dynamically connected. The appearance acts as a screen for the inner dramas, and the dramas protect the appearance from being unmasked.

Let us move on to the remaining metaphysical view, held by Spinoza and many other philosophers, that the universe is a causally determined system, or that every occurrence has a cause. And let us begin by considering the two sentences "Every effect is a caused event" and "Every event has a cause." The first expresses an analytic proposition and the second, according to Kant, expresses one which is synthetic a priori. Like the paradigm usually given of an analytic sentence, namely, "A brother is a male sibling," the first does no more than state features that anything answering to the term "being an effect" must have, or, to put it otherwise, it resolves the meaning of the term into parts, each of which is separately stated. It gives no more than a fleeting impression of expressing a theory about the nature of effects, as it is evident to anyone who for a moment thinks on it that the term "effect" means precisely the same as "caused event": to understand the sentence is to know no more than this linguistic fact. And it would seem only a remote possibility that anyone would be deluded into imagining that these words, any more than the words "Every caused event is an event," expressed a theory or hypothesis, subject to confirmation or disconfirmation.

By contrast the philosophical utterance "Every event has a cause" does appear to state a theory about the nature of events, to the effect that they all without any conceivable exception have causes. Certainly as the words "event" and "cause" are ordinarily used, the meaning of "has a cause" is not part of the meaning of "is an event," and if it is true that the utterance is a priori, then it would appear to express a generalization about events which is logically secure. It looks to express a theory which is both about reality and certifiable a priori. But its appearing to express a theory about occurrences is a deception. For if "Every event has a cause" expressed an a priori proposition, whether analytic or synthetic, understanding it would come to knowing no more than that as a matter of usage the term "has a cause" correctly applies to whatever the word "event" applies to, or that the expression "event which has no cause" has no descriptive use, is not a phrase which describes anything actual or imaginable. To put the matter differently, the claim that the sentence "Every event has a cause" expresses an a priori true proposition entails, and is entailed by, the claim that the sentence "As a matter of usage 'has a cause' applies to whatever 'event' applies to, so that 'uncaused event' has no use" expresses a true empirical proposition. Like the analytic sentence, then, if the philosophical utterance were a priori its purport would be a verbal point with regard to actual usage; [40] it would not express a theory about the nature of events. Now as a matter of fact, the terms "event" and "has a cause" are so used in everyday speech that "is an event but lacks a cause" is a descriptive phrase. It is not the case that *usage* dictates the application of "has a cause" to whatever "event" is correctly applied to, although it may in fact be a true empirical generalization to say that every event has a cause. How then, are we to account for many people over many years thinking and arguing for the claim that the utterance is a priori (since that would imply that they were mistaken about usage while knowing actual usage), and also of thinking it expresses a generalization about a kind of phenomenon? How are we to explain, for one thing, a verbal misconception which, so to speak, has become an inherited piece of property, and how, for another thing, are we to explain anyone's thinking that a proposition could be both about matter of fact and have a truth-value which is logically necessary?

A possible and, in my opinion, plausible explanation of what has happened is that what may be called a *conversion analysis* [41] has been performed, an analysis, that is to say, which calls attention to points of actual usage, not for the purpose of stating the criteria for the application of terms but to justify a *linguistic alteration*. A philosopher like Spinoza, say, who maintains that it is impossible "that something should be made out of nothing," [42] is calling attention to a similarity between expressions which he finds objectionable and which he eliminates by verbal fiat, by an arbitrary change of language. To put the matter briefly, the noun grammar of the word "nothing" in the expression "Something is made out of nothing" makes it appear that "nothing" is being used to name a kind of substance. It would seem that for some philosophers the function of "nothing" looks too much like that of the word "clay" in the sentence "A teacup is made from clay," where the word "clay" in fact is the name of a kind of material. "A teacup is made from clay" actually tells us what the substance is from which a teacup is made, whereas

"Something is made out of nothing" does not say what the substance is from which a thing is made, although the semantic appearance of its doing so is created by its grammar. The sentence "Every event or thing must have a cause" says the same as the sentence "It is impossible for there to be a thing which has no cause," and this in turn says the same as "It is impossible that something should be made out of nothing." On the other hand, the sentence "It is possible for there to be an uncaused occurrence or for there to be a thing which has no cause" says the same as "It is possible that something should be made out of nothing," and the latter is a form of speech that some philosophers find objectionable because of its delusive similarity with statements about what substance things are or may be made from. And to make more pronounced a semantic dissimilarity between types of expressions which their grammar tends to hide, Spinoza deprives "uncaused thing," or "thing made out of nothing," of its ordinary use, by making "Something is made out of nothing" express a logical impossibility. This is what the first series of equivalences achieves. The words "Every event has a cause" do not issue from a mistaken analysis of the actual use of "event" and "cause" but embody a linguistic conversion. The sentence "Every event of necessity has a cause" expresses an a priori proposition by arbitrary verbal decree; and to say the proposition it expresses is synthetic is an oblique way of saying that the sentence is a synthetic or "manufactured" or, perhaps better still, ersatz utterance, one which expresses an a priori proposition only in consequence of *artificial* things having been done with language. The sentence is made to express a proposition it is not ordinarily used to express, by virtue of the philosophical banishment, so to say, the academic exiling, of the expression "uncaused event." And the fact that all this is done in an idiom in which words are not mentioned is responsible for the impression that an esoteric theory about the nature of events is being pronounced, a theory which moreover has the security of a logical truth. A holiday casting out of terminology is made to look like the announcing of a theory about the world by being conducted in the ontological idiom. Instead of saying "the term 'uncaused thing' has no descriptive use in my special language," a philosopher says "It is impossible for there to be an uncaused thing," as if it were a fact that "uncaused thing" has no use in ordinary language. He does unusual things with ordinary terminology, and he does this in such a way as to make it appear that he is using ordinary language in the *usual way* to express an unusual and important *theory* about the world. Thus, by means of a hidden linguistic maneuver, the nature of which he himself is not consciously aware of, he produces at the conscious level of our awareness the false idea that a theory is being stated.

There is still a further and deeper level involved which we can dimly discern. The philosophical words do not express a theory of the sort they appear to be expressing, that is, a general theory about the nature of occurrences; and we are constrained to think that their absorbing and enduring interest lies in unconsciously grasped propositions they are made to express, one of which it would seem is related to a curiosity that went unsatisfied in the infancy of our life. Freud tells us that "the sexual interest of children is primarily directed to the problem of birth—the same problem that lies behind the riddle of the Theban Sphinx." [43] As is well known, children's curiosity is not satisfied by their parents, who give them fairy-tale explanations; and Freud goes on to say, "The feeling of having been deceived by grown-up people, and put off with lies, contributes greatly to a sense of isolation and to the development of independence. But the child is not able to solve this problem on his own account.[44] Freud's description of the character of a person whose childhood curiosity has gone unsatisfied applies perfectly to Spinoza, and we should not be surprised if Spinoza's curiosity also had remained unsatisfied and that unconsciously he was still seeking for an answer. His own words "that all things are in God, and so depend on Him, that without Him they *could neither exist nor be conceived*" [45] give us reason to think this. For in almost undisguised language they express a theory about childhood dependence and procreation. It would hardly surprise us to learn that the word "cause" is unconsciously used to symbolize the father, or his cosmic magnification, God (e.g., The First Cause = God). Spinoza's utterance, "Something cannot be made out of nothing," [46] is evidence of his concern with the problem of birth and his inability to solve it; and his proposition that without God things "could neither exist nor be conceived" expresses a dim realization that his own father played a role in his creation, although what the role was must always have eluded his *unconscious* desire for knowledge. This is shown by the very first definition in his *Ethics:* "By that which is self-caused, I mean that of which the essence involves existence, or that of which the nature is only conceivable as existent," [47] that is, how his father was made remained a mystery to him, and therefore how he was made remained a mystery to him. In short, the philosophical utterance "There cannot be an event without a cause" expresses a proposition which quieted, although it never satisfied, a childhood desire for knowledge: it expresses the proposition that an event, the child, is *somehow* brought into being by his parent.

According to the hypothesis developed here, the *philosophical* sentence "Every event of necessity has a cause" is a subtly contrived, economical structure one part of which is visible to us and the other two parts of which are invisible. The first, the uppermost layer of the structure, is the delusive appearance of words' being used to express a speculation about a familiar type of phenomenon. The other two parts consist of (1) a hidden revision of terminology which expresses (2) a hidden proposition that is important for our unconscious mental life. There can be hardly any doubt that it is mainly for the purpose of expressing this unconsciously grasped proposition that language was remodeled, and it is the unquenchable interest in it that prevents us from drawing close to the deception effected by the changed piece of language.

If the theory developed in these pages about the nature of philosophy is substantially correct, then psychoanalysis is relevant in a very special way to philosophical utterances. It alone can discover for us what they really say, as against what they delusively appear to say. Semantic analysis brings to light the linguistic import of these statements and helps explain how they produce their remarkable intellectual illusions. Psychoanalysis brings to our conscious awareness the nonverbal things they are unconsciously made to express, and it also explains the durability of the illusions.

Notes

1. S. Freud, *A General Introduction to Psychoanalysis,* tr. Joan Riviere (Garden City Pub. Co., 1943), p. 328.

2. F. H. Bradley, *Appearance and Reality* (New York: Oxford University Press, 1930), p. 7.

3. *Ibid.,* p. 6.

4. *Ibid.,* pp. 3–4.

5. In his book *Great Men* (New York: International Universities Press, 1956), p. 28, Dr. E. Hitschmann attributes to Freud the opinion that metaphysics is "a wild goose chase, leaving reliable ground . . . ," an opinion implying that metaphysicians, though unscientific, are seekers after truth.

6. Dr. Michael Balint, "Friendly Expanses — Horrid Empty Spaces," *The International Journal of Psychoanalysis,* XXXVI, 8.

7. Dr. John Oulton Wisdom, *The Unconscious Origin of Berkeley's Philosophy* (New York: Hillary House, 1953), p. vii.

8. *Ibid.,* p. 230.

9. *The Structure of Metaphysics* (New York: Humanities Press, 1955).

10. To prevent possible misunderstanding, it should, perhaps, be explained that by the expression "the illusion of science" is meant the illusion that a factual claim about the existence or nature of a phenomenon is being made. Furthermore, the phrase "illusion of a proposition being stated" is not used to denote a false proposition or a delusive belief; it denotes the false appearance of there being a proposition, the delusion that words are being used to express a proposition when in fact they express none.

10a. *The Foundations of Mathematics* (London: Kegan Paul, French, Trubner & Co., Ltd., 1931), p. 113.

11. *A History of Western Philosophy* (New York: Simon and Schuster, 1945), p. 198.

12. *An Inquiry into Meaning and Truth* (London: G. Allen and Unwin Ltd., 1948), p. 48.

13. *Principles of Mathematics* (New York: W. W. Norton and Co., 1938), p. 448.

14. H. W. B. Joseph, *An Introduction to Logic* (2nd ed.; New York: Oxford University Press, 1916), p. 169 n.

15. *Appearance and Reality,* p. 246.

16. *Ibid.,* p. 486.

17. *Ibid.,* p. 140.

18. *Ibid.,* p. 555.

19. *Ibid.,* p. 140.

20. "Appearance without reality would be impossible, for what then could appear?" (*Ibid.,* p. 487.)

21. *Essays on Truth and Reality* (New York: Oxford University Press, 1914), pp. 253–54.

22. *Appearance and Reality,* p. 448.

23. *Ibid.,* p. 451.

24. *Ibid.,* p. 141.

25. *Ibid.,* pp. 519–20.

26. *Ibid.,* p. 246.

27. *Ibid.,* p. 246.

28. *Ibid.,* p. 486.

29. F. P. Ramsey, *The Foundations of Mathematics,* p. 115.

30. When expressed nonverbally, this grammatical fact presents itself in the guise of a theory. Thus, "No qualities or properties pertain to nothing and . . . when some are perceived there must necessarily be some thing or substance on which they depend" (Descartes).

31. *Appearance and Reality,* p. 246.

32. *Ibid.,* p. 500.

33. *Ibid.,* p. 179.

34. *Ibid.,* p. 192.

35. Thus Schopenhauer: "Death is really the inspiring genius, the *musagète* of philosophy. . . . If it were not for death, people would hardly philosophize."

36. *Appearance and Reality,* p. 528.

37. *Ibid.,* p. 430

38. *Ibid.*, p. 555.

39. *Ibid.*, p. 246.

40. This has been discussed fully in *The Structure of Metaphysics*, Chap. XII.

41. This notion is elaborated in "Moore and Philosophical Analysis," *Philosophy*, XXXIII, No. 126, pp. 193–220.

42. *Ethics*, Book IV, Proposition XX, Note.

43. *A General Introduction to Psychoanalysis*, p. 279.

44. *Ibid.*

45. *Ethics*, Book I, Proposition XXXVI, Appendix. Italics mine.

46. In a communication to me, Dr. M. Balint suggested that this lends itself to the interpretation that the child cannot be born without a mother. He writes: ". . . perhaps you could bring Spinoza's two utterances together because in my mind they belong together. 'Every event has a cause' means as you correctly point out that every child must have a father. In the same way 'Everything is made out of something' means that every child must have a mother as well, that is, that a father cannot create a child without a mother."

47. It would seem plausible that the notion of God as a self-caused being is also a narcissistic projection of Spinoza himself, a projection in which the role played by his father in his creation is denied. I.e., it can be construed as renouncing any indebtedness to his father; and it can also be construed as a denial of anything having taken place between his father and mother. Part of the underlying meaning of the virgin birth would seem to be the denial of the father's role in procreation.

8.

Philosophy and Psychoanalysis

DONALD C. WILLIAMS
Professor of Philosophy
Harvard University

ONE way to take Mr. Lazerowitz's entertaining theory about philosophical theories, perhaps the most natural and genial way, is to suppose it intended to be only entertaining, a parody of the excesses of verbalistic positivism and amateur psychoanalysis. A second estimate is that he proposes it as a wild hypothesis, probably false but worth trying. A third is that he seriously means and believes it. There is, of course, no use asking Mr. Lazerowitz, deep as he is in secret duplicities, for the same indecision would arise about his reply. One is tempted to dodge the dilemma by calculating that, parody or not, it is anyhow best countered with a parody—for example, that Newton's *Principia* was only a play on symbols expressive of the notoriously frustrated yearning of children for the moon. As a mere game, however, this is too easy. My own belief is that Mr. Lazerowitz's intention is serious, and that even if it is not, we should treat it as if it were. It would be pointless to caricature modes of thought whose boldness has long since caught up with any possible burlesque, and our author's persistent advocacy of his principle has shown much less of the tight bright logic of the joke than (shall we say?) of the inimitable inconsequence of consecration. In any event, it is better for us to risk being taken in by a hoax than to re-poison the wells of scholarly communication by a new disingenuousness about disingenuousness about disingenuousness.

Notes to this section begin on page 178.

Deciding to take the Lazerowitz hypothesis seriously is a harsh treatment, inasmuch as for most of us it is tantamount to instant rejection. For indeed I think the theory as wrong as the plain man would deem it, that is, almost preternaturally wrong, so that the only duty I can admit now is to tabulate where its unreasons lie. If the task is especially difficult, this is for no lack of material, but partly because no matter how much old-fashioned sincerity and objectivity Mr. Lazerowitz and I attempt toward each other, the amenities are strained by the very nature of his contention, which is essentially *ad hominem* in that most provocative sense in which a lawyer argues *"ad hominem"* when he abuses the opposing attorney. Mr. Lazerowitz does not say in so many words that metaphysicians and hence their imitators and defenders are knaves and fools, but he does so in the way in which a person who says that there are three oranges in a sack says that there are an odd number of them. The men he diagnoses would rather be half-imbecile delinquents in a reformatory than the kind of "artists" he is good-natured enough to admire. I do not level the common textbook charge that argument *ad hominem* in this mode is in itself a fallacy, for it is not. A proposition may indeed be true or proved though propounded with neurotic and ulterior motives, but it is then so much less likely to be that this will in logic tell more against it than most of the nicer evidence. The rule is that whenever individual x argues for proposition p, and y argues for *not-p*, we must make a rational choice between two dual conclusions: that p is true and y is wrong, and that *not-p* is true and x is wrong. Hence any evidence for or against the general integrity of either champion is logically for or against what he champions. Our procedural question is rather one of the proprieties versus one's tactical obligations to one's cause. I agree in principle with those who would urge that Mr. Lazerowitz by his frankness has invited my party to retort by an unfavorable analysis of his character and purposes (a vein decorously scratched by K. Daya in a review published since our March conference).[1] That I try to avoid such recriminations may be logical malpractice, a cheat on my client, but it stems from what I hope is anyhow an amiable weakness, with at least the excuses that it will save time, and that metaphysicians, being among the few minority groups whom the current mores allow to be defamed with impunity, have thick skins. There are two remarks, however, which I must be permitted. One is to remind Mr. Lazerowitz that his kind of discrediting of philosophies by a claim of some extracurricular insight into their hidden motives is exceedingly dangerous, to be indulged in only when the instance is urgent and the evidence is indefectible, for it was exactly the method of those greatest of practical psychologists, the leaders of German National Socialism, when they argued, with a much bigger show of fact than Mr. Lazerowitz has marshaled, that modern positivism expressed a more or less conscious plot of the Jewish race to avenge itself on and destroy the culture of Europe. The other remark is that, while renouncing the use of Mr. Lazerowitz's method against him, we are not committed not to use his conclusions against themselves. I am honestly in the dark about whether he conceives his doctrine to be of the character which ostensibly he ascribes to the rest of what he calls "philosophy." If he does, it is, and if it is, it actually ascribes no character to anything, and we can chide him only for committing a semantic nuisance. If, on the other hand, he means his strictures to be taken as statements of fact about the business normally called "philosophy," he can preserve an exemption for them only by controverting the fairly patent fact that they *are* philosophy, of a sort. The author is listed on our program as a professor of philosophy, and has made no move, I think, to turn in his badge or to be taken off the philosophical payroll. And this is honest enough, for his discourse, item by item, shows the stigmata it assigns to "philosophy," and he argues with us in just the way which in other philosophers he condemns as febrile and futile. What, for example, could be more obviously offensive to the common usage he canonizes than that when a particularly mordant and austere Idealist said that everything is part of the universe he was reclassifying parts of speech in order both to conceal and to express a wish he were dead? *I* can see how such a verbal freak might be true or false, common usage go hang, and that it is in fact false; but how can Mr. Lazerowitz parley with it at all? If I refrain from pressing this point too, it is because arguments by self-confutation, perhaps on account of their unsporting fatality, are in bad odor, and because this discussion can be kept going only under our oxygen tent of forced amity.[2] That we can't tell whether and how Mr. Lazerowitz hopes to keep his own remarks out of the slough of philosophic deceit, however, is an instance of a substantive fault which we must mention because many fair minds would think his doctrine vitiated by it: that having no foil by way of an account of truth and reason, his charge of self-deception so loses definition that it might be used to gratify a grudge against any mode of discourse. With another spectral grin of magnanimity, then, let us suppose that Lazerowitz supposes, and could defend, that some discourse is not sheer self-deception, and that its content and criteria are approximately such as prevail in the "best" parts of science and common sense.

Though on principle not pursuing the positivistic method which alleges that an opponent's utterance, however well formed by normal standards, does not really say anything, we are entitled to object that Mr. Lazerowitz's positivistic utterances are often not well enough formed by normal standards so that we know what they say. This is unfortunate for a doctrine so largely linguistic, whose credentials depend on the author's showing such consummate mastery of language as no metaphysics requires of any mere metaphysician, and it is unfortunate for us because the idea is strange and devious enough without being veiled in obliquities of expression. I shall not much complain of him, as he does of the hapless Bradley, that his expressions, even in so small a compass, show "compulsive" reiteration. The preciosity, so incongruous with his own professions, which adopts the current technical misuse of "game" and of "language," so that, for example, two men both talking English or Dutch are using "different languages" if they say different things, or say the same thing in different ways, is an affair between him and his conscience. It does, however, multiply the attentive reader's difficulties, already compounded by a literary style which, though of a certain syrupy power, too much delights in modifiers at odds with their principals—as in "forbidden sources," "irresistible stopping place," "the unconscious surrounds us everywhere," "contradictions are introduced into everyday nouns," "the sentence is an invisible description of a grammatically altered language," none of which can well be parsed even as a metaphor. Of even less help, in an essay whose cogency must be in direct proportion to the exactness of its semeiotic, is playing fast and loose with key terms like "reclassify," "names," and "denotes," and with quotation marks.

Turning from these relatively extraneous peculiarities of Mr. Lazerowitz's argument, we confront the solid central question whether there is any good reason to accept what we can understand of it. That he does claim some evidence for his propositions is to his credit in our era when verbalistic and phenomenalistic epistemologies are often presumed to need no evidence, as if they shone enough by their own baleful light. Nor is it quite fair to say that he relies mostly on the two halves of his hypothesis holding each other up: that metaphysics has no literal meaning but is verbal chicanery is explained and supported by the thesis that its real force and origin are pathological, while that metaphysics is pathological explains and is supported by the thesis that intrinsically it is nonsense. Even this is not silly, since the theses would indisputably be less credible if they contradicted each other. The credit they get from such mutual support, however, is insignificant except as relevant data are fed in from outside, and Mr. Lazerowitz believes he has some of the latter. The first, or chicanery, thesis is an old favorite of his which he has elsewhere confirmed by the philosophical record. The doctrines of psychoanalysis, on the other hand, he thinks have been substantiated, I guess, by their therapeutic application. The virtue of the combination of theses, I think he would claim, is that it heals the main hiatus in the first one, being supposed to reconcile us to the otherwise quite incredible implication that God or nature has hidden from the world's greatest and most self-critical thinkers the most elementary fact about their own thinking, only to reveal it to the babes and sucklings of positivism. This onus, I agree with Mr. Lazerowitz, is not one that positivism can lift for itself, and until it is lifted the whole effort of analytic superficialism is indefensible. A single abstract soundness of methodic intention, however, is by no means enough to save Mr. Lazerowitz's endeavor from pretty thorough defeat by the conspiracy of fact and logic against him. It turns out in particular that his two theses are rather liabilities to each other than assets, so we need not be surprised at the scurry both of the advocates of positivism and ordinary language (the first thesis) and those of psychoanalysis (thesis two) to escape the *reductio ad absurdum* that they scent in the alliance he would thrust upon them, nor can those of us who reject both theses fail to take some mean moralistic pleasure in their disconcertion.

Strictly it is impossible quite to separate the parts played respectively by logic and by material fact against Mr. Lazerowitz because, of course, it is only an uncompliant logic that makes any fact hostile, and conversely. We can, however, first take account of what I think is his principal or overarching error, which is so general as to be mostly logical, and then some account of more detailed error in his specific arguments.

Although Mr. Lazerowitz seems committed that a knowledge of the principles of inductive logic is automatically breathed into each of us with his mother tongue, his own grasp of them must have been corrupted enough by professorial communications so that he quite misses the main rules that should have governed his kind of hypothesizing. For a hypothesis is not in general confirmed at all by merely being consistent with some facts; almost any hypothesis is consistent with almost any facts. What count are, first, the antecedent probability of the hypothesis in relation to the funded knowledge of mankind, and secondly, the determinateness and probability with which it might actually have predicted those special current facts normally denominated "the" evidence; and what mainly counts about these is not the absolute values of the probabilities but how they compare with the corresponding ones attached to rival or contrary hypotheses. What we call a "crank" is just such a person as is so absorbed in how his hunch fits a picturesque handful of data that he ignores its status with respect to funded knowledge and to contrary hypotheses.

Now, we could not fairly expect Mr. Lazerowitz to put all his goods into one show window, but what gives his essay its almost unique air of unreality, I think, is that he not only does not mention but seems genuinely unaware of the principal great rival of his theory. This rival may be called "the established hypothesis," for, though frequently contested by subjective and skeptical apriorists, it has been so long and well confirmed that like the belief in George Washington it can hardly be thought of as a "hypothesis" at all. It is, of course, that philosophy, and notably metaphysics, is the candid effort to see the world entire, not in detail but in main outline, using all the resources of thought and perception, gutting and glutting language as need be, ruthlessly analyzing things to their finest structure in order to synthesize to their most embracing system, and conversely—a mixture perforce of wisdom with fatuity, of madness with precision, running enormous risks on the chance of infinite gain; being *human,* in fine. The evidence that such an effort exists, and that it in fact coincides with what is generally called "philosophy," being of the same order as that for George Washington, is so great that it is queer to call it "evidence," and correspondingly easy to underrate it. That there should be such a discipline is antecedently an implicate of any culture that has the concept of truth, for it is inevitable that knowledges should there specialize into nuclei of partial understanding and information with confusion between, and that curious and devout spirits should be always trying to reconcile and round these out into a larger scheme, not merely for the fun of it (though love of the abundant life is as natural as the death instinct), nor even merely because knowledge and understanding of anything are precarious and imperfect save as integrated with knowledge and understanding of all things (though this is a truth of logic), but because life cannot wait the infinite time till specialisms coalesce of themselves, but must be lived right now in the total presence of the world, which will not wait. That this enterprise is "philosophy" is evident to immediate inspection for people who understand and do philosophy. It is confirmed by what the philosophers say, and what generations of amateurs have believed, and by the dictionaries of all European languages—the last being an authority that our linguists gladly admit when they do not pronounce adversely. It is borne out by exactly the convergence of facts that the theory entails: that no definite demarcations ever persist among philosophy, the special sciences, and the plain sense of commerce; that philosophy is the mother of the sciences and the guide of life; that it borrows concepts and results from science and common sense as these do from it; that question after question and hypothesis after hypothesis have moved out of one into another and back again, or been cultivated in all of them at once; that philosophers argue and change their minds by processes and with materials that patently are extensions of those of science and business, and that the methods of all three involve about the same interplay of conceptual and linguistic reform and speculative construction. None of this is absolutely conclusive—there may be revolutions with respect to any inductive topic—but it provides so much antecedent credibility that to neglect it is virtually to disbar oneself so far as our case is concerned. Mr. Lazerowitz would have a claim upon us only if he showed, first, how his theory can explain away the prodigious evidence in favor of the established hypothesis, and secondly, that the established hypothesis cannot explain the facts he adduces for his theory. Neither of these does he seriously attempt, and what he does do rather convinces us that his theory leaves miraculous most of the facts that support the established theory, while the latter not merely is compatible with but positively implies those of his data that are not malobservations (often, I think, by reflections no more problematic than that the most exciting, difficult, and enduring problems are naturally the most enduring, difficult, and exciting).

It is easy enough, in fact, to settle the hash of Mr. Lazerowitz's professed reasons for his two theses, that all philosophy is verbal chicanery and that it is due to secret scatology, so that we might make bold to say the extreme contrary, that no philosophy is tainted either by verbal confusion or by subconscious desires. This is indeed much nearer the truth than Mr. Lazerowitz's contention, and a wholesomer error, but in honor let us register that it is an error. In so far as our ideas are not consciously incubated, they must be unconsciously so; and in so far as we are haggises of impulse and appetite, the appetite for truth must be extremely vigorous to win out. These thoughts, however, are no more than philosophers have drummed into each other and every listener they could get for millennia. What I deny is not that philosophers benefit from a pathology of their subject, but that they need more of it or provide less of their own than other people, and specifically that Mr. Lazerowitz's Freudian diagnoses are true or useful.

When we look now with particularity at Mr. Lazerowitz's argument, it is convenient to redivide what I called his two theses into four stages or articles, increasingly derogatory, idiosyncratic, and psychoanalytic: that philosophies cannot be statements of fact, that they are instead ritual recitations turning on distortions of language, that these are the machinations of an unconscious self, and that this unconscious self is controlled by the peculiarly musty and maudlin obsessions that people with too rough justice call "Freudian." It is natural to leave the last to the last, while we see what can be said for the first three.

While we have agreed that any evidence presented in occasional essays like ours can be only a small sample, it is unlikely that Mr. Lazerowitz picked his worst specimens, so it is ominous for his theory that they are a poor lot: that they so generally mistake his philosophers' intentions, and that both the facts and his mistakes about them are so much more intelligible on the standard theory than on his. His errors, in fact, are just such as we should expect from a person who for years has not looked at any philosophy except from the outside, to "get something on it." His prefatory use, for example, of the question whether things are substantives or adjectives is nonsignificant for anyone who knows that both Johnson and Whitehead believed in both particulars and universals, and so would cheerfully have granted that the question which element is most conveniently identified with "the" thing is indeed a merely verbal one. Having fired his salvo at this innocent unidentified object, Mr. Lazerowitz has no metal left to throw at, and does not notice, the philosophically important dispute between those like Russell who hold radically that things do consist wholly of universals and the nominalists who believe there are only particulars. His other prefatory example, the question whether inductive logic is logic, is devastating for his theory and almost conclusive for the standard one, because it is in plain fact as materially affected by recent studies in the development of probability theory from the same primitives with deductive logic as the similar question whether arithmetic is logic, or logic is arithmetic, was by *Principia Mathematica,* or as the question whether astrophysics is physics was by spectroscopy and celestial mechanics. If there is some justice in his sweeping into the pit of morbidity writers like Carnap and Goodman, who have done so much to teach this kind of hoity-toity disposal of one's metaphysical rivals, it is a justice merely poetic. I am confident he would relinquish his notion that he can anticipate or correct the results of any such logical explorations by a mere feeling of the pulse of ordinary language if he would attempt to use this talent prospectively instead of ex post facto. We observe, by the same token, that his contention that the parties to all these sorts of disputes must really have known the answers already, is not a datum on which he can ground his theory, but simply a reassertion of the theory. We may grant that philosophers are not instantaneously overborne, on the inductive or any other issue, by the impact of specific logical discoveries, but they are certainly not less teachable than, say, psychoanalysts or semanticists. If philosophers take longer to change their minds than physicists and historians, who are not instantaneously unanimous either, this is a proper and predictable function of the greater logical inertia of their wide generalizations. While the inductive question thus nicely conforms to and confirms the established theory of philosophy, Mr. Lazerowitz leaves wholly inexplicable why there is more of a philosophic problem over whether inductive logic is logic than over whether unmarried females are females, for example, which is intrinsically a far more affecting subject.

Much the same futility dogs our author's critique of Bradley. Most of the formulas about the Absolute that he cites from the latter are only portentous ways of declaring the innocent truism, none the less worth statement in a formal system, that the whole contains its parts, which might be discovered verbalistically, by inspecting usage, but which most of us found long since by inspecting wholes and parts. That we can consistently treat all lesser predications as adjectives of the one world sum is a truth that had to be demonstrated, and is no more determinable by verbal fiat, as Mr. Lazerowitz suggests, than whether there are paradoxes in the concept of classes of classes. That the analogies between the way the redness of a rose is "abstract," "incomplete," and "adjectival to" the rose, and the way the rose is "adjectival to" the world sum, are such that everything entails the Absolute, as Bradley thought, is testable by inquiries like those that have lately absorbed the energies of, for example, Professors Goodman and Quine. Mr. Lazerowitz's condescension on this score would have been more instructive if addressed to these gentlemen, for whom it is not too late to profit from it.

It is hard to believe that if Mr. Lazerowitz had had many specimens at hand, or had thoroughly mastered them, he would have taken his only two capital examples from the same kind of philosophy, extreme organic holism, without even observing that this is so. The symptoms he finds in Bradley would have looked very different if he had not treated them as one man's lonely delusion, but had tried to account for them as links in a great chain of absolute monism stretching back through Spinoza to Parmenides. Now, since Spinoza's philosophy is essentially the same as Bradley's, and Bradley thought ordinary linear causation to be delusory, we know that Spinoza could not have had the infatuation with such causation that Mr. Lazerowitz so tortuously claims. One would think, from what he says, that Spinoza obsessively reiterates things like "Every event has a cause" and "It is impossible for something to come from nothing," but so far as I could find by a rapid review, Spinoza hardly broaches either of them. What did obsess him, if you like—somewhat as relativity "obsessed" Einstein and evolution "obsessed" Darwin—was how everything is included in and entailed and glorified by, and how it in turn entails and requires, the system that is Nature or God. Whether something can come from nothing in the trivial sequence of time is sublimely unimportant to him. In the passage that Lazerowitz quotes he is only comparing the obviousness of a moral principle with that of the antique maxim that nothing comes from nothing. The best statement I find that particular things and events have particular causes, on back to infinity, is Proposition XXVIII of Part I, which seems mainly intended to contrast the footlessness of this scheme, accepted by Spinoza from the scientists and the old idea of sufficient reason, with the quite different, more important, incessant, direct, timeless, and immanent causality of God. Offhand as it is, Mr. Lazerowitz goes to the queerest trouble to show there is something queer about this acceptance. Almost everybody, surely, would say not just that things have causes, but that they "must" have causes, so it cannot be an abuse of language; yet contemporary physics says that it is false, so it must be a factual proposition, and not merely a figment of language, either.[3] Spinoza, having accepted the general law of causation because his philosophy had no quarrel here with the philosophic and scientific tradition that it is a universal truth, naturally believed it to be "necessary," in a somewhat inscrutable but dirt-common sense, because his own philosophy not only accepted but greatly magnified the philosophic and scientific tradition that any universal truth, nay, any truth at all, must be necessary.[4] If attributing necessity to any feature of the world is to be explained by obsession with that feature, then most philosophers and scientists have been obsessed by everything—which, I should think, is perilously near a contradiction. An extra pall of fictiveness is cast over the whole affair by Mr. Lazerowitz's custom of wielding his own metaphysics rather more dogmatically than any dogmatist of the past. He cannot understand how any healthy mind can think that "Every event has a cause" is necessary, because he decrees a priori and *ad hoc* that necessary truths must be merely verbal, and this is not merely verbal. A finer modesty might at least entertain that his own obsession on this topic is as fallible, and as likely to be morbid, as Spinoza's, Newton's, and Aristotle's. That he so misreads Spinoza's philosophy at this juncture need not be fatal, since perhaps some other philosophers *have* been obsessed with the special necessity of the causal principle—Lucretius, say, or Freud, whom Professor Jerome Bruner describes as "wedded to" classical determinism.[5] But the fact that he has not found an instance is significant, without putting us under obligation to find one for him.

It would be naïve, of course, to imagine that Mr. Lazerowitz seriously intends to confirm his thesis by his little clutch of cases, even if he were right about the facts; for the thesis itself is rather a deduction from a theory about philosophy and meaning that is mainly a priori. There is a danger that persons whose specialty is psychiatry rather than philosophy will deem the high assured tone of his semantics to have more authority behind it, philosophic or scientific, than it has. The whole shebang is largely Mr. Lazerowitz's own idea, and though this evinces some estimable energy in him, I am safe in saying that it is as underivable from logic, from scientific linguistics, or even from a systematic epistemology of meaning, as we have found it unsupported by the facts about the instances he cites for it. It has the credential of a certain family resemblance to some other antimetaphysical semantics, particularly to the old school of logical analysis and the new cult of ordinary language, but these are generally thought to be inimical to one another, condemning traditional philosophy for the opposite faults, respectively, of excessive regard for and excessive disregard of the proprieties of common sense. Meantime the most sophisticated and influential of the positivistic brotherhood, Carnap, Hempel, and Quine, have had to reject both of the old Viennese hopes on which Lazerowitz pins almost his whole faith, that logical lines can be drawn between science and metaphysics, and between the factual and the merely verbal.

Whatever the inherent worth of the Lazerowitzian semantics, it can be no firmer than the psychology that invests it. That what philosophers must really be doing, since they can't be talking sense, is proposing or adopting changes of linguistic usage though they don't actually propose or adopt any such changes, we may hope to save from self-contradiction by the concept of two philosophers in each philosophical skin, the empirical or conscious $Philosopher_1$, and the noumenal or unconscious $Philosopher_2$. The latter, or *ka* as the old Egyptians would call him, invents the odd usages and foists them on the former. Not having such horror of dualisms, nor of diremptions of appearance from reality, as affects so many of our contemporaries, I am willing to suppose this intelligible, and few of us would dispute that there is more to each of us than is directly observable either by himself or by others. I shall not labor even the oddity of the idea of secret language operations, though this is to impute unexpressed expressions. And it may be only a verbalism, again, to object to calling the *ka*'s antics an indulgence in a different language, on the plea that their effects on $Philosopher_1$ must be supposed to depend on their being a misuse of the *same* language. What well may irk us, however, is being asked to credit a Reality behind the appearances on no better warrant than that the appearances are against it.

Since mathematicians and physiologists must have *kas* as well as philosophers, it would be gullible in us to accept uncritically that only the latter's *kas* play tricks on them. On Mr. Lazerowitz's showing, the purposes of the unconscious obscurantist ought to be much better served by a screen of fake chemistry or anatomy than of fake metaphysics, just because, on his view, the latter is so transparently fatuous and irrelevant that only magic can explain its fooling anybody. It is no answer that scientific expressions are less charged with "affect," for that is just the question: why should expressions about nothing be more effective than expressions about something? The answer, I think, is not that the unconscious *ka* is afraid to tackle the scientists, but that Mr. Lazerowitz is.

Passing over this inability to explain the difference between philosophy and science, we find ourselves possessed of no notion how the *ka* performs any of those feats whose bare description by Mr. Lazerowitz baffles our best conscious attention, nor why they result in metaphysics rather than anything else—space travel, for example, or fits. It is useless for him to say that the process is like artistic creation, because he and we know even less about the occult phases of art than of philosophy, and because its overt phases, which are our only clue to the rest, augur that the latter are very different from those of philosophy, much more different than are those of science. It would help a little if Lazerowitz could show that philosophers generally have other artistic talents, or that artists are good at epistemology, or that the philosophical worth of philosophical works is regularly proportioned to their literary beauty, but of course he attempts nothing of the kind, and we are reasonably confident it cannot be done. Mr. Lazerowitz is likely to reply that his theory does not entail such crude consequents, but if this is correct it is because the theory entails nothing in particular, and has for sole content, I fear, that he is one man who sees nothing in philosophy. He confesses, indeed, that he cannot explain anything by his hypothesis, nor even explicate the hypothesis itself, when he says of the *ka* that "with exquisite skill which rests on the mysterious ability to perceive the innermost workings of language he does invisible magical things with terminology." There never was a braver effort to get something from nothing, for while this seems to praise the subtlety of the philosophic deception, and to prove the subtlety of our author's exposure of it, what it really adds up to is that there has so far been no reason to think a deception has occurred. Mr. Lazerowitz is like a sleuth so perfect that he has detected a murder so perfect that nobody has been killed.

It is at this point that Mr. Lazerowitz invokes psychoanalysis to redeem his own semantics and psychology. But while this may cost psychoanalysis a quantum of credibility that it can ill afford, it can profit Mr. Lazerowitz only a little at best, yielding only some general substantiation that self-deception is a *vera causa,* perhaps, and some notion, however implausible, of a *motive* for the philosophical self-deception, not *how* the unconscious does its sorcery, but at any rate *why*. This is some advantage because so far it has seemed altogether gratuitous that the *ka* should engage in this idiotic deceit rather than providing an honorable metaphysical conscience, say, like the Socratic demon; and psychoanalysis supplies, for what it may be worth, a barrack of dark irrational forces that make it reasonable to expect the worst.

How much psychoanalysis *is* worth, in a scientific and philosophical regard, is debatable enough so that we marvel at Mr. Lazerowitz's abrupt abandonment of skepticism for credulity in its behalf. Even loyal psychoanalysts must be flustered when a man so disillusioned with the charms of diviner philosophy throws himself unreservedly on the bosom of their blowsy daughter of metaphysics and medicine. An unwary professor, to be sure, might from reading Lazerowitz have conceived psychoanalysis to be a thoroughpaced science, as an unwary psychiatrist, we remarked, might from the same source infer the same thing about his semantics. But psychoanalysis is in fact, I think, much more like alchemy, for example, than like chemistry—in its premature practicality, in its informal and anecdotal empiricism, in running to turgid terminology rather than to theoretical system, in its dearth of statistical test and crucial experiment and indeed of any clear logical nexus between principles and observations. That psychoanalysis is a successful business, though it disgruntles some academic psychologists, is nothing against it—so is electronics—but it is not powerfully favorable either. There still seems surprisingly little statistical evidence that psychoanalytic practice has on the whole helped more than it has hurt, or has either helped or hurt more than any rigmarole. And even if it could show a considerable margin of cures, this would be like the successes of faith healing, pilgrimages to Lourdes, and confessions magazines, better explicable by, and hence confirmatory of, other hypotheses than that of the truth of the doctrines officially associated with them.

Philosophically more important than any of the foregoing,

and underpinning it all, including what Bruner calls (*loc. cit.*) "generous addiction to the fallacy of the dramatic instance," is a peculiarity of the whole conceptual fabric of psychoanalysis. The fault is not that its terms are metaphorical, nor that they are abstract, nor that their objects are unobservable, nor even that, like "phlogiston," they happen to have no objects—all these may be healthy traits of live science and philosophy. The fault is that they are not intended to stand for any actual entities at all, but for such powers, potentialities, principles, virtues, essences, or entelechies as William James called "contentless entities" and as Comte relegated to the "metaphysical" stage of thought. For though impertinent to most metaphysics, these descriptions are sufficiently fair to the scholastic metaphysics so that a modern Thomist like Maritain applauds the Freudian mode of conception despite his contempt for Freud's shallow affectation of materialism.[6] The psychoanalytic explanation either of behavior or of consciousness by impulses, repressions, traumas, complexes, compulsions, ids, libidos, and "the play of mental forces," [7] rather than by imaginable neural or spiritual realities, is like the apocryphal Scholastic's explanation of a clock's behavior by an essence of horadicity rather than by wheels and springs. Since the sole real content of this sort of theoretic conception is exhausted in the evidence that provoked its formulation, it "explains" the behavioral or conscious events only, at best, by summarizing them—which is the reason, I think, that psychoanalysts, for all their acuteness and their decades of professional experience, are able to *predict* nothing from their ostensible theory except what good sense and good will could have predicted all the better from the previous phenomena without any theory. It means further, of course, that, like talk about horadicity instead of wheels and springs, the theory is incapable of conjunction with other knowledge to suggest those new *kinds* of explanations and experiments on which true sciences batten. (Ironically, just this futile sort of "metaphysicalness" has been the main effect of the Comtes and the Machs on the physical sciences. The latter, scared off by aspersions on the thing-in-itself and on "picture thinking" from treating of electrons as actualities, like wheels, must think of them as potentialities for sensation and operation, like an id or horadicity, only more occult because not vested, grounded, or embodied in anything actual at all. Physics, as it happens, was so fortified by its own old realistic inheritance that it is only now letting itself be trapped in the impasse where Scholasticism and psychoanalysis were born.)

A general cavil at psychoanalysis as intrinsically unscientific as well as unphilosophical prepares us to find that it can pump little more blood of proof or precision into the depleted veins of Lazerowitzism than the latter can spare for it. Since Mr. Lazerowitz does not yet claim to have made any cures, we may assume that philosophical psychoanalysis is so far no more effectual than he says philosophical argument is, and lacks even that clinical verisimilitude that was attractive in the Freudian original. As a theory, moreover, it incurs some grave special difficulties. One is having to reconcile the Freudian *ka,* postulated as the nadir of brute primitivism, with the exquisite logical and linguistic refinement required of his *ka.* The other difficulty is explaining how your and my deep ulterior motives, which hide the machinations of my *ka* from me and yours from you, manage also to hide mine from you and yours from me—fiercely inimical as the interests of our rival philosophies must be—and to give themselves away only to such rare seers as Mr. Lazerowitz. Must we suppose that subliminal subversives of all parties conspire not to inform on each other?

Our immediate concern, however, is with how Mr. Lazerowitz's philosophic anecdotes fail to back up his psychoanalytic proposals even by the far from exigent standard general in the profession, being mostly untrue, and when true being "explained" only in that weakest way in which the allegation of any outlandish cause or motive "explains"—is psychologically congenial with—any allegedly outlandish effect. He seems hardly to hope for a Freudian explanation of the assertions about things' being adjectives and about inductive logic's being logic, though his theory requires one. But this diffidence is balanced by so great an assurance about the psychic states of Bradley and Spinoza that we almost forget that he knows nothing in particular of "Bradley's inner life," his "pronounced feelings of inadequacy or self-estrangement," nor of Spinoza's problems about reproduction. Where the legitimate analyst would laboriously probe into case histories actually encountered in his consulting room, Mr. Lazerowitz blithely invents the history to match the demands of his theory. It would be a more considerable test of his assumptions if, having inferred the neuroses from his hypothesis, he found some independent way to verify them. (That this effort might unearth something usable in the case of Bradley, I have heard asserted and denied by equally capable and informed persons; any reconstruction of Spinoza's condition is pretty sure to be fruitless.) He would have some substantial confirmation if statistical researches proved a close association between varieties of childhood experiences and adult anxieties, and between types of anxiety and types of metaphysics, but psychoanalysis, I think, has accomplished not even the first, let alone the second.

One does not have to be a psychoanalytic positivist to note that there is some contingency between human dispositions, innate and acquired, and philosophical or indeed mathematical propensities, but it must be slight, for my experience, which is no more but no less reliable than Mr. Lazerowitz's, suggests almost the opposites of the connections he affirms—for example, that absolute idealism is not associated with a feeling of inadequacy, nor either of these with a yearning for death and interment. The last quality that a historian would attribute to the age of Victorian neo-Hegelianism would be suicidal self-distrust; and absolute idealists in general, including Eleatics, Stoics, Vedantists, Spinozists, Hegelians, Transcendentalists, and Christian Scientists, have always seemed an almost offensively complacent and magisterial crew who regard being dead as much less an advantage than a disadvantage. It is open to Mr. Lazerowitz's partisan to say that a magisterial look may cloak a feeling of inferiority, but the nemesis of all such methodology of dissimulation is that it equally permits our party to insist that the inner state of the absolute idealists is in fact a thousand times more complacent than their outer mien.

No less than atrocious is Mr. Lazerowitz's fraternity-house pun on Spinoza's slogan, "All things are in God, and so depend on him, that without Him they could *neither exist nor be conceived,*" in which he discerns an expression of the philosopher's anxiety about the suspected role of a father in his own production. There is no sign that Lazerowitz is aware that Spinoza's is exactly the same principle that in Bradley he took to express the desire to return to Mother Earth, that the phrase his italics leer at is a verbatim repetition of the age-old definition of *substance* in contrast with, not its effects, nor even its parts, but its *properties,* which makes the pun anachronistic and pointless, and that its main purport, as we earlier saw, is to circumvent just the sort of father-to-son relation that Lazerowitz would worry out of it. It should be plain, however, without metaphysical instruction, that of all causal agents the one providing the least similitude to parenthood is the Deity who is self-caused, particularly since, if we must make romantic guesses about childhood, children are much more fascinated with the parentage of their parents than with their own; and of all self-caused Deities, the worst analogue for paternity is the pantheistic God who is Nature, not only most completely impersonal, but, as the quoted passage exults, not preceding but eternally containing his, or its, consequents. Even if Lazerowitz had been right that Spinoza was fascinated by case-to-case causation, therefore, this would much more likely have been due to his known conscious concern with the scientific successes of his time than to his unknown fretting about fatherhood. Since in fact we know that Spinoza began philosophizing by accepting Maimonides on the freedom of the will, and that he made his later rather incidental concessions to determinism as a result of a study of Crescas' revision of the traditional arguments for universal causation,[8] Mr. Lazerowitz's anecdote misses fire all around. I cannot however resist some remark about his logic. One thing certain about the facts of Spinoza's childhood is that they did not alter when he changed his metaphysics. Beyond that we know nothing helpful. A general consideration of the differences between the households of Spanish-Dutch Jews and of small Scottish lairds yields no clear assurance that Hume, who vigorously denied the necessity of the causal law, had fewer unsatisfied curiosities about the principles and practice of human procreation than Spinoza. Any debate would seem sterile anyhow, since even if we granted that philosophies may be engendered by such ignorances, the difference between absolute ignorance and what even the most candid parent could impart on this mysterious topic is so nearly nil as to give no appreciable pause to a person blessed with the gift of wonder. But if we must impose some Freudian interpretation on Spinoza's doctrine of linear causation, we should observe that his Proposition XXXVI, immediately preceding Mr. Lazerowitz's main citation, declares, not that events must have causes, but that they must have effects, so that it is much less likely that Spinoza was wondering whether he had had a father than whether he was going to have a baby.

That Mr. Lazerowitz's procedure is typical of psychoanalysis I am not prepared to say, but any effort to bend the latter to the critique of philosophy, which transcends it as the ocean transcends a dishpan, was bound to be futile. Lazerowitz must be ready to derive from each of a philosopher's two ideas of "causation" that he is obsessed with having had a father, obsessed with having had a mother, obsessed with both, and obsessed with having had neither but being *causa sui*. To brim the cup of fantasy, Professor Lewis Feuer in a rival psychoanalysis of Spinoza has meanwhile produced such arbitrarily variant findings as that Spinoza, usually bracketed with Socrates as one of the two most self-reliant men in history, was a cringing masochist, so far from boasting of being God that he bleated to be a slave.[9] It is not our part now to marvel that men can read through Spinoza to come out with such scraps of junk, but only to comment on the farcicalness of the logic to which philosophical psychoanalysis drives its devotee. It will, so far as the reader can tell, provide a rule of analogy or a rule of contraries as suits the ulterior purpose; it will accept any bit of biography as witness to any sort of neurosis, and any sort of neurosis as source of any sort of philosophy, permitting different neuroses to be matched with the same philosophy, and conversely, not merely on different occasions but on the same occasion; and as if this were not scope enough, it allows the advocate to invent the symptoms, the neuroses, or the philosophies at need. To say the usual thing, that a theory thus coddled fails by being incapable of refutation, is to praise with too faint condemnation. A theory genuinely irrefutable, because all the facts are in its favor, is a fine thing. But the devices that shield this theory from adverse evidence cut it off also from any confirmation, so are themselves a refutation of it.

I should be sorry to have it thought that I am not grateful to Mr. Lazerowitz for the courage and energy with which he has pressed home a repulsive and cumbersome hypothesis that might have been a threat to the traditional understanding of philosophy. A pioneer in his wilderness, he has naturally wrought less elegantly than settled folk would prefer. I hope, however, that he has done just well enough, and ill enough, to show that his travail need not be undertaken again.

Notes

1. K. Daya, Some Considerations on Morris Lazerowitz's *The Structure of Metaphysics,*" *Mind,* XXVII (1958), 236–43.
2. Daya, in the article cited, is less self-denying in this respect too.
3. One of the items discussed at the 1957 sessions of this Conference was the sense, first pointed out, I think, by Russell, in which "Every event has a cause," i.e., determinism, *is* trivially and analytically true—because the only intelligible definition of "causation" is in terms of regularity, and there is no clear-cut way of confining "regularity" so it will not apply, by dint of sufficiently complex

functions, to any world whatever. Since this interesting result is neither a "reclassification" of words nor an observation on common usage, any more than was the discovery of the irrationality of pi, it can be no comfort to Mr. Lazerowitz. To square it with my own concession that the causal principle is synthetic, however, I must suppose we have limited the causal functions to "simple and salient" ones.

4. "It is not of the nature of reason to consider things as contingent but as necessary."—*Ethics,* Part II, Proposition XLIV.

5. In *Freud and the Twentieth Century,* ed. Benjamin Nelson (New York, 1957), p. 280.

6. *Ibid.,* p. 246.

7. Freud, quoted by S. Toulmin, "The Logical Status of Psycho-Analysis," in *Philosophy and Analysis,* ed. Macdonald (New York, 1954), p. 134.

8. See Isaac Husik, *A History of Mediaeval Jewish Philosophy* (New York, 1916 and 1958), pp. 398–99.

9. L. S. Feuer, "The Dream of Benedict de Spinoza," *The American Imago,* XIV (1957), 225–42. Mr. Feuer does make some inquiry into circumstances of Spinoza's life which support other parts of his analysis, though not this.

9.

Philosophy and Psychopathology

ANTONY FLEW
Professor of Philosophy
University of North Staffordshire, England

MAY I begin with a confession? I had hoped originally that we should be doing some philosophy on concepts of psychoanalysis. The expectation was that we should be continuing the work of such recent monographs as MacIntyre's *The Unconscious* and Peters' *The Concept of Motivation,* and of the many oral and written discussions from which these arose.[1] But the offensive which I was planning to mount has been forestalled and overwhelmed by the onslaught of a man whom I had innocently taken for one of us. Professor Lazerowitz has however unmasked himself as an amateur psychoanalyst of the most menacing and aggressive type. We philosophers are to be analyzed now. It is not to be the concepts of psychoanalysis that serve as objects to our metalanguage. We ourselves are to be put on the couch. Nor are the patients to be only the most wayward members of our strange company. The whole profession, including, it seems, even those colleagues who enjoy to the lay eye the rudest of mental health, is to undergo, if only on paper, a group analysis. Well, so let it be. I shall try to follow where Lazerowitz has led.

One reason to welcome this lead is this. While Lazerowitz is, I think, the first to deploy the ideas about the relations of philosophy and psychoanalysis which he develops in "Philosophy and Psychoanalysis" and in *The Structure of Metaphysics,* similar treatments of other intellectual disciplines and of other human

Notes to this section begin on page 196.

activities have been attempted from the earliest days of psychoanalysis. To this day they are assayed both by psychoanalysts and by popularizers of their ideas. So quite a lot of what has to be said about Lazerowitz here will no doubt apply *mutatis mutandis* to some of these other still fashionable moves elsewhere. Though we shall not be engaged in quite the expected sort of philosophy of analysis, we shall none the less in another way be considering the logical relations between disciplines. This is an important task and one which in one form or another has traditionally been assigned to philosophers.

I

"It can come as a surprise nowadays only to very few people to learn that a painting, like a dream, has its origin in forbidden sources in the unconscious and is valued primarily for the thoughts it conceals, its latent content." So Lazerowitz. It can indeed come as a surprise nowadays only to very few people to learn that claims of this sort are made. But whatever light psychoanalytic investigation may be able to throw on questions about the motivation of artistic creation and enjoyment, surely such a drastic claim as this could not possibly be substantiated.

Suppose an art critic maintains that he values paintings for their power, composition, coloring, brushwork, and so on. He would, as Lazerowitz suggests, probably not be gratified to be told: "If you had the advantage of knowing yourself as well as I do you would realize that in fact you value paintings not for any of these things but for the thoughts that the pictures conceal." But if the art critic had his wits about him, and kept his temper, he could reply: "Yes, I suppose it may well be that the reason that I prefer representations of the Crucifixion and the Agony in the Garden to those of the Annunciation and the Madonna and Child is to be discovered by investigations along the lines that you indicate. Yet, at most, this will only show why I like these themes more than those. But if you in your turn had the advantage of knowing as much about art criticism as I do, you would realize that connoisseurs value paintings primarily not for what we call their 'literary content' but rather for their artistic characteristics."

If it is desired to make out the claim that the connoisseur in fact values Botticelli's "Annunciation" or El Greco's "View of Toledo" not primarily for the reasons that he himself would avow but chiefly because their "literary content" conceals some particular "latent content," it would presumably have to be shown that any other Annunciation from the neighbourhood "Religious Objects" store, or any other painting of the same view of Toledo, would be a tolerably acceptable substitute. This contention, applied simply to those now accepted as connoisseurs, is not at all plausible. But even if we were to find that it did hold good we should still have to insist that, precisely to the extent that any representation with all the same elements of literary content was found to be equally acceptable, the original painting was being valued for something other than its artistic qualities. And to that extent those whom we had previously accepted as connoisseurs had not really on this occasion been acting as connoisseurs.

This may suggest an alternative interpretation of the original thesis. So far we have been taking it, as it was presented, as factual. But the sentence following the one quoted above is: "The artist will not, in all probability, be gratified to be told that his work is an externalized form of dreaming, and that the taste, imagination, and skill which enter into it, though admirable on their own account, derive their major importance from the fact that their role is to effect 'secondary elaboration' for the purpose of concealment." Though presented in the idiom of discovery, this surely involves a piece of evaluation. The artist is being told, as if it were a simple fact recently unearthed by psychoanalytic enquiry, that what is of "major importance" is not any matter of artistic values, however "admirable on their own account." But rather it is "to open out to others 'the way back to the comfort and consolation of . . . unconscious sources of pleasure.' " As evaluation this may or may not be acceptable. But what it certainly is not is a finding of psychoanalysis pure.

a) For purposes of dissection we have spoken of alternative

interpretations of the thesis of Lazerowitz. This may mislead. It may suggest that Lazerowitz must himself have distinguished these interpretations as we do, and must on this occasion have had it clearly and definitely in mind to defend either one *or* the other or both one *and* the other. This conclusion may be correct. But I do not wish to imply that it is. Certainly it is not warranted by any evidence internal to this paper, inasmuch as Lazerowitz never in this context suggests the application of any such distinction. It is hard to believe, however, that had he had it in mind at the time of writing he would have been prepared either to offer as a commonplace what we distinguished as the factual interpretation, or to represent as if they were a discovery his evaluative demands. The crux surely is that Lazerowitz was able to say what he did say precisely and only because on this occasion he did not apply the perfectly familiar distinction between the descriptive and the normative; and hence left confused and undissected what we should labor to separate. Thus it would be harder to recognize the extreme implausibility of the factual claim that we *do* value paintings primarily for the thoughts they conceal if one had not sharply distinguished it from the normative demand that we *ought* to. At the same time, of course the value claim that we *ought* to hold the secret consolations provided by a painting more important than its esthetic characteristics must seem irresistible so long as it appears to be the straightforward discovery of a new science. And that delusive appearance is likely to be mistaken for the reality so long as we fail to distinguish in this context between importance from the point of view of esthetic assessment and appreciation; importance from the point of view of psychoanalytic therapy; and, perhaps, absolute importance or intrinsic value. Allowing that the importance of paintings for the psychoanalyst must lie in their latent content, this provides no reason for suggesting that their importance for the connoisseur too must reside in the same place; and no reason either for accepting that their absolute importance, their intrinsic value, must consist in whatever importance is put on them by the psychoanalyst in his professional capacity.[2] The conscience of the autonomous truly protestant individual does not reject the claims of the Vatican merely in order to replace the authority of the priest by the vicarious professional imperialism of the psychoanalyst.

b) It is maybe just worth while to mention the close parallelism between the sort of thing that Lazerowitz was doing in this first paragraph and the sort of attack launched against the integrity, autonomy, and standing of esthetic assessments by those who urge that the really important thing about any work of art is its historical source and social impact. I do not, of course, want to argue to guilt, or innocence, by association: only to suggest that there is this close parallelism between the moves made and to be made on both sides in both sorts of discussion. For just as the discussion of Lazerowitz's thesis derives additional importance from the fact already mentioned that *mutatis mutandis* similar moves have to be made in discussing similar theses about the relations between psychoanalysis and certain other disciplines and activities; so it also gains in interest from this fact, that similar moves have to be made in discussing this sort of thesis about sociology and art, to say nothing of the many related theses about the social significance of other disciplines and activities.

II

"The philosopher is even less likely than the artist to be gratified by being told that his work, like that of the artist, is to give hidden expression to fantasies in a form which makes them a source of pleasure to others; for he fancies himself to be a kind of scientist, a seeker after basic knowledge whose way is 'through speculation upon ultimate truths.' " The first clause suggests that what Lazerowitz wants to defend is an extremely provocative and implausible thesis about the professional activities of all philosophers. It might seem that this interpretation is confirmed by other passages: "There is evidence . . . for supposing that the philosopher . . . gives expression *only* to his unconscious fantasies" (italics in original); and "If the theory developed in these pages about the nature of philosophy is substantially correct, then psychoanalysis is relevant in a very special way to philosophical utterances. It *alone* can discover for us what they really say, as against what they delusively appear to say" (italics mine). But the second clause gives us ground to hope that Lazerowitz would be prepared to accept a substantial and saving restriction on the range of his thesis. For it suggests that perhaps he only wants to apply it to the philosopher who "fancies himself to be a kind of scientist." A similar clause occurs in the passage omitted from the first of the confirming passages quoted above: "the philosopher, despite all appearances, does not use language to express scientific propositions but instead uses it in such a way as to create the illusion of doing so." And again: "the philosopher instead of using language, as he seems, to make factual claims about the world and its various real or only apparent aspects, uses it to create the false impression of stating such claims."

The unsympathetic, purely destructive critic might be inclined to dismiss Lazerowitz's thesis, as he actually puts it here, out of hand—jeering at the sheer absurdity of applying it to the Aristotle of the *Nicomachean Ethics,* to the minute and desiccating contributors to *Analysis,* or to the piecemeal journeymen of the philosophy of science. The more sympathetic commentator might suggest: either, rather mischievously, that Lazerowitz's account of philosophy itself seems to apply at least equally well to his own metaphilosophical contributions in *The Structure of Metaphysics* and in this present paper; [3] and/or, more ponderously, that the very inappropriateness to work such as that of Aristotle and the rest of the descriptions which we have been quoting is to be taken as a reason for asking Lazerowitz whether he might not be prepared to limit his thesis very considerably. It is surely significant that in his penultimate sentence he writes of "philosophical utterances" that: "Semantic analysis brings to light the linguistic import of these statements and helps explain how they produce their remarkable intellectual illusions." The contention "that the philosopher . . . gives expression *only* to his unconscious fantasies" must confound the bourgeois of the philosophical establishment. Yet much of its sting would perhaps be withdrawn if we could be told explicitly how much of the old philosophical order is to be preserved as "semantic analysis"—a new, purified, republican, anticolonialist, democratic, people's philosophy, free of every appearance of pretending to be a super natural, or supernatural, science.

III

"Consider the question 'Is inductive logic logic?' when asked and debated by philosophers." (Surely, by the way, it should be 'Is inductive logic *really* logic?'.) This is the first case examined by Lazerowitz, and perhaps it is one that should be left on this occasion entirely to Professor Donald Williams. Nevertheless there are two basic points that I should like to make.

First, Lazerowitz maintains "that there could be no disagreement over the question, construed as a request for truth-value information about what inductive logic is." Now surely things are not so open-and-shut and so manifest to one and all as this suggests? For there not merely could be, there actually is, rational disagreement about the fundamental nature and hence the status of induction. Some, like Hume, represent the nerve of all inductive argument as consisting in a "failed deduction," an invalid deductive move from particular premises to universal conclusions. Some of these, following K. R. Popper, accept that Hume showed that induction as a method must be irredeemably unsound; but urge that, fortunately, science does not need induction but only hypothetico-deductive methods, which provide a way of learning from experience that is not logically unsound.[4] Others again try to meet the challenge provided by Hume's representation of induction by searching for some suitable very general assumption—about the uniformity of nature or what have you—with the support of which the failed deductive argument may be couched to qualify as a valid proof of (at least the probability of) the universal conclusions. At the same time, yet others urge that inductive arguments can only be justified, and should be represented, as a matter indeed of following a Principle of Induction, but one construed not as a hidden wonder premise supplied perhaps by a leap of scientific faith, but as a rule of procedure. (The rule would run something like this: To be guided by experience, always where all known A's are Φ taking it that all A's are Φ, until and unless some positive reason to the contrary is found in the particular case or cases in question.)

Faced by this kind and this amount of disagreement about the nature, justification, and prevalence of inductive arguments, we surely need look no further to account for the continuing disagreement as to whether or not inductive logic deserves to be awarded the diploma title "logic."

Second, Lazerowitz's conclusion on this case is that: "The question can, without straining the language in which it is couched, be construed as a request for the reconsideration of the current use of the word 'logic,' raised by a person who, for whatever reason, finds himself being impressed by the *difference* between inductive logic and deductive logic" (italics in original). This seems to me to be substantially right. The question should indeed, as we have already suggested, be construed as being about the possible restriction of the award of a diploma title: compare the chestnut example "Was Pope really a poet?"

But even if we accept this interpretation the example gives only very weak support only to the less exciting part of the hypothesis which it is introduced to illustrate: "the hypothesis that a philosophical view is a three-layer structure composed of the illusion of science, an unconscious group of ideas, and an altered piece of language which creates the first and expresses the second." For "the illusion of science" generated by the suggested alteration of a "piece of language" is, even on Lazerowitz's own account, here an extremely weak one, inasmuch as "The question can, without straining the language in which it is couched, be construed as a request for the reconsideration of the current use of the word 'logic,' " whereas there seems to be no reason for dragging "an unconscious group of ideas" in here at all. In his concluding paragraph Lazerowitz urges that perhaps "psychoanalysis is relevant in a very special way to philosophical utterances. It alone can discover for us what they really say, as opposed to what they delusively appear to say." Now suppose we allow that this particular philosophical utterance does indeed delusively appear to say something which might be called in the very broadest sense scientific. Still there seems no reason whatsoever to call for a psychoanalyst to tell us what reality lies behind this appearance. For why should the philosopher not be saying, and be taken to be saying, that the diploma title "logic" ought perhaps to be withdrawn from induction and what has been called inductive logic? And why should we not take it that his grounds are precisely those considerations, about (what he takes to be) the nature and justification or lack of justification of inductive argument, which he deploys in support of his suggestion?

Of course you might find a use for a psychoanalytic consultant if you found that some particular philosopher was pressing this contention in an obsessive, or irrational, or disproportionately heated manner, or if he seemed in some other way to be giving grounds for a suspicion that for him all this talk about the logical inadequacies of inductive procedures was a mere smokescreen, or that for him induction served mainly or entirely as a symbol for something else. Alternatively the psychoanalysts may argue that always, even when the particular case gives no special grounds for supposing that there must be more to the argument than meets the eye, even when reasons and counterreasons are being presented with no more than that degree of affect or lack of it considered appropriate, nevertheless always the discussants are giving—but unconsciously—other and symbolic interpretations to the terms in their discourse in addition to the straightforward common meanings which alone they recognize consciously. But neither of these two possibilities, even were they to be realized, would serve to support Lazerowitz's conclusion as he actually formulated it. For in the first case we should be dealing only with one particular philosopher who happened to be neurotic, while in the second case the analysts would have provided no reason for accepting that the unconscious meaning alone was the real meaning, and the apparent meaning a mere delusion. But Lazerowitz's contention was that perhaps "psychoanalysis is relevant in a very special way to philosophical utterances. It alone can discover for us what they really say, as against what they delusively appear to say."

IV

"The metaphysician's theory is a subtle and remarkable work of verbal art. Its underlying mechanics are a grammatically changed language which is not meant for practical discourse but, like a work of art, is meant only for contemplation. It creates the appearance of a profound theory about the cosmos, while it actually expresses inner psychic dramas." Now if we take the expression "the metaphysician" as in recent years it seems so commonly to have been employed, as a definite description of F. H. Bradley, then we have here, I think, a very suggestive and plausible thesis. For, for the reasons given in Lazerowitz's paper and others, it does seem that in *Appearance and Reality* Bradley is developing a grammatically changed language meant only for contemplation, and creates thereby the appearance of a profound theory about the cosmos. At the same time, precisely because this appearance is only a delusive appearance, it leaves an entry port for the suggestion that what is really being expressed is something else. If we are, following Lazerowitz, to "take it for granted that the unconscious is ubiquitous . . . and . . . assume as substantially correct the basic psychoanalytical tenets," then I think we have a good case here for their application. The remarkable images (some of which Lazerowitz quotes), the curiously obsessive style of the whole book, and the known facts of Bradley's life and character, all add up within this assumed framework to a case considerably stronger than those often accepted as sufficient to justify the sort of interpretation that Lazerowitz is urging. So let us allow that it is reasonable on these grounds and within this framework to entertain as a working hypothesis the idea that the main features of *Appearance and Reality* had their chief importance for Bradley as giving covert expression to his unconscious inner psychic dramas; and that the appearance of a profound theory about the cosmos is delusive.

But to allow this is a very different thing from conceding various other contentions made in this section. Thus Lazerowitz writes: "Furthermore it is hard to think that the deception would have gone undetected without protection from deeper sources in our minds . . . the durability of Bradley's view can be accounted for only by supposing that it has become connected with ideas which are charged with powerful affect." And again: "Ramsey has remarked 'the peculiar incompleteness of adjectives.' This incompleteness, which seems to have rather mystified him, is grammatical. An adjective requires a substantive for it to function in sentences, while a substantive does not require an adjective. And the fact that this incompleteness struck him as being peculiar shows that it has become connected with something in the unconscious."

These two arguments seem to be evidence of a lamentable weakness in historical imagination and in interpretative method.[5] For they take it for granted that whatever is quite obvious now to all of us who have enjoyed a certain sort of philosophical training must have been equally obvious—barring unconscious blockages—to others in the past who were born too soon to have the advantage of this sort of training. They assume, because Lazerowitz now is so quick to transpose philosophical utterances into a linguistic idiom, that others must have been equally able—again of course unconscious blockages and pulls apart—to appreciate what would have been the effect of making such transpositions: even when those others were working before these moves had been invented, or at least before they had become commonplace stock in trade.

Thus, after giving an account of Bradley's argument as presented by Bradley, Lazerowitz provides a second, transposed version "restated in terms of language." From this he proceeds: "It is hardly necessary to point out that the noun and noun phrases descriptive of various phenomena in ordinary language are not contradictory, that they have a use other than in the context of appearance expressions, and that they are not adjectives. Nor is it necessary to call attention to the fact that all this is perfectly well known and cannot be soberly denied by anyone who knows and uses ordinary language." This is all very well. Certainly it is thoroughly trodden familiar ground to what a leading Oxford philosopher has in private mischief called "all the best people nowadays." But of course from this fact that something is obvious to us now we are not entitled to infer that it must have been equally obvious to others earlier, if only they had not been blinded by their deeply unconscious cravings. Again, if we look up the passage in Ramsey from which the phrase quoted is taken we find: "It might also be objected that Mr. Johnson does not make particulars and universals different enough, or take into account the peculiar incompleteness of adjectives which appears in the possibility of prefixing to them the auxiliary 'being'; 'being red,' 'being a man' do not seem real things like a chair and a carpet" (*Foundations of Mathematics,* p. 115). It is surely clear that Ramsey was thinking in a way still semiontological. (Compare the wholly ontological passage which aptly Lazerowitz quotes from Descartes: "No properties or qualities pertain to nothing; and . . . when some are perceived there must necessarily be some thing or substance on which they depend.") But the essay on "Universals" from which our extract is taken is dated 1925, whereas Carnap's *The Logical Syntax of Language,* containing the first version published in book form of his distinction between the "Material Mode of Speech" and the "Formal Mode of Speech" appeared in the original German edition only in 1934. What is obvious depends very much on time and place and person, while the discovery of something which later becomes a commonplace may require enormous painstaking labors, or the insight of genius.[6]

To this Lazerowitz might reply that these deceptions which he considers could not have escaped detection "without protection from deeper sources in our minds," and these mysteries, which he believes could not have appeared to be mysteries but for their connections "with something in the unconscious," could indeed have been detected, or dissipated, by anyone not blinkered and inhibited by unconscious yearnings. To make out this claim, what he would need, and all he would need, is solid evidence of the part played by psychoanalytic therapy in making possible the revolution in philosophy [7] in this century, and particularly in the second quarter of this century. Perhaps there is such evidence from Cambridge or elsewhere. Certainly I know of none from Oxford.

V

". . . The philosophical utterance 'Every event has a cause' does appear to state a theory (*sic*) about the nature of events, to the effect that all without any conceivable exception have causes. . . . But its appearing to express a theory about occurrences is a deception. For if 'Every event has a cause' expressed an a priori proposition, *whether analytic or synthetic,* understanding it would come to knowing no more than that as a matter of usage the term 'has a cause' correctly applies to whatever the word 'event' applies to, or that the expression 'event which has no cause' has no descriptive use, is not a phrase which describes anything actual or imaginable" (italics mine). Here indeed we have a "short way with dissenters."

For the sake of both brevity and simplicity let us leave on one side the possible case in which the utterance under discussion is used to express an a posteriori generalization. Now someone who intended what he said to be in some sense a priori might very well object to this description "a theory about occurrences." Thus he might object to the term "theory" on the ground that he was putting forward the conclusion of an ontological analysis; and that this was an a priori business the conclusions of which could not have either the hypothetical or the explanatory character of a theory. Or he might jib at the expression "about occurrences," on the ground that he was expressing a necessity of reason or a condition of the intelligibility of experience—perhaps part, or one interpretation, of a principle of sufficient reason; and that such an expression was no more a statement about occurrences than a tautology including event words is a statement about occurrences. In either case the considerations urged would certainly constitute grounds for saying that the original utterance only *appeared* "to express a theory about occurrences": but was *really* intended, and should have been taken, in the way which the speaker has since tried to explain. By contrast the consideration that Lazerowitz presents constitutes no sort of ground for saying this; and perhaps only a really extraordinary lack of historical imagination could have made it appear to him that it did constitute such a ground. For in effect what he is doing here is putting forward what he considers to be sufficient reasons for insisting that, if "Every event has a cause" is intended and interpreted in the obvious way, then what it says cannot be known a priori to be true; and mistaking these to be decisive reasons for saying that it cannot really *both* be taken in this way *and* be believed to be known a priori to be true. But this, of course, is grotesque. No doubt to us, and to "all the best people nowadays" it is transparently clear that there cannot be truths which are both synthetic and known a priori: even though to some of us it may seem that considerably more is required in the application of this and associated basic insights to the particular problem case than Lazerowitz would seem to allow.[8] But, as we had to insist in the previous section (IV above), from the fact that something is obvious to us now we are most emphatically not entitled to infer that it cannot fail to have been equally obvious to others in the past (or for that matter to others now), if only it had not been (was not) for the sinister interposition of the dark forces of the unconscious.

a) Furthermore, quite apart from this question about the unsound and unsophisticated methods by which Lazerowitz attempts to derive his conclusion, there are excellent reasons for holding that it is in itself mistaken. His conclusion, it will be recalled, was: "the philosophical utterance 'Every event has a cause' does appear to state a theory about the nature of events, to the effect that all without any conceivable exception have causes. . . . But its appearing to express a theory about occurrences is a deception." We have already suggested that the particular phrases here are not entirely satisfactory. Our present point is that unless this utterance is construed in some fairly straightforward way it cannot begin to play the part for which it has been cast. For it is only and precisely with the aid of this maxim, and with that of other rather more recherché principles of causality, that St. Thomas, Spinoza, and Descartes construct some of their arguments for the existence of God and for other remarkable fruits of philosophy. Now, thanks to Hume the all-destroyer,[9] Lazerowitz is sure—and so am I—that there are no such nontautological principles known a priori; and so all arguments which appeal to any of them must fall to the ground. Yet this has none of it the slightest tendency to show that those philosophers who have claimed, and those who still claim,—for alas there are many both amateur and professional who have not so far attained enlightenment,—to know any such principles to be necessarily true were not in fact claiming exactly what they seemed to be claiming, while it is only in so far as we take them to be saying what they seem to be saying that we can make sense of those of their arguments in which they depend on various principles of causality substantially and not tautologically construed.

b) Lazerowitz, however, persists in taking it that this "appearing to express a theory about occurrences is a deception." This, together with his besetting incapacity to realize that what is obvious to him, having gone through the modern philosophical mill, may not have been, and may not be, obvious to those less happily circumstanced, leads him to ask two new questions: "How are we to explain, for one thing, a verbal misconception which, so to speak, has become an inherited piece of property, and how, for another thing, are we to explain anyone's thinking that a proposition could both be about a matter of fact and have a truth-value which is logically necessary?" This formulation is simply breathtaking in its historical parochialism: and an Oxford-trained philosopher may be tempted to add the adjectives "Cambridge" or "Moral Sciences" to the epithet "parochialism." For how can it seem to anyone with the slightest acquaintance with the history of philosophy, or with the way in which philosophy is done today on the Dark Continent of

Europe, and in darker places in our own more happier lands, that *this* is the problem? For to reach these insights which now to some seem obvious has required enormous toil, and even the contributions of genius. And furthermore, as we have suggested at the end of section IV above, to this enlightenment psychoanalytic therapy seems so far to have been able to make little contribution.

> c) A possible and, in my opinion, plausible explanation of what has happened is that what may be called a *conversion analysis* has been performed, an analysis, that is to say, which calls attention to points of actual usage, not for the purpose of stating the criteria for the application of terms but to justify a *linguistic alteration*. A philosopher like Spinoza, say, who maintains that it is impossible "that something should be made out of nothing," is calling attention to a similarity between expressions which he finds objectionable and which he eliminates by verbal fiat, by an arbitrary change of language. . . . The noun grammar of the word "nothing" in the expression "Something is made out of nothing" makes it appear that "nothing" is being used to name a kind of substance. . . . "It is possible that something should be made out of nothing" . . . is a form of speech that some philosophers find objectionable because of its delusive similarity with statements about what substance things are or may be made from. And to make more pronounced a semantic dissimilarity between types of expressions which their grammar tends to hide, Spinoza deprives "uncaused thing," or "thing made out of nothing," of its ordinary use, by making "Something is made out of nothing" express a logical impossibility.

And so we go on:

> The sentence "Every event of necessity has a cause" expresses an a priori proposition by arbitrary verbal decree. . . . The sentence is made to express a proposition it is not ordinarily used to express, by virtue of the philosophical banishment . . . of the expression "uncaused event."

We have already argued one difficulty of taking it that this sentence is being so used that it merely appears deceptively to say what it seems to say: namely, that this interpretation makes nonsense of the attempts to derive from the proposition expressed the sorts of consequences which Spinoza and others have tried to derive from it. Another difficulty is that it makes what Spinoza and others were *really* saying something rather trifling very perversely expressed, whereas the more specious and usual interpretation represents it as, albeit perhaps in error, at least a substantial important doctrine stated straightforwardly.

d) "The philosophical words do not express a theory of the sort they appear to be expressing . . . and we are constrained to think that their absorbing and enduring interest lies in unconsciously grasped propositions they are made to express, one of which it would seem is related to a curiosity that went unsatisfied in the infancy of our life." We have argued already at length that the premise here is false. So we certainly cannot be constrained by it to any conclusion. I am tempted to go on to examine the suggested conclusion in its own right: wondering whether it would be merely cheap logic-chopping to ask why the child itself is so sure that it cannot have come into existence without a cause, and whether the emancipation of Hume is to be traced to his rare good fortune in being raised on a Scottish farm. But I have gone on long enough. That would make another paper, and one on the sort of subject which I forswore in undertaking to follow where Lazerowitz had led.

Notes

1. Both these monographs were published in 1958 by Routledge and Kegan Paul (London) in their series "Studies in Philosophical Psychology." References to most of the main published contributions to this previous discussion are given by MacIntyre on pp. viii–ix of his book.

2. Sections 3(c) and 5(a) of my "Crime or Disease" in *British Journal of Sociology* for 1954 are perhaps relevant here.

3. See K. Daya's note, "Some Considerations on Morris Lazerowitz's *The Structure of Metaphysics*" in *Mind,* 1958.

4. See his contribution to *British Philosophy in Mid-Century,* ed. C. A. Mace (London: Allen and Unwin, 1957).

5. Richard Robinson's valuable list of simple pitfalls for the historian of philosophy is relevant here: see his *Plato's Earlier Dialectic* (Ithaca, N. Y.: Cornell University Press, 1941), Introduction.

6. Compare H. H. Price, "Hume's Philosophy," *Philosophy,* 1940, *ad fin.,* on "the discovery of the obvious."

7. Compare A. J. Ayer *et al., The Revolution in Philosophy* (London: Macmillan, 1956).

8. See G. J. Warnock on the present case in *Logic and Language* (Second Series; Oxford: Blackwell, 1953); and compare in the same volume D. F. Pears, "Incompatibilities of Colours." A full account of the attractions of the idea that "Every event *must* have a cause" would have to pay attention to the vital part which this and other a priori principles of causation play in the construction of traditional arguments about God. It is still, I think, typical of British philosophers to ignore or underplay the possible logical, or at least psychological, linkages between philosophical analysis and ideology. This is perhaps one of the few weaknesses of G. J. Warnock's brilliant study of *Berkeley* (Penguin Books, 1953): see my review in the *Philosophical Quarterly,* 1955.

9. This title seems to me to fit Hume better than it does Kant.

PART IV

DISCUSSION, CRITICISM, AND CONTRIBUTIONS BY OTHER PARTICIPANTS

These statements were submitted after the close of the Institute Sessions.—*Editor*.

10.

Psychoanalysis As Scientific Method *

JACOB A. ARLOW, M.D.
Clinical Associate Professor of Psychiatry
State University of New York

AN INTERDISCIPLINARY consideration of problems of methodology in psychoanalysis presumes that a knowledge of the psychoanalytic method is shared in common among the discussants. However, from the manner in which the discussion has developed it seems clear that any such presumption was unfounded. Since it is impossible to assess the levels of validity of various psychoanalytic hypotheses or operational concepts without first knowing just what method of investigation psychoanalysis employs, a few simple, yet fundamental, observations, relative to the basis of the psychoanalytic method, are offered in this contribution.

In his presentation Dr. Hartmann mentioned that the psychoanalytic situation is central to the problem of the psychoanalytic method of investigation. The psychoanalytic situation consists of the following: the patient (or subject) lies on a couch not facing the analyst (or experimenter). In accordance with a previously established understanding the subject proceeds to report verbally, as far as he is able, all thoughts, ideas or sensations which occur to him during the session. The subject is expected to report these data of consciousness in an indiscriminate manner, leaving aside all considerations of value judgments. This applies equally to considerations of judgment based on moral standards, the significance of the data for the therapy, the personal nature of the thoughts and even the seeming

* I am indebted to Dr. Charles Brenner for certain suggestions and criticisms.—J.A.A.

irrelevance of what is experienced. To the extent that he finds it possible, the subject is expected to act in the role of an uncritical reporter.

A complementarily objective and uncritical attitude on the part of the analyst towards the productions of the subject is the other major component of the analytic situation. The function of the analyst is to listen in an unbiased, unprejudiced way without introducing any predetermined concept of the origin or meaning of the phenomena under investigation. Every aspect of his manner and the procedure must reflect that his only interest is to help the patient to analyze and understand his thoughts and behavior. This is one of the reasons that the subject lies on a couch facing away from the analyst. This part of technique aims towards eliminating any additional source of possible ambiguity in communication. The analyst may betray a thought process of his own through some physiognomic change, or at least the subject may think he has. An intrusion of this sort constitutes a source of contamination of the field of observation. These are the very same considerations that form the basis for another fundamental aspect of the analytic situation, namely, the anonymity of the analyst. The personal life of the analyst, his private likes and dislikes, his professional, moral, esthetic or political predilections should not be permitted to enter into the analytic situation. By minimizing external sources of mental stimulation the psychoanalytic situation brings under survey data whose appearance is determined primarily or almost exclusively by the mental activity of the subject. This principle would be undermined if the analyst as a personality were permitted to enter the analytic situation, if his values, prejudices, etc., were permitted to operate as stimuli to the subject's thinking. It would be very difficult under such circumstances to know whether we were dealing with some response to the analyst or whether we were dealing with the proper area of psychoanalytic scrutiny, namely, the repetitive behavior patterns of the patient which are autogenously determined. The goal of the analytic situation is to create a set of conditions in the field of observation in which the data are supplied by the subject exclusively.

All events, verbal or motor, which transpire in the analytic situation constitute the data of observation.

The fact that many people can report that analyst A, B or C did not behave in the manner just described or did not set the conditions in the field as indicated is totally irrelevant to our problem, which is to study the validity of the psychoanalytic method of investigation. Reports of breaches of psychoanalytic technique cannot be used in evaluating the psychoanalytic method any more than reports of contamination or sloppy technique in bacteriology can be used to invalidate the findings of that science.

To permit ourselves a brief digression at this point we may exploit the analogy further. In bacteriological investigation contaminants introduce dynamic changes into the experimental situation. When understood through the appropriate technique such "accidents" may yield valuable data leading to further knowledge and development. The discovery of penicillin may be cited as an obvious example of this type of event. Similar situations supervene in analysis. Life provides the contaminations of the field of observation. By accident the patient may come upon some knowledge concerning the analyst, his family or his background. Such events introduce dynamic changes into the analytic situation. To these events, again, the analyst must maintain a detached and observing attitude. He does not respond to the realistic aspects of the material but studies instead the proper area of his observation, namely, the patient's reactions, the effects of the intrusion of this foreign body into the analytic situation. Properly studied, this type of accidental contamination of the field of operation yields valuable data and insight.

These are the main outlines of the analytic situation. Every aspect of psychoanalytic technique is oriented towards preserving the objective, neutral, uncontaminated relationship of the field of observation. The very definite understanding concerning the practical arrangements of time, of appointments, of duration of session, fee for treatment, buttress the atmosphere of the analytic situation.

Psychoanalysts recognize that psychoanalysis is certainly not the only form of psychotherapy, nor does it have to be considered the most efficacious form of treatment of mental illness. Therapeutic efficacy is a related but not a central aspect of the problem of psychoanalytic methodology. Many forms of psychotherapy and other experiences may affect mental illness in a beneficent way, but only psychoanalysis has the methodological tools to investigate and attempt to explain these effects.

Because of the principles that underlie psychoanalytic technique, those who are acquainted in a practical way with the psychoanalytic method are convinced that it constitutes by far the closest approach to a controlled experimental situation that has as yet been devised to study the total functioning of the human mind. Indubitably, it is far from a perfect investigative technique. The context of therapy is a formidable but inevitable hazard. In addition, in common with the study of all dynamic situations, especially biological systems, psychoanalysis suffers from certain very definite methodological disadvantages. Some of these are: incomplete control over many of the factors in the field of observation, the impossibility of reduplicating precisely the events and situations studied, etc.

Although the analytic situation corresponds most closely to the experimental laboratory of other sciences, psychoanalytic methodology is hardly comparable to that of chemistry or physics (perhaps with the exclusion of physiological chemistry). On the other hand, because it considers the unconscious motivations and the genetic background that the subject brings into the experimental situation psychoanalysis has been able to indicate various sources of error in the "laboratory" technique of experimental psychology, a technique which, in academic circles, is apparently held in higher scientific esteem than psychoanalysis.

There is a basic principle or assumption that underlies the technique which has been devised and called the analytic situation. This is the principle of psychic determinism, the assumption that there is causality in the functioning of the human mind. Without such an assumption, psychological investigation of any sort would be meaningless—unless one would be willing to accept as the basis of mental life the crudest type of response to stimuli or the random, though unknown, fluctuation of the metabolic processes in the brain. In any event, such an approach flies in the face of common sense.

Essentially psychic determinism implies the application to the phenomena of mental life of the same criteria for causality and relatedness that apply to the phenomena of nature in other sciences. Once the data of observation have been gathered, the process of correlation and interpretation proceeds as in other fields of science, taking into account consistency of hypotheses, repetitive patterns of sequential relationships, the ability to predict certain phenomena on the basis of a knowledge of these patterns, etc. These principles need no repetition. It seems, however, that there is little conviction that the method of observation and procedure outlined above is actually followed in psychoanalysis. To become convinced of this, one has to observe the psychoanalytic process at first hand or else study detailed expositions of correlation and interpretation of data as utilized in psychoanalysis. Expositions of this sort appear in Freud's *Interpretation of Dreams,* in *The Pyschopathology of Everyday Life,* in *Wit and its Relation to the Unconscious,* in the *General Introduction to Psychoanalysis,* and in some of the classic case histories by Freud. It is true, unfortunately, that in many psychoanalytic writings authors have not been as precise in the exposition of their methodology as was Freud in his pioneering work. There are many reasons for this, but perhaps the main one is the fact that in writing for a group of colleagues, analysts assume that the method employed is well known, and for purposes of convenience employ a "shorthand" of exposition which does away with the necessity of detailing elaborate reports at great length.

What was, and perhaps still is, one of the most controversial of psychoanalytic concepts, namely, the notion of mental functioning occurring outside of the scope of consciousness, becomes a necessary and inevitable conclusion if the principle of psychic determinism is applied to the phenomena of mental life in an unbiased and objective fashion. The study of slips of the tongue constitutes perhaps the easiest and most convincing method of demonstrating this principle. It does not require too much effort to demonstrate that slips of the tongue are motivated, and that sometimes the person who makes the slip is perfectly aware of the motive at the time he makes the slip; or that the person was not aware of the motive at the time that he made the slip of the tongue but after some reflection could understand that such motivation could actually exist; and finally there are those instances where the motivation for the slip of the tongue remains completely unknown to the person who made the slip and he resists any implication of motivation, although the motivation appears quite clear to others who heard the slip of the tongue in the context in which it happened. For illustrations of this point one is referred to the works mentioned above.

The regular and consistent patterning of the data of observation permits the analyst to make predictions which can be confirmed by further observation. In his discussion Dr. Loewenstein described how a supervising analyst is in a position to make and, in fact, does make many predictions on the development of the case and on the appearance of certain specific material. It should be noted that these predictions are made on the record of a patient whom the supervising analyst has not even seen. The frequency and specificity of predictions is far beyond chance relationship. Phenomena of this sort must be observed at first hand by critics of analytic methodology. It is possible that a fruitful interdisciplinary study of psychoanalytic methodology might be developed by having a student of methodology sit in on a supervised psychoanalytic case.

The fact is that analysts are always making predictions, which they submit to confirmation or invalidation by the further study of their data. A simple clinical illustration may be introduced at this point to illustrate this method of operation. During an initial interview I asked a patient how long he had been married. He answered, "Sixteen months, three weeks." The overly exact quality of this response aroused in me the suspicion that I was dealing with a person whose character structure was colored by obsessional thinking and compulsive traits. To confirm my suspicion I asked further, "How long did you know your wife before you married her?" He answered, "Two years, three months." At this point, inwardly, I made a further set of predictions concerning this individual's mental traits. I guessed that he would be especially concerned with money, that he would have a passion for accumulating it, keeping meticulous records of his financial transactions, and that he would be most reluctant to spend it. A further set of predictions concerned his relationship to cleanliness. I could guess that he would be excessively neat regarding his person and his clothes, tidy in his surroundings, orderly in his manner, and vigorously punctual regarding appointments and the fulfillment of financial obligations. Questioning confirmed each of these predictions in minute detail. But even further predictions can be made on the basis of the minimal hints given by this patient. In the course of detailed psychoanalytic investigation it could be predicted that a specific type of childhood experience regarding bowel training and interest in excrement would emerge. Such predictions in psychoanalysis are beyond the probability of a guess. These are predictions that have been validated regularly, hundreds of times in psychoanalytic investigations. Thus, we can see how a pathognomonic detail may enable the trained and experienced psychoanalyst not only to predict a whole set of correlative conditions but to hypothesize correctly concerning the genesis and development of certain mental characteristics. Naturally, there is a hierarchy in the predictability of phenomena in psychoanalysis just as there is in the phenomena of other sciences. The example given above is one of the best known and best validated relationships observed in psychoanalysis.

An historical note might be of interest here. The correlation between certain traits of the individual's character and a specific set of childhood experiences was hypothesized by Freud on the basis of data obtained from the analysis of adult patients. Utilizing this data, he was able to hypothesize the genetic elements in the individual's early childhood which were related to these character traits. Subsequently, these retrospective reconstructions were substantially validated by direct observation of the behavior of children. Direct observation on children confirmed the hypotheses concerning the age at which the characteristic conflict concerning bowel training and excremental play took place. In addition, the quality of the relationships, exactly as predicted from the data of the analyses of adults, could be observed *in statu nascendi*.

The distinction between data of observation and hypotheses should be kept in mind in connection with the so-called Oedipus complex. It is by no means a matter of chance that precisely this aspect of psychoanalytic theory aroused the interest of the group —but this is not the time to discuss this special interest. To begin with, a distinction should be made between the oedipal phase and the "Oedipus complex." The reason for placing the phrase "Oedipus complex" in quotes will be discussed later.

The oedipal phase refers to the period of the child's life which falls roughly between the ages of three and six years. The significant characteristic of this period, so far as certain aspects of the emotional development of the individual are concerned, relates to sexual and aggressive feelings towards the parents or towards those who fulfill the corresponding role for the child. Sexual and aggressive feelings are directed toward both parents. The quality of these relationships differs in the little boy and in the little girl. Little girls undergo a longer and more complex set of oedipal reactions. Also, the oedipal reaction differs from one boy to another depending upon the specific structuring of his life situation and all of the antecedent vicissitudes of his development. The *most frequent* pattern for the usual kind of boy during this period consists of *predominantly* tender sexual feelings towards the mother and rivalrous feelings of hostility towards the father. The word "predominantly" must be emphasized and underlined because we are dealing here with a phase of development in which both tender and hostile feelings are felt for both parents. In unusual situations, which may develop for a variety of reasons, the predominant pattern described above may be reversed. The little boy may prefer his father and have tender sexual wishes directed toward him, feeling at the same time hostile rivalry toward his mother.

The term "oedipal phase" rather than "complex" is used

here because what is being discussed is a regular developmental phase to be observed in children reared in family patterns in civilized society. The existence of the relationships which give the characteristic quality to this phase is not a matter of conjecture or reconstruction. It is a matter of observation. If one listens to children, watches them, plays with them and studies them, one will be able to hear expressed in various forms—directly, through play activity, through fantasy, through the dreams which may be told—precisely those wishes which are characteristic of the oedipal phase. (Why these observations were not made or understood before Freud is another problem, irrelevant to the methodology of psychoanalysis but pertinent to the resistance to psychoanalytic findings.)

Thus, psychoanalytic concepts concerning the existence of the oedipal phase are of one order of validity. It corresponds to a description, a summary of observed data, not to any reconstruction or hypothesis. It is quite a different matter, however, when one turns to the "Oedipus complex." An entirely different order of methodology is involved at this point. In effect, an hypothesis is advanced concerning the significance, the interpretation of data acquired during psychoanalytic investigation of adults. In a condensed and simplified form, the hypothesis may be put into the following words: "In his current life the subject (or patient) is behaving in response to the sexual and aggressive wishes which he felt towards his parents during the ages of three to six, i.e., during the early oedipal phase." The subject is usually unaware of any such processes occurring in his mental life. He may have substituted other figures for his parents and his expression of his sexual and aggressive feelings may have undergone certain distortions, disguises and transformations. One can see at a glance that the validation of such an hypothesis involves methodological considerations and problems of quite a different nature from the observation of children during the oedipal phase. A host of data has to be interpreted, integrated and correlated before the reconstruction and the validation of the specific features of the Oedipus complex in the adult subject are possible. This is accomplished within the analytic situation following the principles of psychic determinism and the available canons of causality as outlined at the beginning of this contribution.

Professor Sidney Hook raised the following question: "On what specific evidence would a psychoanalyst decide that a child did not go through the oedipal phase?" In response to this question we may say that such cases have been described. From what has been said above it is possible to understand that in such an instance we would be dealing with an anomaly of emotional and mental development. Phenomenologically, the little boy who does not achieve the oedipal phase of development would express no tender or romantic feelings or fantasies regarding his mother. He would not express any wish to grow up and marry her, nor try to oust his father as the rival from the marriage bed. Manifestations of a wish to exhibit his penis to the mother, to press his penis against her, to have her admire and fondle his penis would not appear. Evidence of pleasurable manipulation of the penis and concomitant fantasy as observed in normal development would be minimal in such a case. Such a child would hardly regard the other individuals in his environment as distinct entities or personalities. They would be important to him only in so far as they could grant immediate satisfaction of his bodily wants or needs. Once they had fulfilled these functions he would lose interest in his parents or nurses. He would hardly refer to them, conjure up few images or memories concerning them, and have no concern about their personal feelings or individuality. Considerations of masculinity or femininity would be minimal and completely subordinate to preoccupation over dependency, passivity, sleeping, eating and bowel function. We would anticipate in such a child impulsive emotionality and very meager identification with the standards, the ideals and behavior of his human environment. These are only a few features of the picture of a child who does not develop an oedipal phase, but sufficient features have been mentioned to indicate that the concept of an oedipal phase is not a procrustean bed into which psychoanalysts wish to force all the data of observation. The existence of an oedipal phase in the development of the young child is based upon definite, observable patterns of behavior, upon a concrete set of interpersonal relations and upon a host of other mental phenomena. Definite criteria of a positive and negative nature must be available before one can say whether a child has or has not achieved the oedipal phase of development.

In summary, it should be acknowledged that psychoanalysis is not an esoteric cult in which the analyst foists upon gullible neurotic patients a preconceived mumbo-jumbo inherited from Freud. Psychoanalytic therapy is a meticulously painstaking investigation into human mental processes. It is by no means a perfect experimental tool, but it is, nevertheless, a rational and objective procedure, governed by strict methodological considerations and operating within accepted canons of the scientific method.

11.

Science and Mythology in Psychoanalysis

SIDNEY HOOK
Professor of Philosophy
New York University

JOHN DEWEY once remarked that although he was critical of dualistic elements in Freud's psychology, especially of his concept of a substantial unconscious, he was deeply impressed by Freud's extraordinary powers of observation of human behavior. This judgment can be paralleled by many other tributes paid to one or another aspect of Freud's work by thinkers who in general have been critical of psychoanalysis as a scientific theory. John B. Watson, for example, who believed he could induce neurotic behavior in any animal or human being purely by environmental conditioning, wrote:

> The scientific level of Freud's concept of the unconscious is exactly on par with the miracles of Jesus. I say this despite my reverence for Freud and my admiration for his courage in insisting upon the role sex plays in the lives of all. I say this in spite of the fact that Freud's teachings have stimulated the thought of all psychologists and of all psychiatrists.[1]

A similar appreciation is expressed in the more recent judgment of one of the most caustic critics of psychoanalysis, Dr. H. J. Eysenck, Professor of Psychology at the University of London:

> The answer to the question which forms the title of this chapter—What is wrong with psychoanalysis?—is simple: Psychoanalysis

Notes to this section begin on page 224.

is unscientific. It is only by bringing to bear the traditional methods of scientific inference and experimentation that we can hope to reap all the benefits of its founder's genius.[2]

These expressions of admiration for Freud and his work combined with skepticism of the large claims he and his disciples have made for his theories are characteristic of the reaction of many, if not most, academic psychologists. It certainly is not prima facie evidence of resistance. It has led some devotees of psychoanalysis to retort, paraphrasing words recently used by a sociologist about his own discipline, "Psychoanalysis may be unscientific, but it is true." It is indisputable that we have a great deal of common-sense psychological knowledge about people which has not the status of exact scientific knowledge. But the knowledge psychoanalysts claim to have about human beings, especially about their unconscious desires, is hardly common-sense knowledge, outraging as it often does not only the language of common usage but the assurances of common belief. There is a sense in which something can be said to be "true" without being "scientific" in the preferential connotation of the term. This is acknowledged whenever it is recognized that there is an inescapable continuity between the world of common sense and the world of science.[3] But it cannot be the same sense in which an assertion is made that something is true and *un*scientific.

However, our concern is not with definitions of truth or knowledge in the first instance but only with the question of the status of psychoanalysis as a scientific theory. The difficulties which at present stand in the way of its acceptance, so far as I can see, are primarily intellectual. The Freudian conception of man no longer has any terrors for us. Human beings have become so case-hardened to shock and cruelty and celebration of the absurd in our century that they could hardly be more disturbed if all the reports of psychoanalysts about what they have dredged up from the depths of men's minds turned out to be true. In the case of critics like Dr. Eysenck, it seems unlikely that men who have no hesitation in accepting the findings of parapsychology as scientific, despite the fact that belief in the alleged phenomena of telekinesis challenges traditional physics, would have any compunctions in accepting the assertions of psychoanalysis if sufficient evidence could be adduced for them.

Logically, the question concerning the scientific status of psychoanalysis depends upon an answer to a prior question, viz., What makes any subject scientific? Fortunately, this prior question was not raised focally by any participant in the discussion. Had it been, the Conference might have bogged down trying to formulate the necessary and sufficient criteria of a scientific discipline—a very thorny problem on which no consensus has been reached by philosophers of science. The actual question was not so much one of characterization as it was one of classification or comparison. Is psychoanalysis more like meteorology, medicine, or agronomy, to which only a purist would deny the adjective "scientific," or is it more like phrenology, chiropractice or Christian Science? So far as I know nobody has ever denied scientific status to psychoanalysis on the ground that it is not like physics. For we would then have to rule out the whole of biology as a science, which would be absurd.

A subject is usually regarded as unscientific if in principle no observable state of affairs could falsify its claims, so that by *ad hoc* modifications its assertions can be made compatible with any state of affairs whatsoever. It was in order to pinpoint the discussion on the possibility of falsifying one of the central doctrines of psychoanalysis that I asked the psychoanalysts present to describe what kind of evidence they were prepared to accept which would lead them to declare in any specific case that a child did not have an Oedipus complex.

This question has a history. I have asked it innumerable times since I read Freud in 1919. The history of the answers I have received would make interesting reading. Three responses stand out in my memory. The first was from Dr. Ernst Kris, who, after some thought, replied that a child lacking an Oedipus complex would be one who acted like an idiot. This was hardly satisfactory because it was not clear whether the possession of the Oedipus complex was being taken as a criterion of normality or whether it was associated with its presence. At any rate there are different degrees and types of subnormal children, and what differentiates them from normal children seems much more general than the behavior frequently interpreted as part of the oedipal behavior pattern. The second response was made by Dr. Sandor Rado, who at first questioned the validity of the question but who after discussion manifested a genuine perplexity quite rare in the circumstances. The third memorable response, at a meeting of the Conference on Methods in Science and Philosophy at the New School in New York was made by a leading practitioner whom I will identify only by an initial—call him Dr. Z. It consisted in the charge that I was quite clearly a misogynist and in a histrionic denunciation of troublemakers who lure psychoanalysts into traveling long distances to meetings and then needle them with sophistical questions. Making up his facts as he went along, he asserted that psychoanalysts no longer used the term "complex" (this was in the early fifties), and therefore the question was meaningless. Although an extreme illustration, until recently this typified, I am sorry to say, the most frequent generic response to my question.

In asking this question I was *not* assuming that an Oedipus complex can be seen or touched or directly observed any more than intelligence can be seen or touched or directly observed. I was not even assuming that it was an observable. All I was asking for was the evidence on the basis of which one could legitimately deny its presence. This is not a tricky question but one often asked to specify the meaning of terms, the statements that contain them, and the conditions under which the statements are warranted. For example, we hear that someone is "intelligent" or "friendly." Many types of behavior can be cited as evidence for the presence of "intelligence" or "friendliness." But unless we are also told what we would have to observe to conclude that an individual is not intelligent or not friendly, the terms could be applied to anyone in all situations.

In asking this question I was making no assumption that its answer would be the citation of an atomic simple or an isolated feature independently of a gestalt, context, or systematic connection. The situation may be as complex as one in which we attribute to an individual the absence or presence of moral courage. A specific trait is rarely if ever decisive when we are describing a pattern. None the less, no one particular trait, in and of itself, can count as evidence for *both* the presence and absence of a particular pattern.

Finally, in asking the question I was not demanding that someone describe a crucial experimental test that would decisively confirm or refute the hypothesis that any particular individual had an Oedipus complex. This may be as unfeasible as a crucial experimental test of whether an individual is a true friend. Some tests, however, are more significant and reliable than others; and unless one can describe what would count as unfriendly behavior, even if he never lives to see it, one does not really understand the meaning of friendly behavior.

The Second Annual Meeting of the New York University Institute of Philosophy will always remain memorable to me because after waiting forty years I received something of an intelligible answer to my question. In the discussion Dr. Charles Brenner undertook to describe the behavior of a child who would show no signs of the presence of an Oedipus complex. And Dr. Arlow, in his contribution to the present volume, develops this reply a little more explicitly, making a distinction, unessential for our purposes, between "oedipal phase" and "oedipal complex," using the former expression to designate what is usually intended by the latter. Dr. Arlow's reply will repay close study. I content myself with just a few observations. He writes:

> Phenomenologically, the little boy who does not achieve the oedipal phase of development would express no tender or romantic feelings or fantasies regarding his mother. He would not express any wish to grow up and marry her, nor try to oust his father as the rival from the marriage bed. Manifestations of a wish to exhibit his penis to the mother, to press his penis against her, to have her admire and fondle his penis would not appear. . . . Such a child would hardly regard the other individuals in his environment as distinct entities or personalities.

> They would be important to him only in so far as they could grant immediate satisfaction of his bodily wants or needs. He would hardly refer to them, conjure up few images or memories concerning them. . . . Considerations of masculinity or femininity would be minimal. . . . We would anticipate in such a child impulsive emotionality and very meager identification with the standards, the ideals and behavior of his human environment. These are only a few features of the picture of a child who does not develop an oedipal phase, but sufficient features have been mentioned to indicate that the concept of an oedipal phase is not a procrustean bed into which analysts wish to force all the data of observation. The existence of an oedipal phase in the development of the young child is based upon definite, observable patterns of behavior, upon a concrete set of interpersonal relations and upon a host of other mental phenomena.

In this passage it is noteworthy that Dr. Arlow leaves it unclear whether the evidence of any one of these traits is sufficient to justify the inference that the oedipal phase of development has not been achieved, or whether all of these traits must be observed to warrant the inference. The reference to "a host of other mental phenomena" leaves open the possibility that even if all the traits enumerated above have been observed, which point to the absence of the oedipal phase, it may still be manifested if some of the "host of other mental phenomena" are present.

Secondly, Dr. Arlow seems to be explicating Dr. Kris's statement that a child without an Oedipus complex would be an idiot. Yet some children classified as idiotic exhibit some of the traits whose presence Dr. Arlow may regard as sufficient to indicate the achievement of the oedipal phase, for example genital play.

Thirdly, if one takes Dr. Arlow's description at its face value, I believe that an unprejudiced observation of the behavior of children who are not judged idiotic by reference to psychoanalytic criteria alone, will show that the oedipal phase is far from being universal. Many normal children do not manifest it. This would seriously invalidate one of Freud's central hypotheses. It would tend to indicate that the absence of the oedipal phase as well as variations in the extent, intensity, and mode of its expression are determined by social and cultural institutions. It suggests that the *significance* of the child's unlearned behavior depends upon the responsive reaction of adults and the institutional framework within which it is interpreted and channeled.

Fourthly, if we follow the lead of this last point, acute doubt arises as to whether Dr. Arlow's reading of infantile behavior is not already determined by his theoretical prepossessions. He is *not* giving a phenomenological description of children's behavior, properly bracketed off from causal imputation, but presupposes that the child's expression of "tender or romantic feelings" towards its mother contains a predominantly sexual component. There is a profound difference in the elements enumerated as evidence of the oedipal phase, between saying of the child that (a) he expresses tender and romantic feelings, (b) he expresses a wish to grow up and marry his mother, etc., and (c) he manifests a wish to exhibit his sexual organ, etc. At most (c) is a clear expression of a libidinal impulse; (b) may be a highly questionable reading of the child's language or a misinterpretation of attention-getting behavior when a habit pattern set up by the mother (or anyone in the same role) is disrupted; (a) may be a perfectly "innocent" imitative reaction to the behavior of the parent. Whatever significance may be found in a mother's caress, it is the sheerest dogmatism to read the same or similar significance in the returning caress of the child. As well argue from the almost reflex-smile with which the infant responds to a beaming countenance that it is committed to a principle of cosmic benevolence.

Fifthly, the same question-begging assumptions seem to me to be involved in the inferences Dr. Arlow makes concerning behavior which is allied to the absence of the oedipal phase of development. Why does it follow that a child who has not achieved the oedipal phase "would hardly regard the other individuals in his environment as distinct entities or personalities"? Because such a child is an idiot? This is much too broad a base for the inference; even objects may not be clearly distinguished by such a child, and persons are sometimes better distinguished than objects. Or is it the case that Dr. Arlow assumes that the differentiation in the child's environment is based primarily upon different sexual responses? But this is precisely what is in question.

As grateful as I am to Dr. Arlow for his patient attempt to reply to my query, I must confess that I still am not satisfied that I understand from his account in what circumstances the behavior of a nonidiotic child would be necessary and sufficient evidence that he had not achieved the oedipal phase of development. A further specification of the behavior pattern of such a child would go a long way towards resolving our methodological perplexities on this key point.

II

Since psychoanalysis does claim to function as a therapy, its clinical successes and failures seem to me to be highly relevant in evaluating the truth of its theories. If it has no clinical successes and if it is not confirmed by experimental findings, then it has no more scientific standing than any other consistent mythology. Since the experimental findings are unclear, it seems to me of the first importance, as difficult as it may be, to assess the clinical experiences of psychoanalysts. I am sorely puzzled that some psychoanalysts seem inclined to dismiss the question of therapeutic efficacy as an irrelevant intrusion into the evaluation of its truth claims. It is as if a meteorologist dismissed the significance of his daily weather predictions as irrelevant to his science. After all, medicine made great strides in developing scientific theories of disease through its clinical practices. One can distinguish between scientific and unscientific clinical approaches.

Unless psychoanalysis has better clinical or experimental successes than alternative theories, it can hardly aspire to scientific status. The difficulty is that even if it has these successes, this is not sufficient evidence for its validity. It must find ways of eliminating other hypotheses compatible with the same results. If, as a priest of some Mithraic cult, I give an ailing penitent mouldy bread and say a prayer over him, he may recover. If the recovery takes place several times when penitents are treated in this fashion, I am justified in continuing to use this technique. But the success of the treatment is not decisive with respect to the validity of the theory that prayer is efficacious unless I can deduce from my theoretical assumptions something specific not otherwise known, and not explicable by any other supposition.

That the clinical successes of psychoanalysis, however modest, may be explicable without assuming the validity of psychoanalytic theory is a point made with increasing frequency by students of scientific methodology today. This criticism was made long ago and sometimes by psychoanalysts themselves. After sixteen years of psychoanalytic practice, Dr. Trigant Burrow wrote:

> I have come to feel that what we have called analysis in the sense of our present personalistic system is just another application of the method of suggestion, and that with us analysts, as with others, the method involves a situation in which we are as truly the unconscious dupes of the suggestive process we employ as are the unconscious subjects upon whom we employ it.[4]

It is not surprising that Dr. Burrow holds this position in view of his contention that "the attitude of the psychoanalyst and the attitude of the authoritarian are inseparable." [5] I am not endorsing this judgment but merely reporting it as an illustration of the fact that therapeutic successes by an analyst may be accounted for in theoretical terms other than those of psychoanalysis.

I suspect that the humility of psychoanalysts about their therapeutic successes has been reinforced by recent claims of Dr. Eysenck and others that the proportion of recoveries or improvements among neurotics who have not received psychoanalytic treatment is as great as among those who have. Without denying that clinical results are usually more questionable than experimental laboratory findings, it seems to me that what is called for is not an apologetic attitude but a more systematic and critical one. And not alone for psychoanalysis. In a sense the Catholic church has been running a clinic at Lourdes.

Perhaps the whole history of the religious confessional can be considered a clinic prolonged over the centuries. There is a great deal to be learned from its checkered pattern of successes and failures provided we approach the record critically, not as devotees, and follow up the subsequent histories of those declared cured or improved after some exciting or dramatic experience. Titchener once vehemently denied that "the cure of sick souls" was a proper pursuit of scientific psychology. This piece of dogmatism seems to me no more warranted than the belief that "the cure of sick bodies" is not a proper pursuit of scientific biology or that "the cure of sick societies"—if we can give that phrase a meaning—is not a proper pursuit of scientific economics or sociology. It may not be *the* proper concern; it certainly is *a* proper concern. The distinction between pure and applied science, and all intelligent clinical practice is a species of applied science, is a vague and shifting one. Anything the scientists in a field concern themselves with in the course of their inquiries is *a* proper concern, especially if they make new discoveries and advance the frontiers of knowledge.

III

Many have been the attempts to offer psychological interpretations of philosophy. The only justified criticism of Professor Lazerowitz's psychoanalytical hypotheses about the relation between the philosopher's personality and his doctrine is that they are false. According to him, "it [psychoanalysis] alone can discover for us what they [the philosophers] really say, as against what they delusively appear to say." I find that I can as a rule understand what a philosopher says better than I can understand what a psychoanalyst tells me he is really saying. When I am in doubt as to what he is really saying, logical analysis is immensely more helpful than psychoanalysis. To be sure I find that taken literally some philosophers seem to be talking nonsense and that those who talk about the absolute seem to me to be talking absolute nonsense. In such cases, since I do not believe that human beings really get excited about nonsense, I try to find out what general problems or conflicts are involved in the maze of syntactical and categorial confusion. Usually I find that what is at issue is some cultural or social or political problem. And if for the term "real" we substitute the term "reliable" or "valuable," many expressions that are difficult to construe make sense.

The attempt to explain or classify philosophies by the temperament of philosophers is older than Freud. One recalls Nietzche and William James in this connection. There may be some correlation or even causal connection between temperament and philosophy, just as there may be some correlation or causal connection between the temperaments of scientists and their inclination to support corpuscular theories of light over wave theories. One would like to know what relevance such connections have wherever the questions of truth or validity or adequacy or predictability arise concerning the assertions made by a proponent of a scientific theory or philosophical doctrine. Someone observed at the Conference that the philosophers who believed in the scientific validity of Freudian theory were those who had been psychoanalyzed and who were striving to defend their not inconsiderable investment in their therapy. Whether true or false, surely this has no bearing on the evidence. Accepting determinism as a postulate, I am prepared to admit that there are causes for a man's belief in what is true just as there are causes for a man's belief in what is false. This does not invalidate the distinction between the true and false, whatever the proper analysis of such terms may be.

To the extent that philosophy is denied cognitive significance and assimilated to art, I find psychoanalysis no more illuminating when applied to the interpretation of great works of art than to the great systems of philosophy. The *explicans* is always more problematic than the *explicandum*.

All attempts to correlate or explain philosophical beliefs by psychological temperament and/or childhood experience seem to me to suffer shipwreck on two stubborn sets of facts. The first is that every system of philosophy has been fervently believed by individuals of the most diverse temperaments and psychological histories. This conclusion is reinforced by an historical study and psychological analysis of the master-disciple relationship in many fields. I doubt whether Jesus would have converted another Jesus or Freud another Freud. When a psychological lion and a psychological mouse both espouse the same doctrine, it is hardly illuminating to explain belief in the doctrine in terms of temperament. To be sure, lion and mouse will believe the same thing in different ways, they will perhaps interpret or see different things in the same formal doctrine, and they certainly will act as differently as lions and mice do when they live or die for their doctrines. All this means, however, is that they will do most things in different ways. It will not explain what they believe in common. And it is a set of common beliefs that defines a doctrine or philosophy.

The second set of facts is the evidence that many thinkers have profoundly changed their basic philosophical views in the course of their lifetime. A man like Bertrand Russell has boxed almost all points of the philosophical compass. John Dewey started philosophical life a convinced Hegelian. A. E. Taylor, who died in the odor of sanctity, began his intellectual career as a naturalist. Since they had only one childhood and since there is no evidence that their patterns of personality changed, psychology, and particularly psychoanalysis, seems as irrelevant to explaining any specific philosophical doctrine they hold as the milk they imbibed as infants.

Freud somewhere says that "before the problem of the creative artist, analysis must lay down its arms." It must lay down its arms, I believe, not because the mysteries of creation are necessarily beyond explanation, or outside the scope of material determination. It must lay down its arms because the monistic dogma of psychoanalysis is palpably inadequate to account not only for the varied achievements of creative artists and philosophers and scientists but also for the work of poetic mythologists like Freud himself.

Notes

1. *The Unconscious,* ed. E. S. Dummer (New York: 1928), p. 93.
2. *Uses and Abuses of Psychology* (Edinburgh: 1953), p. 241.
3. Cf. John Dewey, *Logic: The Theory of Inquiry* (New York: 1938), chap. 5, *passim.*
4. *The Social Basis of Consciousness* (New York: 1927), p. 3.
5. *Ibid,* p. xvii.

12.

Remarks on Dr. Kubie's Views

ADOLF GRÜNBAUM
Professor of Philosophy
Lehigh University

DR. KUBIE rejects as ill conceived the request of Professor Hook for a specification of at least some of the overt behavioral traits which psychoanalysts would be prepared to construe as evidence for the *absence* of an Oedipus complex. The reason he gives for this contention is that, in the nature of the case, the refutation of the existence of a *subconscious* state or process cannot legitimately be grounded on a criterion requiring evidence drawn from *overt* behavior.

Instead of exhibiting the credentials of psychoanalysis as a rational discipline, this view, if maintained, undermines whatever scientific status the hypothesis of the Oedipus complex might otherwise enjoy. For in rendering that hypothesis *proof against disproof* (ex post facto), Dr. Kubie's conception makes it *irrelevant* to the explanation of observable human behavior. It may be instructive to note that Dr. Kubie's argument has an exact analogue in the reasoning of those who espoused the existence of an absolute rest system which is, in principle, undetectable observationally, and who rejected the demand of the special theory of relativity for falsifiability on the basis of evidence. In the manner of Dr. Kubie's defense of the status of the thesis that all children have an Oedipus complex, the proponents of the absolute aether rest system sought to render their thesis proof against disproof by claiming that the failure of that rest system to become manifest through the "apparent" length and time determinations made in moving systems cannot reasonably be construed as a basis for denying its existence.*

* For details on the relevant issues in physics, see A. Grünbaum, "Logical and Philosophical Foundations of the Special Theory of Relativity," *American Journal of Physics XXIII* (1955), pp. 460–64.

13.

The Experimental Investigation of Psychoanalysis

MICHAEL SCRIVEN
Department of Philosophy
Swarthmore College

1. Introduction

"WE CAN SAY, without any lack of appreciation for what has been accomplished, that psychoanalysis has been prescientific. It has lacked experiments, having developed no technique for control. In the refinement of description without control, it is impossible to distinguish semantic specification from empirical fact." So writes E. G. Boring in his definitive history of psychology [1] and no judgment could be more objective. Psychoanalysis occupies a favored but dangerous position in our intellectual fortifications; we must sometimes regard it as the citadel of reason against the forces of superstition, while at other times it is a redoubt to be conquered in the name of science. It is becoming increasingly difficult to defend the first attitude except when looking at the past history of the warfare between science and religion. The sociological reasons for this are interesting, but I want to indicate here the main logical reason for the failure of psychoanalysis to retain its status as a great scientific achievement. As a set of hypotheses it was a great achievement fifty years ago; as no more than a set of hypotheses it is a great disgrace today. The logical reason is that experimental design in this area is difficult. It is far from being impossible, however, and we have the resources, the need, and the absolute moral obligation to execute such experiments before encouraging or condoning the further practice of psychoanalysis.

Notes to this section begin on page 251.

You may feel these are strong terms, but I beg you to examine the considerations I shall adduce before supposing that one can talk about the "inherent plausibility" or the "proven success" of psychoanalysis. It is in fact the most sophisticated form of metaphysics ever to enjoy support as a scientific theory.

The design I shall describe is, in its simplest form, an asymmetrical test of psychoanalysis; negative results count heavily against that theory, positive results count weakly if at all for it. But it can be elaborated in the directions indicated, to the point of becoming a symmetrical test. Our need to establish even the most elementary facts about psychoanalysis is so great that I have concentrated upon making clear the simpler and less contentious design.

The test is based on an important consequence of the fact that psychoanalysis is in part a therapeutic enterprise. Any therapist with scruples is committed to a certain probability statement whenever he accepts a patient (possibly after several diagnostic interviews). The statement is that the patient can probably be helped. There may be some cases where this is quite dubious and therapy is undertaken in the charitable belief that it offers the only hope, albeit a very slender one. This can hardly be the general rule, however, since psychoanalysts are quite willing to claim in retrospect that they have *substantially* helped *most* of their patients. It is very difficult to see how they could possibly justify the removal of some ten million dollars a year from sick America if this were not the case (800 now practicing, averaging at least $12,500 each).

It is therefore relevant to test their claim that they do effect some substantial improvement in most of their patients, by some kind of "before-and-after" study. If we find no such improvement we have evidence of a very weighty kind against psychoanalysis. Since it is a complex system of hypotheses, some of them may well continue to be true, the erroneous claim being due to others. But we shall require strong evidence for this view, and evidence is very much harder to get for the so-called dynamic or "process" hypotheses of psychoanalysis by comparison with the therapuetic-result or "outcome" hypotheses: if the latter turn out to be false we shall have little reason—though still perhaps some—to suppose that the former are well founded.

If we discover a substantial improvement in the patients who have undergone analysis, we have by no means shown that this is due to their treatment, let alone to those aspects of the analysis that spring from psychoanalytic theory—the transference, interpretations, etc. It may well be that they have recovered spontaneously, or because of some incidental feature of the therapeutic environment—perhaps the mere fact of being able to discuss personal problems with an interested and noncensorious listener, or, at a later stage, the need to terminate the heavy financial burden of analysis. Further refinements on the basic design are required to identify the particular factors which produce the cure. Nevertheless, even with the simplest design, we *can* find out whether psychoanalytic therapy, which involves many such factors, actually produces a significant improvement. This is a matter of extreme urgency, and one concerning which we are wholly ignorant. I repeat, *wholly* ignorant; for not only has no experiment of the kind to be described ever been done, but the design is of such minimal stringency that any weaker form, (and, a fortiori, any practitioner's individual "clinical experience") must be regarded as virtually irrelevant.

2. Relation to symposiasts' views

Let me conclude these introductory remarks by relating them to those of the symposiasts. It will be seen that I am not denying Hartmann's claim that the most important or the largest volume of evidence for psychoanalysis is to be found in the analytic sessions. This may be true, but it is quite certain that psychoanalysis is committed to certain claims which can be evaluated without the least consideration of the patient's conversation or behavior during therapy. I may add that one can, with a little ingenuity, extend the present design to deal with process hypotheses and protocol data; and that no other kind of design or observation *can* deal with such data. One may maintain one's faith in the libido theory or the dream theory until such experiments are performed. But it will be quite impossible to claim they have been scientifically established until that time.

I feel great sympathy with Nagel's position but think he is perhaps requiring a more direct kind of supporting evidence than it is fair to insist on. Kubie's remarks about the tragedy—for psychoanalysis—of the early therapeutic emphasis seem to me particularly poignant; the tragedy being not only that it diverted attention from process validation studies but that analysts undertook half a century of unvalidated therapy. It will be clear from my earlier remarks why I hold him plainly mistaken in regarding (therapy) outcome studies as an irrelevant or impractical approach to the investigation of psychoanalytic claims.

3. The general problem of testing causal claims

Experimental design is a creative enterprise in the sense that a design will support an interpretation of the results only in so far as the designer has been able to think up other-than-the-desired explanations of the results from weaker designs, and has built in appropriate safeguards. Hence, the design is only as good as the designer's capacity to create alternative theories about certain data. We want to know if psychoanalytic therapy "works," i.e., improves the condition of the neurotics (and some others) with whom its practitioners claim to succeed. Suppose we know several people who went to analysts and seemed to be better after treatment. Would this not constitute *some* evidence for the success of psychoanalytic therapy?

In the first place, it would *not,* because, as we have already mentioned, any of the incidental features of the therapy may be responsible, or the recovery may be spontaneous. It is a mistake to be too worried over the first of these possibilities: for we are certainly interested in answering the question whether *any* feature of the therapy is remedial. Still, it is of great importance, eventually, for us to identify the specifically useful factors. If only we could tell by studying the treatment very closely which factors were operative, we could achieve this more difficult goal;

yet in the treatment many factors are present and the ones that are effective do not wear any identifying label. The natural solution is to arrange a comparison between the original therapy, and treatment of a comparable patient by a slightly different method, involving only some of the same factors. If this other treatment is just as effective, the differentiating factors may be ignored. If not, we may suppose they are of some importance.[2]

It is possible, in very simple situations of science and everyday life, to tell which of a number of concurrent factors produces a certain result, e.g., the breakdown of an automobile, without doing a special comparison study. This is because we sometimes have previous knowledge of the independent causal efficacy of many of the factors present; e.g., we know that having gasoline in the carburetor is not in itself a cause of malfunction, that blown fuses do cause malfunction, etc. In dealing with psychoanalysis we cannot call on such evidence because it has never been established; hence we *must* turn to comparative studies.

4. The particular problem of testing claims of effectiveness

In fact, we must use comparative methods, not only in order to find out which factors are curative, but in order to find out whether the therapy works *at all.* For the difficulty of telling by inspection which factor works extends even to the problem of telling whether any of them works. Suppose we work on a stalled automobile for some time, changing the plugs and cleaning the points, etc. At last it starts. Did our activities produce the cure? Not necessarily, for it may have been due to the engine or the atmosphere's cooling off, thereby allowing a vapor lock or an expanded bearing to return to normal. Thus, even to establish the bare claim of curative efficacy for the therapy as a whole, we shall require *some* independent test of spontaneous recovery rate. We thus see it is central to a sound design to use control groups of at least one kind. It is wholly uninteresting for an analyst to claim 44 per cent or 70 per cent success unless he can also tell us how many of these people would have recovered to the same extent, given the same lapse of time, without treatment. It is perhaps worth mentioning that the few (and fairly unsatisfactory) studies made of spontaneous recovery give rates ranging from the 37 per cent of Laslow and Peters, to the 68 per cent (in *one* year) of Eysenck; and that the 44 per cent previously mentioned is the average improvement rate claimed for psychoanalysis in a survey of 24 articles. Claims about the curative effect of psychoanalysis are therefore entirely speculative until some figure for spontaneous recovery rate of comparable patients can be established. Even if psychoanalysis showed slightly better results on this score, there remain (a) the question whether the slight improvement would be worth the enormous extra cost, and (b) two further difficulties, each of them potentially sufficient to invalidate *any* conclusions from the first part of the experimental design: the question of the permanence of the cure, and the question of the justification of the term "cure." The first part of the design, however, consists in establishing a spontaneous recovery rate by study of an untreated control group—and, if we are interested in a more exhaustive study, the establishment of recovery rates for control groups undergoing various simplified forms of treatment.

5. The problem of selecting a control group

A great deal of fuss is always made over the problem of selecting a control group. It is largely unnecessary. Analysts rightly argue that even within a symptomatically identical group, dynamic differences may be enormous and the indicated treatment totally different. But we are not trying to match treatments, only symptoms; for we are mainly interested in the question, Can a psychoanalyst actually help a patient with such and such symptoms? And this is also what the patient is interested in, of course. It is perfectly legitimate for psychoanalysts to claim they cannot treat certain members of a group of patients all of whom appear essentially similar to a psychiatrist with no psychoanalytic training; so let us allow the psychoanalyst or psychoanalysts we are using as therapists for the experimental group to select those patients who appear curable to them, perhaps after several interviews. And then let us divide these patients up into two groups (or more, in the case of the extended experiment) either randomly, or first on the basis of their symptoms (and perhaps age, sex, beliefs about psychoanalysts, in the extended study) and then randomly within these subgroups. We shall furthermore keep a careful record of the proportion of the original group of patients that was rejected by the therapists as uncurable, and make some independent assessment of the proportion that psychoanalysts in private practice reject; for we would like to be able to say how likely it is that a sick person in the ordinary population, not just in the experimental group, will be (a) accepted for treatment and (b) cured by psychoanalysis, if accepted.

The answers to the first of these questions will help us to decide whether we should allot effort and funds to research on other methods of therapy for neurotics even if psychoanalysis is 100 per cent successful with the patients analysts select. There would still be some reasons for this, even if the analysts accepted all neurotics who come to them (as Ferenczi indicates he did), since the duration, expense, inconvenience, and frequent unpleasantness of analysis are not ideal. The precaution of a secondary survey to compare the behavior of the therapists while participating in this experiment with their behavior in ordinary practice, applies not only to selection procedures but at every stage. It does not indicate mere suspicion, but recognition of the difference in the kind of patients involved and the circumstances. In so far as we are concerned with the extended program, i.e., positive support for, or detailed refutation of psychoanalysis as commonly practiced, we shall certainly need these data, and of course we can get them if we take the trouble to use tape recorders and independent observers of the intake procedure in private practice, etc. We do not need them for the minimum design which is our primary concern here, except in so far as it is possible that the therapists will select and perform *less* well on test than in practice. There being no reason that their own offices cannot be used and the experimental patients mingled with their own, it would be somewhat surprising if this effect appeared. One reason that it *might* is important. The neurotics in the experimental group differ from their ordinary patients in one respect: they did not voluntarily select, though they do voluntarily participate in, psychoanalysis. It is quite possible that the acceptance—and cure—rates amongst the therapist's own patients are higher than among the group he is allotted in the proposed design. This group is selected either from the intake of a general hospital or in some other way, e.g., by the uniform application of certain criteria for "neuroticism," etc. (these are discussed below) to a selection from the population at large. Studies suggest that by comparison with the analyst's patients the experimental group will include a larger proportion of people from nonprofessional classes and lower economic groups, people with weaker verbal skills, less education, and less susceptibility to belief in Freudian doctrine. We may suspect that the most important relevant factor in the self-selection of patients for psychoanalysis is some belief that psychoanalysis is or may be correct or successful. But we are mainly interested in the possibility of psychoanalysis of people with certain symptoms regardless of their intellectual orientation, and analysts have not usually restricted their claims. However, it may be that our experiment would yield null results, whereas believers in the possibility of psychoanalytic therapy do receive some benefit. This would show up in a variation of acceptance rates if, and only if, the psychoanalyst recognizes the value of belief; and it would support a "faith healing" interpretation which substantially weakens the scientific claims. Such an interpretation is also testable, e.g., by comparison studies involving neurotic Catholics receiving "treatment" by their priests, etc. Even the basic design could be restricted to patients voluntarily applying for psychoanalysis, provided we face certain ethical difficulties. Our *control* group would also have to be individuals who wanted psychoanalytic therapy, and putting them in the control group would involve keeping them out of therapy for a long time. It is true that there are several analysts who have to turn away very many patients, and one might suppose a control group could be formed of these; but they are usually referred to, or discover, another therapist.

6. The notion of "spontaneous" recovery

Thus there arises a general problem that even applies to the standard control group, i.e., that selected from the neurotic population at large or from the neurotic intake of a large hospital (the important difference between these being that the latter have already identified themselves—or accepted their identification—as in need of help). For at least in the latter case members of the control group are going to seek other therapy rather than stay sick and do nothing about it for several years. Even if they do not seek other therapy as such they will do something that they would not otherwise have done, which will constitute a therapy-surrogate. Hence we shall not be comparing psychoanalysis with the *spontaneous* recovery rate, but with a conglomerate "therapy" of divorce—changing jobs—marrying—adopting religion—drinking, etc. Now this is not a very serious objection since we really are interested in the improvement psychoanalysis offers over self-help rather than sitting around; and it seems unfair to deny the control group its instinctual and possibly therapeutic responses to illness, in the cause of preserving spontaneity. In the social sciences, the best standard reference condition is often the uncontrolled one rather than the highly controlled one. Even in the automobile example, *spontaneous* recovery does not mean *uncaused* recovery.

Nevertheless, there is a way of improving the information yield of the design and at the same time solving the practical problem of keeping in touch with the control group, which we must do in order to judge its improvement. This can be done by arranging for the controls some standardized, regular, interviewing procedure which will probably be regarded by the patient as therapeutic. For example, the patient may be instructed to come in once a fortnight and may be dealt with, by someone deliberately chosen for extreme ignorance of psychoanalytic thought, in the following way. The interviewer will ask a series of rigidly standardized questions beginning always with an inquiry about progress over the preceding two weeks, proceeding via questions from a group about jobs, marital relations, etc. (selected antecedently to any interviews, as circumstantially appropriate to the individual patient) to a group of more specialized—but not individually "tailored"—questions about symptoms and attitudes, e.g., How are you sleeping? The question supply will be large enough so that a few different ones from the latter group will usually occur in each session; but the main object will be to encourage the patient to talk. A few anecdotes of an ambiguous kind may be provided for the interviewer to use in filling in awkward gaps, and as a stimulus for comment; or he may be instructed to terminate the interview when conversation runs dry. The same noninterpretative, nonsymptom-oriented procedures may be prescribed for dealing with requests for opinions and advice, e.g., the use of standardized remarks such as "Think over your previous experience before deciding." (Naturally such interviews must be monitored, or recorded for later monitoring, to avoid emergencies.) A generally sympathetic attitude will be encouraged in the interviewer, and fees will be charged (refundable later). Of course, this arrangement may well prove therapeutic by comparison with a less supervised group, and ideally we need both. And if psychoanalysis proves substantially better we shall be one step *nearer* supporting psychoanalytic *theory,* though still so far that I doubt one could even say one had raised the probability of that hypothesis appreciably. One should rather say that one possible disproof of part of it had failed. Now there is a risk inherent in using such a control-group arrangement; it may encourage dependence and discourage what are possibly more efficient self-help procedures. The only effect of such a possibility would be narrowing the gap between the results of psychoanalytic therapy and no therapy at all, assuming psychoanalysis shows up better than this control. But once more, the *absence* of a significant distinction would count heavily against psychoanalysis.

7. The choice of therapists

In an extended experiment, it would of course be well worth having a series of control groups along the spectrum of therapist methods; but the first necessity would be the use of other psychoanalysts to form several primary experimental groups, since it is not at all clear that even the self-called Freudians provide a more homogeneous kind of therapy than, e.g., a group formed of those therapists who charge more than $24 an hour. Some studies have indicated that a group of "good" therapists from a wide range of schools (chosen by peers' ratings) are more alike in their methods than are the therapists of any one school; others have indicated the contrary. Substantial conclusions would be made easier if several psychoanalysts participated; and it would be advisable to select those highly regarded by their peers. If these perform very differently, and some of them no better than the control, we shall have a consideration against the idea that peers' judgments (let alone laymen's) can identify good therapists. If they perform at the same level, and this is markedly different from the primary control's level, we shall begin to see grounds for supposing psychoanalysis does help therapy; although this could be reliably shown only by the use of other comparison groups.

There might profitably be the one previously suggested where a priest is allowed to select and treat patients of his or similar faiths. There might be one involving a completely new and wholly nonsensical system of therapy with elaborate trappings, vocabulary, ritual, and postural exercises; another by analysts (or analytically oriented therapists) involving highly accelerated treatment with a maximum of twelve sessions. The work done in this direction is already encouraging. Again, there could be some therapy along the lines Mowrer has suggested, in which strong "character-building" recommendations are inserted just as soon as they can be related to the patient's problems, perhaps in the first session. Each of these groups will contribute a little by elimination to deciding which factors are producing the improvement in psychoanalysis—if indeed any are. They also partially guard us against the possibility that some factors in psychoanalysis are beneficial but that others have a detrimental effect (e.g., the common Freudian attack on attempts at the abstract reasoning-out of a philosophy of life as "intellectualization," a form of resistance to therapy), the net result being zero. But I remind you that each of these further comparisons can well form an experiment in itself, and that we do not need them in order to ascertain something of the first importance: does psychoanalysis as practiced produce a worth-while improvement compared with either self-help or an opportunity to unburden problems to an untrained but neutral listener?

8. The duration of the effect

We may now pass to the second great *practical* difficulty for the design, leaving aside for the moment the great *conceptual* problem of defining and identifying "sick," "well," and "improved." In one sense the second difficulty is an aspect of the third; for one part of a worth-while definition of "cure" must be a reference to the *durability* of the cure. We should regard the claims of psychoanalysts with great suspicion if their "cures" were highly transitory, a sort of "propping up" of the character which rapidly collapses when the prop is withdrawn. It is the usual defense of psychoanalysis against other therapuetic approaches, especially short-term therapy, that other methods only "treat the symptoms," i.e., that only psychoanalysts can deal with the real underlying causes and thereby make the cure last. "Treating the symptoms" is said to result merely in "converting them" into other and perhaps more serious manifestations of disorder. Indeed, this may be so, but we have unfortunately no grounds for supposing that psychoanalysts, even given their great advantages in dealing with a self-selected clientele, from which they may themselves make further selection, and in curing which they may take several years, can succeed in producing more *temporary* cures at the end of that time than unskilled interviewing of the kind mentioned. The purpose of the *second* part of the design, however, is to establish something about the relative *permanence* of any improvements displayed in the groups being compared.

It is important to understand just how seriously handicapped the psychoanalyst is in trying to make some estimate of the permanence of his own "cures" (i.e., the patients who get well in the course of, and perhaps because of or in spite of, treatment by him). Suppose one of these patients has a relapse after termination of treatment. What will he do? It is quite likely he will *not* return to the therapist who has discharged him as cured, for at least two reasons. He has been treated by this therapist for a very long time at enormous expense without a permanent cure's being achieved, and he knows there are many other therapists and therapies available; perhaps it is time for a change. Second, there is always the embarrassment involved in confronting someone with proof of his failure when he thought he had succeeded; common enough to make most of us uneasy even about returning defective and guaranteed merchandise when doing so requires face-to-face discussion.

There is also very understandable possibility that some patients feign improvement in order to terminate, either through boredom or through desire to cease the payments. This connects with the alleged neurotic defense called the "flight into health" and will not be easy for an analyst to identify, lacking—as he usually does—direct evidence about improvement in home life, vocational problems, etc. It should by now be clear that the analyst is in an extraordinarily insecure position when he talks about permanent cures. What is required is a follow-up of the discharged patients extending at least over a length of time commensurate with that of the treatment, in order to pick up any cyclical changes in the individual's condition. For the patient may be a so-called "upswing terminator," i.e., a cyclically neurotic individual who enters treatment at or before the trough of the cycle and looks very good towards the next peak; all the analyst will see is a sick man coming in and a well man leaving. Certainly there should also be readily observable changes in his capacity to interpret his own actions and attitudes, but it is possible to claim that these are just *concomitants* of the improvement, and *consequences* of acquisition of the psychoanalytic approach and vocabulary, rather than *causes* or *symptoms* or *proof* of the "cure."

Follow-ups are notoriously difficult to arrange in practice, because the patient lacks motivation for keeping in contact. A financial incentive can be provided here by research funds or rebate of therapy fees; but we must take care not to accept the analysands' reports of their condition at their face value. (We shall discuss this judgmental problem in more detail under the next heading.) It must be faced from the start that a follow-up is not a frill but an expensive and exhausting part of the inquiry. The major interest of the follow-ups—which must naturally be performed on the control group as well—is, of course, to see whether any apparent gain by one group, in terms of patient's condition at termination of therapy, is offset or increased by subsequent developments. We need to see how a new and severe environmental stress, two years after termination, will affect the man who used once, but is no longer able, to talk it over with his analyst.

Among the difficulties which make the design a challenge to complete is the question of terminating the "pseudo-therapy" control groups. If they produce "cures" before the analytic group does, there is no problem. But an analyst will sometimes and rightly terminate an uncured case because progress is not being made. How long should the pseudo-therapist keep trying without improvement? As long as the average psychoanalyst? Until he has reached a total time equal to the average length of a psychoanalysis? The same probiem arises in determining the appropriate duration of a follow-up. But we can certainly reach a useful compromise here: apparently unsuccessful pseudo-therapy should—where possible—be continued as much longer than psychoanalysis as it can be before it has used up its advantages in terms of cost, convenience, pleasantness and hours-per-month, and its follow-up should continue for a comparable period. The fact that this difficulty does not arise for a nontherapy control is an advantage for its use.

9. The nature of the effect

The moment has now come to deal with the great conceptual problem of the design. What is a cure? And what are its correlative notions of "the goals of therapy," neuroticism, and improvement? (A definition of any one will readily yield a [pretty complete] definition of any other.) One of the favorite moves of the psychoanalyst dealing with this question is to argue that only a psychoanalyst is really able to judge a cure. It should not be supposed that such a claim is a priori unscientific. It is perfectly correct to argue that only a radiologist can judge whether an X-ray shows tubercular indications, and the reply that we have an independent check via autopsy or surgery is rather too simple, since tubercular indications are not said to be *infallible* indicators of tuberculosis. But there must be some connection, even if only a *statistical* one, between the signs and the *independently* testable reality. Similarly, we may concede the need of expert advice in making reliable judgments of cure, but we can identify the experts only on the basis of their success in doing some related task that we *can* independently judge. This is not a result of any limitation on their skill, but a required property of any skill, such as the one they claim; we know very well what we want done in *general* terms and we know how to identify experts at doing it. We may then be willing to accept in some cases the experts' refinements on our rough categories, just as long as their *overall* success improves and they meet the usual test-retest reliability criteria (or interjudge reliability, if claims of a scientific kind are involved).

To listen to the analysts one would suppose they have little agreement about the goals of therapy, i.e., the definition of a cure. Balint has given a good survey in his 1934 paper (reprinted many times, most recently in Clara Thompson's anthology *An Outline of Psychoanalysis,* Random House, 1955, under the title "The Final Goal of Psycho-Analytic Treatment"). There is Freud's triple definition: making the unconscious conscious, removing infantile amnesia, overcoming the resistances. There are the more emotionally and less structurally centered definitions referring to the abreacting of the strangulated affects (ah! that marvelously rich and suggestive vocabulary). There we range from Rank's desire to see the birth trauma abreacted to Reich's attainment of orgastic potency, with Kovács' mention of the desirability of unwinding the repetition factor providing a semi-structural criterion. To top it all, Balint rejects the lot in favor of the achievement of the capacity to love (which to our ears today sounds very schizophrenic-based). Now, in face of these diverse suggestions, how can we ever test *the* process of psychoanalysis? We shall always be dealing with a minority's view, and the majority may well be immune from our carefully established criticisms or support.

As I have tried to emphasize throughout this discussion, it is important to keep a firm grasp of the problem with which we begin and refuse to be talked into supposing it does not exist. The possibilities of inconclusive results are legion, and a crucial experiment does not exist; but a good design will make it as likely as possible that the results will increase our knowledge *substantially,* and *ensure* that our knowledge will at least advance by the exclusion of one possible and interesting result, together with its associated family of hypotheses. In the present case, our primary problem was whether a psychoanalyst can help a neurotic. If we remember to look at this from the patient's point of view, we see that a null result with an analyst or two selected as good by their peers means there isn't any reliable way for him to get help from psychoanalysis. He would probably have difficulty getting treatment from the "top" analysts anyway, outside the experiment, but if *they* can't do anything, to whom should he turn? The *possible* existence of others who can do better is no more interesting than the possible existence of a religious sect which might cure him if he adopted its faith and contributed to its coffers. In an important sense, i.e., in so far as it is, as practiced, scientific, psychoanalysis is correctly judged by the performance of those *it* regards as skillful.

But would there be any agreement among psychoanalysts about such a selection? In my experience the answer is yes (which suggests that the apparent differences in outcome goals may not have—at least, are not *believed* to have—very much practical effect). But it matters very little whether there is such agreement or not. For its absence merely shows the absence of any known objective criterion for judging "skill" even amongst the allegedly "skilled," or possibly the absence of any capacity for the employment of such a criterion.

Either alternative constitutes a severe indictment; and it will be necessary for us only to make a random selection *among those therapists not judged incompetent by their peers* in order to duplicate the experience of the best-informed patient in search of analysis. Indeed we may thereby miss the "good" analyst, but this is no more a criticism of the design than is the fact that it does not investigate the Rosicrucians. For our main problem is whether there is a set of *teachable, identifiable* skills that are of some value; and a null result will certainly show this to be false. Naturally, in the absence of a consensus about professional skill, even more than in its presence, it will be an improvement in the design to use as many therapists as possible. And in making judgments of what constitutes a cure, it will be worth using and testing several alternative ones to discover whether they actually yield a difference in practice. But in judging how serious these qualifications are it is important to see that (a) even if we cannot, for practical reasons, cope with more than one or two analysts, we shall be able to draw some important conclusions of the kind mentioned, provided we select our analysts as indicated; (b) most of the apparent differences over the aims of therapy are wholly irrelevant for reasons to be discussed in detail below; and (c) it is of course *possible* that every proposition Freud formulated was correct (except in so far as it contradicted some other propositions he formulated), and yet no practicing analyst is achieving any therapeutic success; but we may certainly conclude that psychoanalytic theory *as now understood* is faulty if it has neither reorganized nor explained this very striking refutation of its own claims. Indeed the situation envisaged is really impossible, for Freud certainly claimed cures, and there would be no reason to suppose he actually brought them about if current psychoanalysts are incapable of doing so; hence, *some* of his own claims would have to be judged false. In reply to the more reasonable suggestion that ego psychology or dream theory may be valid though the therapy inefficacious, we must point out that they are based on even less substantial evidence than the therapy and indeed originated as part of a theory to explain alleged therapeutic success. The reason that disagreement over the goals of therapy amongst the psychoanalysts is of negligible importance for our design is readily stated. We are mainly interested in therapy for people who are very plainly sick, and successful therapy will consist in getting them to the stage where they are no longer plainly sick, and where they can maintain this improvement. If there is much room for debate whether therapy is still required we may reasonably feel that the case is not one for serious concern; and certainly the psychoanalytic claim of successful therapy applies in the cases of severe sickness too. Thus we may legitimately, as well as sensibly, confine our study to that group. Lest this sound naive about the difficulties of identifying unsound mental conditions, let me indicate in more detail the criteria I regard as adequate (and necessary) for identifying the "very plainly sick." The patient's report must be given heavy weighting. If he feels fine, we shall probably have to scratch him from the class of candidates for a psychoanalyst's treatment, because he will not be accepted by them without a desire for treatment: of course, he may nevertheless be as sick as a happy psychopath can be, but we must look elsewhere when we are considering claims of successful treatment. However, the old observation that Freud never recognized the psychopath as a clinical entity because he lacked data from independent observers, sounds a warning for us in dealing with neurotics. The pseudo-neurotic malingerer, the hypochondriacal symptom-fantasier, the "flight into health," can be reliably identified only with the assistance of observations by the family, workmates, supervisor, neighbors, offspring's schoolteacher, etc. Patients are *not* sick just because they say they are or display anxiety; they may be lying for good reasons or genuinely misinformed about sex mores or philosophically puzzled. An objective judgment requires a skilled and probably repeated medical inspection, a cross-checked report by a social worker on interviews with the environmental neighbors mentioned; and of course the individual's own reports interpreted by some one or several people. The arguments are mainly about the last problem—evaluation of interview material. The simple and important way to deal with them is to say this: if someone can't convince *one* of two or three independently evaluating but nonanalytically-trained general practitioners that he is seriously ill, don't accept him. If he can, run the background check and see if he is manifesting signs of malfunction, incapacity to relate, loss of character, etc., in his normal environment. If he passes this, he's sick. If not, put him in a group to be re-examined at intervals to see whether the cut-off level is being set too high on either of the tests mentioned. To pick the cut-off level on the second test, use a panel of patient-intake interviewers from hospitals with a shortage of therapists. One could add a condition that at least 25 per cent of the original group be rejected, to further narrow the field towards serious neuroses. Also run a battery of tests like the Multiphasic, the self-describing Q-sort, and the discomfort quotient, and validate a regression formula based on them using the other data as criterion, eventually giving this formula equal weight, if it earns it on the usual test-evaluating standards. Now we have something like a thorough procedure for picking the sick, and it must be thorough because we have to apply it to the much tougher problem of picking the unsick at the end. It is extremely important to realize from the very beginning of a study like the one I am proposing here that no one part is "the main part." The therapy sessions, in the present design, even though there are several years of them, are probably going to cost less and take less time to operate than either the controls or the follow-up, and quite likely less than the evaluation procedures. But no part is of the least use without the other parts; there are no concessions to "conventionally accepted standards" of evidence or the "statistical approach" here. No justification of the claim we are considering can be given *at all* except in so far as each part of the design is implemented. I do not mean that the *details* I have mentioned are immune to improvement; I mean that *some* detailed treatment of *each* of the three sections is required. It might be supposed that we could dispense with all these environmental investigations of the patient's condition at the termination of therapy if he gave a clear statement of improvement. Maybe we would miss a few cases of liars, "flight into health," bored dilettantes, etc., but at least we would know how many people who begin by feeling sick finish up well enough to say they are not sick. This is a feeble reply; what if their behavior at home is now intolerable, their work relations are reaching a crisis and their insomnia is increasing? They may have a number of reasons for saying *to the analyst* that all is well, and they may have acquired enough sophistication to convince him of it, but they are of little interest to the searcher for therapeutic *assistance*. Now, just how many of these cases are there? A silence greets us; the journals' pages are blank. We have no idea. There is a more serious trouble, however. What of the patients who genuinely feel they are better at the end of three years, who show great "insight" into their symptoms and an apparent lack of anxiety about them; but *still have them,* e.g., impotence, masochistic involvements, homosexuality, or masturbation? They can hardly be regarded as "cured" in the *desired* sense. My experience includes more of these than of the first kind, enough at least so that I know we must discover how many there are before we can accept the patient's report on anxiety level as of central significance. We have some indications, from studies such as that of Kogan Hunt and Bartelme, that even the best-looking criteria for cure fail to correlate in practice. In their case it was: patient's report, experienced neutral judgment of patient's condition, and the Discomfort Relief Quotient (a reasonably valid questionnaire). Thus, our general suspicions find substantial support in so far as they have been investigated.

The fact of a cure is thus impossible to pin down using only one indicator; but by employing multiple criteria we shall at least be able to locate a number of clear-cut cases, and our study can rely on them and not insist on decisions where substantial conflicts of criteria exist. Underlying the debates that arise over conflict cases, however, is a pervasive conceptual difficulty we cannot wholly ignore. Whereas we can regard something like the excoriation syndrome, or sudden loss of the capacity to love one's children and friends, as a virtually indisputable indicator of neurosis, what are we to say of suicidal attempts by a Jewish boy rendered desperately unhappy by the rejection and persecution of his anti-Semitic fellow students, or a similar attempt by a Japanese man shamed by his failure to find husbands for his sisters? What are we to say of the adoption of religious beliefs? Of homosexuality? The real issues here are not trivial; even though we can certainly test psychoanalysis on the basis of cases which are much more clear-cut, and we can be sure that its failure there would represent a serious defeat for it, we must at some stage in the development of scientific therapy make decisions about the difficult cases such as these. The psychoanalysts, of course, are themselves divided on these issues, Rado from Jung, Bergler from Klein, on issue after issue. The answer—and the explanation of the divergence of beliefs—lies in the realms of philosophy and the empirical study of human needs and values, and neither is very conspicuous in the training of a psychoanalyst today. They have no skill in discussing the "problem of evil" or the basis of a deontic ethic, none in the calculation of a correlation coefficient. For solving problems that involve estimates of the *value* of life, religion, and heterosexual interests they are severely handicapped (as their output on these subjects indicates), although perhaps able to make important piecemeal contributions.

I am arguing that one of the problems with a general definition of cure is its essential involvement with moral questions; and with questions of the relative value of, e.g., a creative-nonconformist-anxious pattern of life compared with a noncreative-conformist-nonanxious pattern; and with genetic and empirical questions of an unsettled and nonmedical kind, in short with problems for which psychoanalysis cannot possibly have the right answer since it lacks the data, even if it had *one* answer to offer. There are serious enough practical problems in judging cases apart from these, to which I shall turn in a moment, but these are the ineffable philosophical-empirical barriers which can be scaled only by hard work in the appropriate field, no longer by the amateur. These problems alone give a philosopher the right to work in and a duty to watch the field.

Using the plainly sick, plainly well groups alone, and using control groups and follow-ups, there are still interesting problems of evaluation. Suppose the psychoanalytic group looks better at termination than the control, but a year later is indistinguishable. Have we shown psychoanalysis to be a worthless endeavor? Not necessarily; it depends on how much value the patient places on those months of relative superiority. The use of electric shock on manic-depressives in the depressive phase yields similar results; a short-term gain but no long-term change. Yet in that case a worth-while treatment is established, because it is cheap and short, has quick results, and can be painless. The problem would be less easily settled in the case of psychoanalysis.

Another problem: how and by whom are the criteria for cure (or improvement) to be applied? The difficulty is that using psychoanalysts to judge improvement introduces (if psychoanalytic theory is correct) a potential unconscious bias; not using them represents something of a bias in the other direction. The latter point is not a serious objection in one sense; for the patient and his wife, doctor, boss, etc., are not psychoanalysts, and if they cannot agree on any improvement, psychoanalysis is in bad shape. Yet it might become important in an extended or process study, especially if doctors *antagonistic* to psychoanalysis were used. In many such cases, where potential bias is involved, the standard methodological device is the use of "uncontaminated" judges. We can use analysts or antianalysts, as long as we do not inform them whether they are judging members of the control group or of the experimental group.

Furthermore, we can sometimes profit by throwing a few highly normal people, picked from the better-adjusted staff, faculty or alumni, into the hopper. In this way we may see whether an interpretation of "neurotic" is being employed that includes virtually everyone. Suppose this is so at the pretherapy evaluation. We have an awkward problem on our hands. If the judges know their second rating is posttherapy (and for rating "improvement" as opposed to "well," they have to know this) then *this fact alone* may make them rate more leniently, i.e., look harder for "signs of improvement" (or for the reverse), manifesting a pro-therapy (or antitherapy) attitude. How can we distinguish this bias from a genuine improvement in the patients? Because this bias will also operate in judging the control group, it will not give a false impression of psychoanalytic superiority, as does the "contamination" bias, but it will give a false impression of improvement in *both* groups.

The introduction of a batch of subjects consistently judged normal by other judges, in the posttherapy (as well as the pre-therapy) evaluation groups, will tell us the answer; for we can compare the number of actually normal people rated neurotic by the judge at the beginning with the number he rates neurotic at the end, and correct his other ratings for this "bias-line drift." We can in fact use the same normals at beginning and end, and in rating "improvement" this will be necessary in order to avoid any detection by the judge of the introduction of new patients. However, this device has its deficiencies which render preferable the use of validated written tests and separate panels of judges or strongly restricted interviewing methods at each end. For the normals will not be able to recount details of their neurotic symptoms and thus be identified. If they are restricted to yes-no answers or the judges are restricted to requests for descriptions of specific behavioral patterns (Do you sleep well? Do you find the children trying most of the time?), then we can do better with a questionnaire. This may be excellent; even though many of the same problems are involved in validating any inferences from it, these can be conquered piecemeal. Another move would be to use as normals, nonneurotic patients from the allergy, dietetic and rehabilitative wards of the hospital; they would have some symptoms to discuss.

Even the basic idea of the uncontaminated judges suffers from a similar problem here: for the experimental group which has undergone psychoanalysis will unfortunately carry some of the trademarks of that treatment in the form of the Freudian vocabulary, ease in discussing symptoms, etc., which will provide a foundation for unconscious prejudice in their favor or against them. Indeed, it *is* a kind of progress that the patient has "learned to live with" his symptoms, but it is hardly as good as an improvement in the unpleasant symptoms. The moral of all this is that, apart from the conceptual problems of the concepts of "cure," "improvement," etc., there are great practical difficulties in arranging for these concepts to be applied objectively. One sees once more the attraction of such definitions as "the approach of the patient's self-concept to his ideal concept" which we can get by statistical analysis of a forced Q-sort (i.e., an ordering of a list of traits into a preassigned number of groups with a preassigned number of traits in each group). But this is just one more subjective rating by the patient, and its merits within that category do not get it out of the category.

Once more, we must make an effort to retain our sense of direction. These are difficulties, not primarily for us in testing psychoanalysis but for psychoanalysis in justifying its claims; for the testing comes after the claims are made. Without any attempt to deal with the difficulties mentioned, how in the name of Roger Bacon could a psychoanalyst imagine that his own hopelessly contaminated, uncontrolled, unfollowed-up, unvalidated, unformalized estimation of success has ever established a single cure as being his own work? At least the people who claim that the earth is flat are giving a *nearly correct* account of a *large part* of their experience.

But we may say this. Just in so far as an objective test of improvement is possible—and the use of the most neutral judges we can discover by general study of their views, behavior and research, plus the precautionary procedures and background investigations mentioned, provides a very plausible approximation—so far we can check on this claim of psychoanalysis and so far as we can not in this way verify their therapeutic claims, so far we must be clear that there is no reason at all to believe in them.

10. Acknowledgement and Postscript

My debt to Paul Meehl's writing and conversation is apparent in every paragraph of this paper and in very nearly every line, although my conclusions are perhaps rather more sceptical than his own. He has commented on these topics particularly in the Psychotherapy article in *Annual Review of Psychology, 1955;* in *Clinical vs. Statistical Prediction* (Minneapolis: University of Minnesota Press, 1954); and in "Construct Validity in Psychological Tests," reprinted in *Minnesota Studies in the Philosophy of Science,* Volume 1, *The Foundations of Science and the Concepts of Psychology and Psychoanalysis* (FSCPP), ed. Feigl and Scriven (University of Minnesota Press, 1956).

It is of the greatest importance not to read this paper as an attack on psychoanalytic *hypotheses as such.* I myself believe the dream theory and the theory of the defense mechanisms (to give only two instances) to be brilliant conceptions. They have the loose texture and possibly excessive fertility of many embryonic scientific theories, but I have elsewhere argued forcefully for their methodological legitimacy *as hypotheses* (in FSCPP). I think it probable that they embody genuine insights. But that is only a bet, and without studies of the kind illustrated here they cannot possibly be regarded as established. However, there are some reasons for supposing that the experience of psychoanalysts is a better basis for those hypotheses than for outcome hypotheses. The therapeutic claim of psychoanalysis, i.e., the claim that psychoanalytic therapy has some specific advantages due to the truth of psychoanalytic theory, is more easily dealt with experimentally, and it will be seen from the design that *it* can hardly be said to have been founded on the only kind of experience that can support it.

Notes

1. *A History of Experimental Psychology* (2nd ed.; New York: Appleton Century, 1950), p. 713.

2. Not absolutely, but relatively to the set of common factors. An exhaustive study would require a comparison of the results just mentioned with those from a study (or preferably, studies) using a different "basic therapy," i.e., set of factors common to both groups, but the same differentiating factors.

14.

Psychoanalytic Theory and Evidence

WESLEY C. SALMON
Assistant Professor of Philosophy
Brown University

THE distinction between considerations which are in a broad sense logical and those which are empirical is a fundamental one for the philosophy of science; indeed, this distinction constitutes the basis for differentiating philosophy from the empirical sciences. It is the business of the philosopher of science to investigate and explicate the logical criteria a scientific theory must satisfy and, in cooperation with the empirical scientist, to determine whether a particular theory does satisfy them. Failure to meet these logical criteria would be an insuperable objection against any scientific theory. If it satisfies the logical criteria it must still pass the test of empirical confirmation. The logical criteria are within the domain of philosophy, but the actual empirical confirmation is not. The collection, evaluation, and interpretation of the evidence is strictly the business of the empirical scientist.

It is not the aim of the present essay to formulate and discuss the general philosophical principles which are applicable to all of the empirical sciences. Rather, the attempt will be made to apply some of the more familiar and relatively noncontroversial principles specifically to parts of psychoanalytic theory.[1] The general area of investigation will be the logical relations between observational evidence and hypothesis or theory. No attempt will be made to deal comprehensively with the nature of the evidence which supports psychoanalytic theory as a whole. The

Notes to this section begin on page 266.

discussion will take up some restricted but important issues concerning the confirmability of psychoanalytic theories and hypotheses.

I

Freud and his followers have repeatedly emphasized the fundamental role of a principle of determinism in psychoanalytic theory.[2] Since the concept of determinism has had a long and varied philosophical history, it may be useful to distinguish several of the more important philosophical doctrines of determinism, indicate the roles these doctrines have been intended to fulfill, and show how the psychoanalytic principle differs from them in content and function.[3] I hope to show that the philosophical interpretations of determinism are inappropriate to psychoanalytic theory, and I hope to present a formulation which will be appropriate. In reformulating the psychoanalytic principle I am not attempting to state what Freud or any other psychoanalytic theorist had in mind when he referred to a principle of determinism.[4] I shall be attempting to state with reasonable precision a principle which will have the theoretical import required by psychoanalytic theory. This formulation bears directly upon the problem of evidence, the subject of this essay as a whole.

(1) Philosophers have often taken determinism as an a priori principle. Some of these philosophers have used the principle to circumvent the Humean problem of the justification of induction. To avoid the circularity of using inductive reasoning to establish a principle which would serve to justify induction, the principle of determinism has been regarded as a priori. In psychoanalytic theory there is no problem of the justification of induction; like any other empirical science, it makes use of inductive methods without involvement in the problem of their justification. The problem of induction is a problem in the philosophy of science, and one that should in my opinion be taken seriously, but it is not a problem in any one of the empirical sciences. Hence, no

empirical science need include a special a priori principle to secure for itself a justification of the inductive method.

If the principle of determinism were a priori, either it would be a synthetic a priori metaphysical presupposition of science[5] or it would be an analytic a priori truth of logic. It has been argued effectively by many authors that neither science in general nor any particular science has need of metaphysical presuppositions.[6] On the other hand, if the principle of determinism were a truth of logic it would be tautological and therefore empirically empty. In neither case would it be required as a basic principle within the empirical discipline of psychoanalytic theory; it could be deleted from the theory without affecting the empirical content of the theory in any way.

In psychoanalytic theory the principle of determinism is a posteriori. In Freud's work it is supported by a large body of empirical evidence taken, for example, from the investigation of slips of the tongue or pen, dreams, and neurotic symptoms. Whether or not this evidence can be regarded as conclusive, it is the kind of evidence upon which the principle rests.

(2) The philosophical doctrine of determinism has often been stated in a very general way which may be rendered somewhat inaccurately as "Every event has a cause." Apart from the fact that determinism in the inanimate world is irrelevant to psychoanalytic theory, there are two important reasons why this sort of formulation misses the psychoanalytic principle. First, it need not be taken as a basic postulate of an empirical science that every event in the range of the subject matter of that science be subject to causal determination and explanation. Even if we adopt the dubious assumption that it is the business of science to discover causal relations, we do not need to postulate beforehand that such relations exist. The most we need is a regulative principle that the discovery of such relations is important to the scientific discipline in question—that it is worth while hunting for such relations. A regulative principle would be a directive for the conduct of science, not part of the content of a particular science. Whether such relations exist need not be decided beforehand; it may be left to the investigators to see whether they can

be found. There is nothing logically peculiar in looking for something even though we cannot be given iron-bound assurance that it exists. We merely need to know that it would be worth finding if it did exist. Of course, we would not undertake the search if we knew ahead of time that the object did not exist. But we are certainly justified in the search if we simply do not know whether it exists or not. Furthermore, even if it were not true that every event is subject to complete causal determination, it might still be true that some very interesting causal relations exist. The investigation of these relations would unquestionably form an appropriate part of a scientific discipline.

Second, psychoanalytic theory is not content merely with the statement that certain events, such as slips of the tongue, have some cause or other. For psychoanalysis it is important that these causes be psychic causes. If such events were completely determined by physiological causes, this would not be sufficient for psychoanalytic theory. Psychoanalytic theory holds that such events as slips, dreams, and neurotic symptoms have as their causes such occurrences as conscious or unconscious impulses, wishes, desires, etc.[7] This point will be discussed more thoroughly below; here it is sufficient to point out that the psychoanalytic principle specifies the *kinds* of causes involved whereas a philosophical principle would not.

(3) The philosophical doctrine of determinism has often been related to ethical issues, and often in conflicting ways. It has sometimes been argued that determinism excludes freedom and moral responsibility; at other times it has been held that determinism is a necessary condition of freedom and moral responsibility. Philosophical disputes of this sort are perennial; there is no need to enter upon them here.[8] We need only remark that such ethical issues are irrelevant to the methodology and empirical content of psychoanalytic theory. We cannot countenance the acceptance or rejection of a fundamental principle of an empirical theory on grounds of alleged desirable or undesirable ethical consequences.

(4) In philosophy of science the controversy over determinism has often been a controversy over the kinds of laws

that are fundamental in science. Those who reject determinism hold that statistical laws are fundamental and that events are determined probabilistically. At least, the opponent of determinism holds we have no good ground for asserting that deterministic laws must be fundamental and that all probabilistic relations must be explainable in terms of deterministic ones. The determinist, on the other hand, maintains that all events are governed by unexceptionable and nonstatistical laws. We may use statistical laws because it would be impractical to trace out all the causal determinants of some events or because of our ignorance of some of the causal laws, but the determinist maintains that complete causal determination obtains in the real world nevertheless.

The issue of determinism is widely discussed in the philosophy of quantum mechanics, but it is doubtful that psychoanalytic theory needs to make a commitment on this sort of issue. It is one thing to deny that certain events are completely haphazard and unrelated to previous events. It is quite another to claim that events of a certain kind are related to their predecessors by deterministic laws. It is a distinct possibility that there are stable probability relations between events and their predecessors in which the degree of probability is sometimes high. There would hardly be grounds for complaint if psychoanalytic theories could be shown to be well-confirmed statements of probabilistic relations which would enable us to explain any event as following from certain predecessors with a high degree of probability. In such a case we would have every right to deny that events such as slips, dreams, and neurotic symptoms are haphazard and meaningless, and this is what the psychoanalytic principle of determinism is concerned to deny.

The foregoing discussion has not been intended as an exhaustive survey of philosophical principles, doctrines, or controversies; it has been intended to show that these are quite irrelevant to the psychoanalytic principle of determinism. We might characterize the psychoanalytic principle provisionally in the following way: it is an empirical postulate subject to confirmation or disconfirmation by empirical evidence; it asserts the existence of definite relations among events; but the relation may be either deterministic or probabilistic; and it specifies that the "causes" involved are of a rather specific sort. Perhaps it is misleading even to call a principle that fits this description a "principle of determinism"; however, the usage is so well established it would be futile to recommend a change at this point. It is better to emphasize the difference between philosophical determinism and psychoanalytic determinism and hope that confusion will be minimized. It is probably advisable always to speak of psychic determinism when the latter principle is involved.

There is a good deal to be done before we can state the principle of psychic determinism in a satisfactory form. It is not sufficient to say that all psychic events have psychic causes, even if we understand the statement probabilistically. In many cases, at least, when we apply the principle of psychic determinism, only the determinants are psychic while the event which is probabilistically determined is an event of behavior—a movement of the body, for example. On the other hand, we do not wish to say that every event of human behavior has psychic determinants; blushing has, but flushing often has not. Nor will it do to say merely that voluntary behavior has psychic determinants. In the ordinary sense of "voluntary," such behavior as a nervous tic is not considered voluntary, yet we would hold that it has psychic determinants. Rather, what we want to say is that the organism's responses to stimuli fall into two classes; first, responses which are mediated only by constitutional mechanisms, i.e., mechanisms which cannot be modified by stimuli (except perhaps of a physically traumatic sort), and second, responses which are not thus mediated by constitutional mechanisms. Psychoanalytic theory says that there are psychic mechanisms in such cases, whether or not there are neurophysiological mechanisms. Roughly, if there are neurophysiological mechanisms, they can be modified by experience.

Stimuli and responses are publicly observable phenomena.[9] In addition, there may be certain privately observable psychic phenomena such as conscious wishes, feelings, and emotions; this is a matter of controversy with which we need not become involved here. However, on any theory whatsoever, unconscious psychic phenomena are not directly observable by anyone, subject or other observer. They are inferred entities or events.

If we begin by thinking of the organism as a container whose surface and environment we can observe but whose interior cannot be directly observed, then our problem can be regarded as that of understanding the output of the organism.[10] It becomes obvious that the output is conditioned by the input; there is a relationship between stimulus and response. In some cases the relationship is constant—a certain type of stimulus is followed by a certain type of response with a high degree of probability, unless a definite physical pathology can be discovered. In such cases we have simple reflexes and the like—stimulus and response are mediated by a constitutional mechanism. Perhaps it is possible to give a completely physiological explanation of this mechanism; whether it is or not is beside the point here. In other cases a psychic mechanism can readily be found; at least, the organism can report the existence of such a mechanism which he claims is an object of his immediate awareness. "He called me a fool, and this made me angry so I left the room." Conscious anger is the mechanism according to this report. It may be desirable to investigate this mechanism further, since being called a fool does not always lead to conscious anger, and conscious anger under these circumstances does not always lead to leaving the room, but at least we have a good start toward an understanding of the behavior when we realize that conscious anger occurred. When behavior occurs which is not the result of a stimulus setting off a constitutional mechanism and which cannot be explained in terms of a psychic mechanism which the subject can report, then, according to the principle of psychic determinism, there is an unconscious psychic mechanism which causes the behavior in question. The existence of this unconscious psychic mechanism cannot be established by direct observation (including introspection); it can only be inferred on the basis of indirect evidence. In order for the principle of psychic determinism to be empirically meaningful, then, it is necessary that there be independent evidence for the existence of this psychic mechanism, apart from the specific item of behavior it is supposed to explain. If no such independent evidence were possible, then the assertion of the existence of the mechanism would add nothing to the statement of the behavior to be explained. Other parts of psychoanalytic theory indicate what the independent evidence is. The theory gives a limited list of inferred entities such as unconscious feelings, desires, impulses, conflicts, and defense mechanisms. In some cases, at least, the theory states that such entities are created (with a high degree of probability) under certain specifiable conditions. The occurrence of such conditions constitutes independent inductive evidence for the existence of the entity. Furthermore, according to the theory, if one of these unconscious psychic entities exists, it is possible under specifiable conditions to elicit a certain kind of conscious entity (which may go under the same name without the qualification "unconscious"). Free association, hypnosis, and narcosynthesis are ways of eliciting the conscious entity. It is not that the subject becomes aware of an unconscious entity—there is a sense in which this is impossible by definition. Rather, according to the theory, the occurrence of the conscious entity (or the report of it if one insists upon excluding introspective evidence) under the specified conditions constitutes inductive evidence for the existence of the inferred entity at an earlier time. Other items of behavior such as slips, dreams, and neurotic symptoms constitute further inductive evidence for the existence of the inferred entity. It may be, and often is, the case that none of these items of evidence is by itself very conclusive, but we must keep in mind that inductive inferences often involve a concatenation of evidence each item of which is quite inconclusive. Nevertheless, the whole body of such evidence may well be conclusive.

In view of the preceding discussion, then, we may attempt a formulation of the principle of psychic determinism. It will be quite different from any formulation of a philosophical doctrine of determinism.

Every item of human behavior constitutes indirect inductive evidence concerning the inferred mechanisms by which the or-

ganism mediates between stimulus and response. Particularly, behavior which cannot be explained on the basis of constitutional mechanisms alone constitutes indirect inductive evidence for the existence of conscious or unconscious psychic mechanisms for which other indirect inductive evidence is also theoretically available. In short, no item of behavior is inductively irrelevant as evidence concerning the mechanisms by which the organism mediates between stimulus and response.

I offer the foregoing formulation, tentatively, as an adequate statement of the principle of psychic determinism. Whether this is what psychoanalytic theorists have always meant is beside the point. It is offered as an empirically verifiable statement which will fulfill the required function in psychoanalytic theory. It is empirically verifiable in the sense that it asserts the existence of certain objective probability relations. These relations are fundamental to psychoanalytic theory.

II

In the preceding section I have spoken of psychoanalytic theory as a theory of the mechanisms which mediate between stimulus and response. It is a theory which postulates the existence of certain unobservable events, entities, and mechanisms. In that section I spoke of indirect inductive evidence for the existence and nature of these unobservables. The charge has sometimes been made that all of this is vacuous because the relationship between observables and unobservables is stated in such a way that *any* evidence supports *any* hypothesis about the unobservables. In this section I wish to examine such criticism.

The kind of situation I shall take up is this. A subject X is observed by a psychoanalyst. On the basis of his observation of X and on the basis of psychoanalytic theory the psychoanalyst hypothesizes that X has a certain unconscious feeling. For example, from his knowledge of X's childhood he may hypothesize that X has an unresolved oedipal conflict. On the basis of this hypothesis he may derive the conclusion that X has unconscious hostility toward his father. This latter statement is another hypothesis, for unconscious hostility cannot be observed directly. When it comes to confirming this hypothesis, trouble may arise. Suppose X is observed to treat his father with a great deal of affection and solicitude. Rather than withdrawing the hypothesis that X has unconscious hostility toward his father, the psychoanalyst may say that X also has unconscious fear of hostility and exhibits behavior of the opposite extreme in defense against his own feelings of hostility. At this point the critic will very likely rise in objection and say that the psychoanalyst is making his hypothesis about unobservables immune to any negative observational evidence; hence the hypothesis is empty. If affectionate behavior is not evidence against hostility, the critic might say, then nothing could be.

If it were true that the hypothesis is compatible with any conceivable evidence, then it would be empirically empty and thus useless from the point of view of empirical science. In order to be nontautological a hypothesis must be falsifiable in principle. If it is impossible consistently to describe observable conditions which would, if they occurred, falsify or render improbable a psychoanalytic hypothesis, then the hypothesis could not be considered an empirical one.

There are at least two ways to answer the objection in the specific instance cited above. First, we might point out that overt hostility and extreme affection and solicitude do not exhaust the possible modes of behavior of X toward his father. The modes of response cover a continuum ranging from the one extreme to the other and including more moderate forms of behavior such as appropriate filial affection, indifference, and covertly hostile neglect. One way to answer the above objection is to maintain that behavior at either extreme of the continuum is evidence for the existence of hostility, while the more moderate forms would constitute evidence against the hypothesis. This answer can be made rather plausible by citing a great deal of clinical and everyday evidence for the fact that behavior at one extreme of a continuum often replaces that of the other extreme.

A second and better answer can be given. Rather than maintaining that a few restricted items of behavior can constitute conclusive evidence for or against the hypothesis, we can point out that a large range of facts is relevant to the hypothesis and the hypothesis must be judged on the weight of total evidence. Any single item of behavior or any small sample may be compatible with the hypothesis that X has unconscious hostility. We know that conscious hostility can be expressed and handled in a wide variety of ways. According to psychoanalytic theory, unconscious hostility can be dealt with in an even wider variety of ways. The unobserved mechanisms are extremely complex, and this means that the variety of modes of response is large. But it does not mean that every total behavior pattern is compatible with the hypothesis of unconscious hostility. It does mean that a good deal of evidence is required to determine whether the unconscious hostility exists, and this evidence must be taken in conjunction with a complex set of theories and hypotheses. A dialectically clever psychoanalyst might be able to argue rather convincingly that any given behavior pattern is compatible with any hypothesis concerning unconscious entities, but such forensics are no part of psychoanalytic theory and are not sanctioned by it.

What, then, is the character of the total evidence bearing upon the hypothesis that X has unconscious hostility? What counts as evidence for the hypothesis, and, more important, what would count as evidence against? It is, of course, impossible to give a complete and detailed answer to these questions, but it is not too difficult to give a fairly clear indication of what the answer must be. Here are some kinds of relevant considerations. How does X generally deal with anger and hostility? Does he express conscious anger or does he suppress it? Do situations which would arouse conscious anger in most people arouse conscious anger in X? If X generally avoids the expression of conscious anger and tends not to feel conscious anger in situations which would ordinarily arouse conscious anger, then this would tend to confirm the hypothesis that X's hostility will be unconscious if he has any. On the other hand, if X does not show tendencies to suppress and repress anger, that would tend to count against the hypothesis. Does X have dreams in which violence occurs, and in which the object of the violence is associated by X with his father? Does X make slips of the tongue which are associated with anger toward or abuse of his father? Does X "unwittingly" hurt his father's feelings? Does X "accidentally" break things belonging to his father? In the process of psychoanalysis does X develop conscious hostility toward his father? If the answers to all the foregoing sorts of questions are negative, then the hypothesis of unconscious hostility toward his father is disconfirmed; if there are a fairly large number of affirmative answers, then the hypothesis tends to be highly confirmed.

If criteria like those roughly indicated above are applied to a large number of subjects and it is found that with a high degree of probability a subject with a certain type of background turns out to have unconscious hostility toward his father, this tends to confirm the larger theory which would yield the prediction of hostility in such cases. When the larger theory has been confirmed, then the very fact that the subject X has a certain background lends weight to the hypothesis of his unconscious hostility. Indeed, if the larger theory is well enough confirmed, this may be the greatest evidence there is for the hypothesis of unconscious hostility. Then, the fact that a subject Y whose background is similar to that of X developed conscious hostility toward his father in the course of psychoanalytic treatment will lend weight to the hypothesis that X has unconscious hostility.

The ideal that the theory attempts to approach is, of course, to be able to predict with a high degree of reliability which individuals will have unconscious hostility toward their fathers and which will not, and then to predict, with respect to those who do have such hostility, the exact mode in which they will deal with it. Some progress has been made in this direction, but a good deal is left to be done.

The whole point of this section of this essay is well illustrated by an example taken from Freud's work. In Chapter IV of *The Interpretation of Dreams* Freud attempts to defend his thesis that all dreams are wish fulfillments. He explains how many dreams which appear not to be wish fulfillments can be shown to be wish fulfillments upon analysis. But there is one type of dream that he calls "counterwish dreams." These can be explained as wish fulfillments only by interpreting them as fulfilling the wish to produce a dream which does not fulfill any wish, that is, as fulfilling the wish to refute the theory that all dreams are wish fulfillments. The critic of psychoanalytic theory may look upon this as almost a paradigm of the interpretation of any evidence, however adverse, as compatible with or even supportive to psychoanalytic theory. Surely, the critic might say, the hypothesis that every dream is a wish fulfillment is a tautology if we are allowed to count as wish fulfillment dreams any dream which cannot be the fulfillment of any other wish than the wish to have a dream which is not a wish fulfillment. Any possible evidence contrary to the theory is thus automatically made compatible; negative instances are automatically transformed into positive instances.

Such a criticism would be superficial and unjustified. First, we must note that the wish to refute a scientific theory is a genuine wish in every sense of the word. It would be an unexplained peculiarity in the theory if it held that this particular type of wish is somehow incapable of being expressed in a dream. When we consider the emotional fervor that rose in opposition to Freud's theories during his lifetime, and when we consider, in terms of psychoanalytic theory, how important it must be to patients in psychoanalysis to deny the existence of certain wishes, such an exception would seem even stranger. The wish to deny the thesis that all dreams are wish fulfillments is no casual wish. However, this does not answer the critic's charge. In order to answer his criticism we must state what would constitute evidence against the theory: First, if one of these dreams which cannot be explained as any other kind of wish fulfillment were to occur to someone who had never heard of Freud's theory, this would be most damaging. Second, if a counterwish dream were to occur to someone who had not been negatively inclined toward Freud's theory, that would count as negative evidence. Freud points out carefully that every such counterwish dream occurred to someone who gave ample independent evidence of being negatively disposed toward the theory. In particular, these dreams were had by persons hearing Freud's lectures for the first time and reacting negatively to them, and by patients in analytic treatment who were experiencing strong resistance. Freud said he could almost predict when a patient would have such a dream. Third, if such a dream occurred to someone who was negatively disposed towards Freud's theory, but at a time when the issue was not under consideration, that also would count as negative evidence. Freud explicitly states that events of the previous day constitute the occasion for a dream. Furthermore, he points out that oftentimes the counterwish dreams occur the very night after the individual first heard Freud's theory. In other cases, perhaps, this happens when the issue has arisen during the day. But, according to the theory, these dreams can occur only to those who vehemently reject the theory and only when the day preceding the dream has occasioned resistance to the theory. Such a dream, occurring under any other circumstances, must count as negative evidence.

Psychoanalytic theory has been discussed as a theory of the unobservable mechanisms which mediate between stimulus and response in the human organism. According to the theory the mechanisms are complex, and they undergo changes which constitute a complex history. The main point of this essay has been to indicate the wide range of evidence which is relevant to the inference concerning these mechanisms, and to show that it is in principle possible to state the kind of evidence which should count as positive and that which should count as negative. In so far as this kind of case can be made for the various parts of psychoanalytic theory, to that extent the theory is shown to be empirically meaningful. Whether it is empirically *confirmed* is an entirely different question, and one which can be answered only by empirical investigation.

Notes

1. Terminological note: In this essay the term "psychoanalytic theory" will be used to denote the empirical theory in a general way and to distinguish it from psychoanalysis as a therapeutic technique. I make no attempt to state precisely what I take to be the content of psychoanalytic theory—that in itself would be a colossal task. I appeal only to those parts of the theory which are accepted by analytic theorists of a relatively orthodox Freudian kind. "Hypothesis" is used to refer to statements about individual cases; presumably such statements result from the application of the theory to these cases. Hypotheses are not directly verifiable by observation; they are indirectly confirmable on the basis of observational evidence. "Theory" is reserved for the generalizations which are supposed to hold for all cases and which constitute the substance of the scientific discipline. "Logical" is used in a broad enough sense to comprehend both inductive and deductive considerations as well as semantic ones.

2. Statements to this effect abound. For example, see Sigmund Freud, *A General Introduction to Psychoanalysis* (Garden City, N. Y.: Garden City Publishing Co., 1943), pp. 27, 95 n.; Sigmund Freud, *The Psychopathology of Everyday Life* in *The Basic Writings of Sigmund Freud* (New York: Random House, 1938), pp. 150 ff.; and Charles Brenner, *An Elementary Textbook of Psychoanalysis* (Garden City, N. Y.: Doubleday and Co., 1957), chap. I.

3. Two of the most famous classical statements are those of Kant and Laplace: *Immanuel Kant's Critique of Pure Reason*, ed. Norman Kemp Smith (London: Macmillan and Co., 1933), p. 218; P. S. Laplace, *A Philosophical Essay on Probabilities* (New York: Dover Publications, 1949), pp. 3–5.

4. Quite possibly Freud associated the psychoanalytic principle of determinism with a philosophical doctrine; indeed, he seems to regard determinism as a presupposition of empirical science. See

Sigmund Freud, *A General Introduction to Psychoanalysis,* pp. 27, 95–96.

5. Kant is probably the most important historical representative of this point of view.

6. Herbert Feigl, "Scientific Method without Metaphysical Presuppositions," *Philosophical Studies,* Vol. 5, No. 2, February 1954; Arthur Pap, *Elements of Analytic Philosophy* (New York: The Macmillan Co., 1949), chap. 16.

7. Antony Flew, "Motives and the Unconscious" in *Minnesota Studies in the Philosophy of Science,* Vol. I, *The Foundations of Science and the Concepts of Psychology and Psychoanalysis,* ed. Herbert Feigl and Michael Scriven (Minneapolis: University of Minnesota Press, 1956).

8. For discussions of this topic see *Determinism and Freedom in the Age of Modern Science,* ed. Sidney Hook (New York: New York University Press, 1958).

9. This seems to be the point of departure adopted by Ellis, who, incidentally, emphasized the probabilistic character of his reformulations. Albert Ellis, "An Operational Reformulation of some of the Basic Principles of Psychoanalysis" in Feigl and Scriven, editors, *op. cit.*

10. For a discussion of such models see Egon Brunswik, *The Conceptual Framework of Psychology, International Encyclopedia of Unified Science* (Chicago: University of Chicago Press, 1955), Vol. I, No. 10, Part IV. See also Otto Fenichel, *The Psychoanalytic Theory of Neurosis* (New York: W. W. Norton and Co., 1945), Part I-A.

15.

An Observation by an Experimental Psychologist

HOWARD H. KENDLER
Professor of Psychology
New York University

I SHOULD like to comment as an experimental psychologist. I believe the psychoanalysts are making a strategic error in assigning priority to clinical data when formulating their theory. Clinical data are of necessity a function of many interacting variables which cannot be isolated and controlled. As a result, the best one can hope from clinical data are crude empirical uniformities. Such crude uniformities cannot serve as the foundation of a highly abstract theory that seeks to encompass a wide range of apparently dissimilar empirical phenomena. If one looks at scientific theory in physical sciences, one discovers that abstract theories with broad empirical implications are primarily based upon data from highly controlled experimental situations.

Psychoanalytical theory as it is now formulated seeks to explain empirical phenomena that cover a wide range. But as Professor Nagel clearly shows, they fail. One reason for their failure is that their theoretical formulation does not possess any firm empirical foundation. Psychoanalytical theory would profit much by deciding to restrict the empirical scope of its theoretical formulations, and by paying more attention to experimental facts. Perhaps a more modest approach, with ingenious experimentation, might produce a psychoanalytical theory that would not suffer from the many defects it now possesses.

16.

Psychoanalysis: Protoscience and Metapsychology

GAIL KENNEDY
Professor of Philosophy
Amherst College

IN THESE comments I shall limit myself to Freud's own version of psychoanalytic theory. During the opening session on Psychoanalysis as a Scientific Theory it was asserted that this theory could not be considered "scientific" for at least three sets of reasons: (1) It has the stigmata of a theory that is so formulated as to be by its very nature irrefutable; (2) no adequate methods for establishing the data on which the theory is based, or the predictions from the hypotheses formulated, are provided; and (3) Freud's metapsychology depends on speculative conceptions which are, in crucial instances, inconsistent with well-established results of other sciences, or are beyond the range of scientific confirmation.

I

Is psychoanalysis an "irrefutable" theory and therefore pseudo-scientific? Irrefutability may take several forms: (1) Such a statement as "All events are due to Divine Providence" cannot be disproved. It precludes inquiry by begging the question. (2) A theory may be irrefutable because its proponents always admit what is favorable to the theory, and deny whatever is adverse. (3) A theory may be irrefutable because its proponents resort to *ad hominem* arguments when it is attacked. (4) It may be irrefutable because its concepts are so vague that they can

Notes to this section begin on page 280.

always be extended in a way that will yield an *ad hoc* explanation of any apparent exception.

None of this first group of objections is, I think, of much importance. Of course, psychoanalytic theory might be so formulated as to preclude the logical possibility of negative cases. That it need be so formulated, or that the theory as it is actually used corresponds to such a formulation, is questionable enough to throw the burden of proof upon the critic. A proponent of psychoanalysis might use the theory in a way that presupposes conclusions which *should* be open to question. This is something that with a certain amount of logical ingenuity can be done in defense of any theory. No doubt in the heat of the controversy over psychoanalysis it has occurred. Freud himself may have lapsed on occasion into question-begging arguments. But is there something in the psychoanalysis theory which especially lends itself to this sort of reasoning, or which logically requires it? I do not think so. Is it a *typical* mode of reasoning in this field? I do not think that it is. Again, a proponent of psychoanalysis might be the sort of person (as Huxley said of Herbert Spencer) whose "conception of tragedy is the murder of a beautiful theory by an ugly fact." Also he might "have you going and coming" by explaining your objections away as due to your "resistances." Karl R. Popper charges that both these kinds of argument are characteristic of Marxism, psychoanalysis and Adler's "individual psychology." Speaking of his student days, he says:

> These theories appeared to be able to explain practically everything that happened, within the fields to which they referred. Their study had the effect of an intellectual conversion or revelation—of opening your eyes to the truth hidden from those not yet initiated. Once your eyes were thus opened, you saw confirming instances everywhere: the world was full of *verifications* of the theory. Whatever happened always confirmed it. Thus its truth appeared obvious; and unbelievers were, clearly, people who did not want to see the truth—either because it was against their class interest, or because of their repressions which were still 'unanalysed,' and crying aloud for treatment.[1]

What this amounts to, however, is saying that the individuals Popper has in mind subscribed to these theories as articles of faith. It is not the theories themselves but their uncritical adherents who are here condemned as pseudo-scientific.

Finally, do proponents of psychoanalysis habitually resort to the device of explaining away apparent difficulties? Often it is difficult to draw the line between an *ad hoc* explanation and the legitimate extension of a concept. No doubt, proponents of psychoanalysis have sometimes failed to hew to the line. But in a young science *many* concepts are bound to be vague; in any science *some* concepts are bound to be vague; and in any science concepts must be either abandoned or amended to take account of novel data. An idea, as Peirce remarked, is "a little person," and any live theory is a growing body of ideas. Freud himself understood this well. In one of his rare comments on scientific method he said:

> The view is often defended that sciences should be built up on clear and sharply defined basal concepts. In actual fact no science, not even the most exact, begins with such definitions. The true beginning of scientific activity consists rather in describing phenomena and then in proceeding to group, classify and correlate them. Even at the stage of description it is not possible to avoid applying certain abstract ideas to the material in hand, ideas derived from various sources and certainly not the fruit of the new experience only. Still more indispensable are such ideas—which will later become the basal concepts of the science—as the material is further elaborated. They must at first necessarily possess some measure of uncertainty; there can be no question of any clear delimitation of their content. So long as they remain in this condition, we come to an understanding about their meaning by repeated references to the material of observation, from which we seem to have deduced our abstract ideas, but which is in point of fact subject to them. Thus, strictly speaking, they are in the nature of conventions; although everything depends on their being chosen in no arbitrary manner, but determined by the important relations they have to the empirical material—relations that we seem to divine before we can clearly recognize and demonstrate them. It is only after more searching

> investigation of the field in question that we are able to formulate with increased clarity the scientific concepts underlying it, and progressively so to modify these concepts that they become widely applicable and at the same time consistent logically. Then, indeed, it may be time to immure them in definitions. The progress of science, however, demands a certain elasticity even in these definitions. The science of physics furnishes an excellent illustration of the way in which even those 'basal concepts' that are firmly established in the form of definitions are constantly being altered in their content.[2]

All this first group of alleged faults are different ways of begging the question. They are fallacies to which impassioned believers are peculiarly prone. The real issue raised by those who criticize psychoanalytic theory on this ground is not one of the validity of the theory as a set of statements which might eventually be confirmed or disproven as a whole, or in part, but about the attitude of its proponents. Have they been partisans, or inquirers, or a mixture of both? Earlier controversies in the history of science, where powerful emotions are aroused,—for example the one over evolution in the sixties and seventies of the last century—show that highly competent individuals, such men as Agassiz and Owen, Huxley and Gray, may be both, and yet, on the whole, act as scientists, not propagandists, in carrying on the argument. Is this true of Freud and of many of those who have extended and developed the theory? I do not see how anyone who has tried to read without bias in the extensive literature of this field can fail to arrive at the conclusion that psychoanalysis is an attempt by responsible inquirers to establish a new branch of science.

II

The second charge is that psychoanalysis is an elaborate theory depending on wholly inadequate methods of confirmation. Neither the data on which the theory is based nor predictions derived from the theory are subjected to public and repeatable tests which meet the canons of scientific method. This assertion is made on two major counts: (1) psychoanalysis developed as the consequence of experiments in the therapy of mental illness, yet there is little correlation between claims made for the theory and actual therapeutic results; (2) the psychoanalytic method has to be employed in an atmosphere of privacy, even secrecy, which precludes an objective judgment of the results.

It is true, of course, that many analyses are unsuccessful or but partly successful, and it is also true that there are many alternate ways of being "cured." Some persons recover from a mental illness "spontaneously"—that is, we do not know why nor how they got well. Religious conversion, and other kinds of experience with sufficient emotional impact to produce a secular conversion, may mobilize latent resources within the individual powerful enough to effect a "change of heart." [3] Other reputable methods of psychiatric treatment produce their cures. And many a patent quack can claim his quota of successes through the use of auto-suggestion, electrotherapy, hydrotherapy, a sugar-free diet combined with breathing exercises, or whatnot.

Psychiatry is not the only branch of medicine where statistics of "cures" and "failures" are unreliable. In tabulations of cases treated by psychoanalytic methods the number cited is small, and there are so many variant factors entering into the treatment of each one that the crude statistics have little probative force. At most, they may suggest problems for more detailed and circumstantial investigation. There is, then, a gap between the theory and the therapeutic results of its application to the treatment of mental illness. Yet, its status as a scientific theory is not necessarily invalidated by this discrepancy. To Freud himself the practice of psychoanalysis was largely a means; he was not inclined to be unduly optimistic about the future of psychoanalysis as a mode of treatment and was primarily interested in it as a method of investigation. His real goal was a better knowledge of the structure and mechanisms of the human mind. And it is psychoanalysis as a method of research with which we are here concerned.

A more serious objection than the gap between theory and therapeutic results is that the method is inherently unscientific because of the way in which it must be used. How in the private, even secret, relation between analyst and patient can the subjective element possibly be eliminated? Statements of the patients themselves cannot always be taken at face value—Freud early discovered that many of the "memories" disclosed were false, that in some crucial instances patients were unable to distinguish their fantasies from what had actually occurred. Worse than that are the effects of the transference which develops in the analytic situation. When the analyst makes interpretations, the patient's unconscious may all too willingly comply by furnishing associations in the form of fantasies, dreams, and selected memories which serve either submissively to corroborate the interpretation (though it may be wrong) or defiantly to corroborate the interpretation *because* it is wrong. And under the influence of the countertransference the analyst himself may be seduced into accepting the patient's own subtly and indirectly proffered interpretations, or he may project his own unconscious conflicts on to the patient and end up by treating the wrong person. How is it possible to get out of this quagmire?

When we consider the multitude of theories that can always be "thought up" to explain supposed "facts" and the variety of dissident theories both psychoanalytic and nonanalytic in the field, why not regard the Freudian version of psychoanalysis as just one set of conjectures among many? Why take its pretensions seriously? Yet there are, I believe, good reasons for regarding psychoanalysis as a protoscience—the beginnings of a science that is still in the *clinical* stage of development (as described by Freud in the passage quoted), the stage in which there is constant interaction between a rapidly growing body of observations and theories that are continually being altered in order to accommodate new discoveries.

First, the evidence is not *all* private. There are mitigations. Predictions made in the course of an analysis, such as those that the patient must have had an early traumatic experience of a given sort, can often be checked.[4] Case histories are reported. Recordings of whole analyses (a Gargantuan task) have been made. Psychoanalysis has infiltrated the field of psychiatry.

Medical schools, hospitals, clinics and established institutes for the training of analysts provide opportunities for systematic observation and discussion of neurotic and psychotic patients from the psychoanalytic point of view. An increasing consensus has thus grown up within the medical profession. The belief in psychoanalysis may be a group illusion of these practitioners—phrenology and mesmerism once had large numbers of reputable and experienced adherents—but none the less this substantial consensus is relevant, and the systematic observations may well be important indirect evidence for the essential validity of the theory.

Moreover, as is the case with any comprehensive theory, psychoanalysis can be broken down into a large number of subsidiary hypotheses. There is available a large body of circumstantial evidence, drawn from a wide variety of fields, which is relevant to the testing of these hypotheses. Among the sources from which this evidence may be drawn are: detailed studies of the overt behavior of neurotics and psychotics; the use of drugs, in narcosynthesis, and of hypnotism to investigate repressed emotions and memories; the controlled use of drugs which produce a temporary simulation in normal persons of neurotic and psychotic states; the experimental production of neuroses in animals; experiments on animals and with human subjects dealing with such basic mechanisms as repression, displacement, fixation and regression, dream symbolism, etc.; [5] studies of children raised as orphans or in other abnormal situations; [6] the comparative study of child-rearing practices in different cultures; [7] the comparative study of institutions, of rituals and myths, of art works and literature, etc. From all these diverse sources, and others as well, converging evidence may be drawn that is relevant to the accuracy of the data upon which psychoanalytic theory is based and the confirmation of specific hypotheses which may be derived from that theory.

If then, psychoanalysis is susceptible to piecemeal confirmation or disconfirmation through circumstantial evidence drawn from many diverse fields, it should be an embryonic science, a system of hypotheses as yet not fully unified but testable by ordinary scientific methods. That, I think, it now is—a proto-science.

III

The third set of criticisms is that Freud's metapsychology depends on speculative theses which are, in crucial instances, inconsistent with well-established results in other sciences, or are beyond the range of scientific confirmation.[8] Three of these, in particular, are open to this charge. They are (1) that certain basic inhibitions, which Freud thinks of as now being generic human traits, the prohibition of parricide, cannibalism and incest, are the result of early racial experiences, traumatic in character, which have been inherited through the id; (2) that the Oedipus complex is a recapitulation by each individual, under the stimulus of emotional attachments to the parents (or parent surrogates), of this traumatic experience undergone by his remote ancestors; (3) that there are two basic sets of complementary and opposed instincts, the erotic or life instincts and the aggressive or death instincts, and that this basic dualism pervades all of organic nature.

Freud willingly admits that he cannot prove these assertions. His account of the initial organization of society and of the revolt of the brothers in *Totem and Taboo* he calls a "scientific myth," and in *Beyond the Pleasure Principle,* where he first advanced his conception of the universal polarity of erotic and death instincts, he says that it is so highly speculative "I am neither convinced myself, nor am I seeking to arouse conviction in others." None the less, Freud did come increasingly to "believe" in these three propositions as basic to his metapsychology.

Two separate contentions are involved in the first of these statements. One is the inheritability not only of instinctual dispositions, "the ability and tendency to follow a certain direction of development and to react in a particular way to certain excitations, impressions and stimuli," but also of archaic memory traces. The inheritance of "dispositions," however, they may have originated, is not in doubt. What seems implausible is the inheritance of memory traces and Freud's explanation of the way in which it came about. A memory, he says, enters into the archaic inheritance "when the experience is important enough, or is repeated often enough, or in both cases. With the father-murder both conditions are fulfilled." [9] This seems contrary to established findings of present-day genetics. Freud makes no attempt to answer this objection, nor to supply any alternative explanation. His attitude, as indicated in other contexts, seems to be that psychology and ethology are *prior* to the biological sciences in the sense that they describe behavior for which the biological sciences must ultimately give an explanation. Similarly, he believes that the anthropologists (who as a body have rejected his theory of the primal group) must eventually explain somehow what he regards as psychologically well grounded facts.[10] There are, I think, alternative ways, perhaps more plausible, of attempting to explain the archaic memory trait: (1) If the primal murder occurred often enough it might be explicable through the operation of natural selection.[11] (2) By social inheritance the archaic memory might be directly transmitted from the unconscious of parents to the unconscious of children. Freud believed that there could be communication at the subconscious level without any conscious awareness, but he did not consider this possibility.

On the universality of the Oedipus complex, whether or not it be a recapitulation of ancestral experiences, Freud gets more support. Ethnologists believe that some form of "nuclear family" exists in every human culture, and many would agree that an Oedipus complex, or some complex which would be an equivalent for that type of social organization, occurs as a result of the prolonged dependence of the human child upon the care of parents or parent surrogates.

Freud's dualistic theory of instincts when stated at the level of Empedocles' principles of Love and Strife is clearly beyond the bourne of science. What is important for psychoanalytic theory is the question: Are there two basic sets of instincts, the erotic and the aggressive? Freud thought it easier and more plausible to explain such phenomena as the repetition compulsion, ambivalence, sadism and masochism, and melancholia as manifestations of a partial defusion of these two normally fused sets of original instincts. To say that aggression is a product of frustration ignores the question: Where does the aggression come from? To argue that an aggressive act is the deflection of an initial positively toned (possessive) drive toward the barrier still leaves the problem of how a drive is changed into its qualitative opposite. A simpler and more plausible hypothesis is to suppose that the original drive is a fusion of erotic and destructive impulses. To possess is originally to incorporate, it is both a having and a destroying of the object. And all "creative" exercise of energies involves an element of destructiveness. Something must be done away with or else forcibly remolded (incorporated) in whatever we make.

There is some evidence from physiology for this dualism. Certainly the erotic drives depend upon mechanisms of the body, and the now classic research of Walter B. Cannon did a good deal to disclose the physiological basis of aggression. More recently it has been found that the adrenal medullae of "constitutionally" aggressive animals such as the lion contain a relatively high amount of noradrenalin, while in animals such as the rabbit whose safety lies in flight adrenalin predominates. The drug meprobamate (Miltown) apparently blocks the secretion of adrenalin. Tweak the whiskers of an ordinary mouse and he rushes off in panic, but the "tranquilized" mouse when tweaked maintains his equanimity. Men are not mice, but there is evidence that outwardly directed anger accompanied by aggressive behavior is associated with the production of noradrenalin, whereas aggression directed inward accompanied by fearfulness, anxiety, and depression is associated with the production of adrenalin.[12]

These highly controversial theses are not the whole of Freud's metapsychology. Other parts of it, such as his topological division of the psyche into an id, ego and superego, are more immediately derived from clinical data, and less doubtful. And by far the greater part of psychoanalytic theory consists of what I have called protoscience. One *can* get along without these far-reaching contentions in the form Freud stated them. They are not essential, many practicing analysts would say, to therapy, nor even to the formulation of a logically coherent theory of the etiology of neurotic and psychotic disturbances. Yet Freud found them indispensable. When even the faithful Ernest Jones expressed scepticism concerning his ideas on the erotic and death instincts, Freud replied in a letter that "he could no longer see his way without them, they had become indispensable to him." [13] This is a revealing statement. The parts of Freud's metapsychology which are most speculative and implausible were not just the divagations of a genius who could also be a cautious and uncannily sensitive observer; they do not indicate, as some critics have thought, that Freud was rather inept when it came to the construction of theories. What Freud meant—quite literally, I am sure—was that he could not see his way in a hitherto uncharted field without them. Without imagination the perceiver is blind. Without an increment of excitement there are no fresh perceptions. As Carl Hempel has pointed out, it is "the fictitious concepts rather than those fully definable by observables" that stimulate predictions and thus afford *new* observations, of something that was not previously discerned. Hence, Freud was tentative, yet also tenacious, about these hypotheses. They were essential to him in the way a set of working plans is to the creator of any novel construction. Throughout his life Freud altered the plans as he went along. Subsequent inquirers may and should modify them in accordance with their needs. Eventually they may present a more fully developed, more precise, even more plausible metapsychology as the framework of psychoanalysis. It is easy, then, to conclude that Freud's metapsychology is "unscientific"; but could he have founded psychoanalysis without it?

Notes

1. "Philosophy of Science: A Personal Report," *British Philosophy in the Mid-Century*, ed. C. A. Mace (London: 1957).

2. "Instincts and Their Vicissitudes," *Collected Papers* (London: 1925), IV, 60–61.

3. There is an example of this in *As You Like It*. The cruel Oliver, who had tried to kill his younger brother Orlando, has been rescued by Orlando from a savage lioness. When he tells Celia of this, she says, "Was't you that did so oft contrive to kill him?" And Oliver replies: " 'Twas I; but 'tis not I. I do not shame / To tell you what I was, since my conversion / So sweetly tastes being the thing I am."

4. An example of this sort of verification is given by Marie Bonaparte in "Notes on the Analytic Discovery of a Primal Scene," *The Psychoanalytic Study of the Child* (New York: 1945), I, 119–25.

5. For a brief recent survey and discussion of this particular type of experimental work see Ernest R. Hilgard, "Experimental Approaches to Psychoanalysis," *Psychoanalysis as Science*, ed. E. Pumpian-Mindlin (New York: 1952; second edition, 1956), pp. 3–45.

6. Cf. Anna Freud and Dorothy Burlingham, *Infants Without Families* (New York: 1944).

7. Cf. *Childhood in Contemporary Cultures*, ed. Margaret Mead and Martha Wolfenstein (Chicago: 1955).

8. There is an oddity here. If the metapsychology is refuted by facts, then surely *it* is not untestable. And if the metapsychology is testable, then how is it related to its allegedly untested, perhaps untestable, psychology? Can one have a testable metapsychology for an untested, even perhaps untestable, psychology? I owe this point to my colleague, Professor Joseph Epstein.

9. *Moses and Monotheism* (New York: 1955), p. 129.

10. Cf. *Moses and Monotheism,* p. 169. Recently F. D. Klingender has published an article, "Palaeolithic Religion and the Principle of Social Evolution," *The British Journal of Sociology* V (1954), in which he says (p. 150): "Human society did not therefore, on this hypothesis, begin with the act of revolt to which our children still secretly aspire, while they are in the grip of the Oedipus conflict, but with its far more difficult sequel: the renunciation and redirection of natural impulses which put an end to what was virtually a state of perpetual revolt in the primate group. This way of looking at the matter may imply a shift in the emphasis generally placed on Freud's theory, but the main burden of my argument was published forty years ago in *Totem and Taboo* (1913)."

11. An interesting hypothesis which might explain how instinctive patterns of behavior have gradually evolved from what were originally learned responses is suggested by W. H. Thorpe in Chapter 8 of his *Learning and Instinct in Animals* (Cambridge, Mass.: 1956).

12. Daniel H. Funkenstein, "The Physiology of Fear and Anger," *Scientific American,* May, 1955, pp. 74–80.

13. *The Life and Work of Sigmund Freud* (New York: 1957), III, 276.

17.

Comments

PERCY W. BRIDGMAN
Higgins University Professor, Emeritus
Harvard University

A PHYSICIST is so remote from most of the issues of interest to this conference that the most he can hope is to observe what is involved in the detached spirit of a man from Mars. There are two comments that I would like to make. The first is, that in spite of the apparently unsatisfactory status of some of the constructs of the psychoanalyst it would appear that there is nothing fundamentally unsound at the foundations, but that if one takes the necessary trouble and care everything can be put on a completely "operational" basis—it is not necessary to postulate unprovable principles or essences such as the vitalist does, for example. The second comment is that perhaps some of the features which distinguish psychoanalysis from other disciplines can be explained by the prominent role that introspection plays. This role is fundamental, because without the introspectional report that the analyst is able to draw from his patient some of the basic concepts of the analyst are merely verbal constructs—they have no "reality" because there is no second method of getting to the terminus.

18.

On the Empirical Interpretation of Psychoanalytic Concepts

ARTHUR PAP
Associate Professor of Philosophy
Yale University

I

It is a truism of scientific methodology that a theory cannot serve as an explanation of observable phenomena unless it is empirically testable, and that it is not empirically testable unless its abstract vocabulary is, directly or indirectly, completely or partially, interpreted in terms of observables. The methodologists who participated in the second NYU conference evidently felt that psychoanalytic theory is still far from meeting this requirement of empirical testability. Professor Nagel properly emphasized that a careful formulation of "correspondence rules" connecting such abstract terms as "unconscious incestuous desire" with observational vocabulary (whether physicalistic or not) is needed before one can decide whether the impressive body of evidence cited by psychoanalysts as confirming their theories does or does not confirm them. And Professor Hook, in the same spirit, challenged the psychoanalysts to describe the sort of evidence which they would accept as a refutation of Freud's theory of the Oedipus complex: if any conceivable sort of child behavior can be reconciled with the theory that the male child is sexually jealous of his father and unconsciously wishes his father were dead and he himself were his mother's lover, then this theory is, of course, as unscientific as the theory that whatever happens is caused by the will of God.

Notes to this section begin on page 297.

In the following I shall suggest an analysis of psychoanalytic concepts as *disposition* concepts that might satisfy the demand for empirical testability though at the same time it raises a grave question about psychoanalytic *explanation*. The word "unconscious" has several meanings,[1] and I shall consider at least one meaning of it which is not characteristically psychoanalytic (viz., mistaken introspective analysis). Its characteristically psychoanalytic meaning, however, seems to me to be dispositional; or more accurately, this is the meaning that remains after it is divested of misleading metaphorical connotations.

First a few preliminary remarks about the nature of disposition concepts. Roughly, the sense of "disposition" in which dispositions are ascribed not only, as in ordinary language, to people and animals but also to inanimate objects may be explicated as follows: to ascribe disposition D to x is to assert that x has some intrinsic property K such that anything which has K reacts to a stimulus S in fashion R provided certain environmental conditions (often not reliably known in detail) are fulfilled. For example, if D is solubility in water, K may be whatever chemical property is definitory of "sugar," S immersion in water, R dissolution in water, and one obvious environmental condition the absence of a cellophane wrapping around the lump of sugar. In some cases the implication connecting S and R is probabilistic rather than strictly causal; one might then speak of a "probabilistic" disposition. Thus a psychologist may ascribe to a rat a certain probability (i.e., relative frequency) of response as a dispositional property: if a rat has undergone a certain conditioning, then there is a probability p that if confronted with the choice between running down a path leading to food or another path leading to a sex partner, it will run down the path leading to food. In this example K is the relevant kind of conditioning (past reinforcements) plus the present intensities of certain "drives" (hunger, sexual drive). As indicated by the property variable K, dispositions are ascribed to things in so far as they are of a determinate kind. Without specifying the *kind* of thing which is acted on by S in such and such circumstances, one cannot reliably predict a definite response R.

But in making dispositional statements we *anticipate* discovery of a causal law rather than asserting a causal law: we express the belief that there is a property K which jointly with S and certain other conditions is causally sufficient for the occurrence of R, but we do not know as yet *which* property it is. When I ascribe to a man the disposition to be frightened by dogs I am saying that, generally, his perception of a dog causes him to be fearful. But since other people remain undisturbed by similar perceptions, this causal statement would be false unless it implicitly referred to some relevant property of that man which distinguishes him from people who are not frightened by the sight of a dog. What seems to be meant by the dispositional statement, then, is that the man has some (unspecified) property such that any man who resembles him in that respect would react similarly to similar stimuli. Subsequent inquiry might enable me to specify this property: he was dangerously bitten by a dog in his childhood. Thereafter I am in a position to supersede the dispositional statement with a specific generalization: anybody with such and such a background will (other things being equal) feel frightened in the presence of a dog. Again, to say that turpentine is inflammable is to say that anything which is turpentine has certain (unspecified) physico-chemical properties K such that anything which has K and is exposed to fairly high temperature (in the presence of sufficient oxygen, etc.) will burn. But once K is *specified,* the anticipatory dispositional statement can be replaced by a specific causal generalization.

The purpose of these sketchy remarks on the analysis of disposition concepts [2] is to suggest that dispositional talk is characteristic of the *pretheoretical* stage of a science, since to ascribe dispositions is, to borrow a suggestive metaphor from Herbert Feigl, to issue promissory notes. One "promises" future discovery of a generalization which will, together with relevant singular statements, explain an observed regularity; but this is not equivalent to explaining the latter. The law that anything with a structural microproperty K dissolves in aqua regia, together with the premise that these objects have K, explains the observed regularity that these and similar objects (pieces of gold) dissolve when immersed in aqua regia. But the dispositional statement that objects with these surface characteristics are soluble in aqua regia does not explain it; it only says that the explanation which it is hoped will be discovered is one in terms of (at the time of the dispositional assertion unknown) *intrinsic* properties of the objects, not one in terms of a fortuitous collocation of circumstances. The same holds for the "explanation" of observed regularities of behavior in terms of instincts. The statement that the observed regularity is due to some kind of instinct is not an empty tautology, but it is not an explanation either; it is a promise of a forthcoming explanation. To give a dispositional analysis of the typically psychoanalytic meaning of "unconscious," therefore, is to suggest that psychoanalysis is so far to a large extent a pretheoretical science.

That a dispositional statement cannot occur in the *explanans* of a causal explanation may be formally shown as follows. The statement that an object y has the disposition to react in circumstances C, C′, C″ . . . . C^n in fashion R has, on the suggested analysis, the form: $(\exists\theta)\ [\theta y \cdot (t)(x)(\theta x \cdot Cx,t \cdot C'x,t \ldots\ldots C^n x,t \rightarrow Rx,t)]$. But it is impossible to deduce from such an existential statement, conjoined with $Cy,t_0 \cdot C'y,t_0 \ldots\ldots C^n y,t_0$, the description of the actual response, Ry,t_0. Such a deduction can be made only from a specific law of the form $(t)(x)(Px \cdot Cx,t \cdot C'x,t \ldots\ldots C^n x,t \rightarrow Rx,t)$. The complete causal explanation then takes the form:

$$\frac{\begin{array}{l} Py \cdot Cy,t_0 \cdot C'y,t_0 \ldots\ldots C^n y,t_0 \\ (t)(x)(Px \cdot Cx,t \cdot C'x,t \ldots\ldots C^n x,t \rightarrow Rx,t) \end{array}}{Ry,t_0}$$ [8]

(The "intrinsic" predicate P may itself carry a time argument, but this would not affect the logical point here made.)

II

If to ascribe an unconscious desire or wish to an organism is to ascribe to it a dispositional state, then unconscious desires are not causal antecedents of overt behavior, and it is a mistake to suppose that an item or pattern of overt behavior has been causally explained when one says that it expresses such and such an unconscious desire. Suppose that a person A regularly acts with respect to person B as though he disliked B; that is, *if* A disliked B he could be expected to act with respect to B just the way he is observed to act with respect to B. We say to A "obviously you dislike B," but A in apparent sincerity denies this. Now, what does it mean to say that, nevertheless, A *unconsciously* dislikes B? If it meant "A acts as if he consciously disliked B but he does not consciously dislike B," our explanation of A's actions would have the curious form: q, because (if p, then q) and not p. According to the dispositional analysis of "unconscious dislike," however, this means that A's apparently unfriendly or discriminating actions towards B are not just the result of an accidental collocation of circumstances that are independent of A's relevant attitudes, but depend on some intrinsic property of A: A has some intrinsic property such that any person with the same intrinsic property would probably react similarly in similar circumstances. The intrinsic property in question may be A's belief that B threatens his professional position, for example. Once such a property is discovered, a genuine causal explanation is at hand, but the word "unconscious" will have disappeared. In many cases no immediate causal antecedents can be detected on the molar level in terms of which observed responses, mental or physical, could be uniquely explained. In that case the intrinsic property to be discovered consists in certain aspects of the person's past experience (problem of *mnemic* laws in biology and psychology) or —at a utopian stage of physiological psychology that fills the day-dreams of physicalists—in brain modifications resulting from such past experience. Thus psychoanalysts often succeed in tracing neurotic adult behavior to certain kinds of traumatic experience in childhood. Also Freud's famous case of the bride's disappointment during her wedding night leading to a strange form of compulsive behavior falls into this category. Here we have genetic laws, of an imperfect probabilistic character, indeed, and so far wholly unexplained in terms of a general theory of psychopathic behavior; but they can legitimately be used for probabilistic and in principle confirmable explanations of abnormal behavior patterns. What I am suggesting is that the word "unconscious" cannot appear in any genuine causal explanation, whether rigorously deterministic or probabilistic, whether in terms of the postulates of a rigorous theory of human behavior or, more modestly, in terms of pragmatically reliable empirical generalizations, because its function is only to *mark,* not to *solve,* a problem of explanation.

It is often said that Freud and his followers are concerned with explanations of pathological behavior in terms of *motives,* specifically *unconscious* motives, hence not with *causal* explanations. Freud reports that his patient did not know why she performed that ritual every morning until he made its "meaning" clear to her: it was a substitute fulfillment of her (unconscious) wish that her husband might have proved potent during that traumatic night. Now, let us first see what is meant by "motive" in an uncomplicated context like "what motivated him to marry the unattractive old widow was the desire to inherit her considerable fortune." Ryle is, I think, wrong in contending that such an explanation of behavior is "analogous to the explanation of reactions and actions by reflexes and habits, or to the explanation of the fracture of the glass by reference to its brittleness" (*The Concept of Mind,* p. 90). To say that a person is in the habit of doing such and such in circumstances X is, indeed, to assert a hypothetical lawlike proposition, but the statement that he desired to inherit her fortune is not of this sort. It is true that a state of desiring something is not "occurrent" like a state of seeing, hearing or smelling something. One can desire, or intend, something at a time when one is not actually aware of such a desire or intention, while one cannot, in the same sense, smell a foul smell without being aware of it or see a red patch without being aware of it. But given some stimulus occasioning an introspective act—like the question "Why do you marry that woman?"—the man will become aware of (a) desiring to inherit her fortune and (b) being impelled to marry her in order to satisfy that desire, in a sense in which one cannot be aware of a hypothetical fact, a fact like "whenever I taste pure lemon juice, I shiver." Motives of the familiar sort, then, are desires, intentions, purposes which causally determine human behavior and of which the agent becomes aware when certain normal conditions of self-examination are fulfilled.

Now, it seems to me that Freud and Freudians commit a serious "category mistake" in treating unconscious motives as still causal antecedents of human, especially neurotic, behavior which are like motives of the familiar kind except that, due to repression, they cannot under normal conditions become objects of the agent's awareness. If to ascribe an unconscious wish to the patient is to predict that under therapy the patient will eventually become aware of such a wish (provided certain essential conditions, like cooperation with the analyst, etc., are realized) and acquire the beneficial belief—whatever it may mean—that his neurotic symptoms served the purpose of its "substitute" fulfillment,[4] then an unconscious wish is a dispositional state of an organism. In that case the "explanation" of neurotic symptoms in terms of an unconscious wish is, to borrow Ryle's example for use in a more appropriate context, like explaining the breaking of an object in terms of its brittleness and unlike explaining it in terms of the antecedent event of its being released. As I argued above, to ascribe the fracture to brittleness is to assert that the observed event is to be explained in terms of some intrinsic property of the object; that is, we express the belief that the antecedent event (release) would be followed by the same effect under a wide variety of circumstances *provided* the object involved resembles the given one in certain (as yet unspecified) intrinsic properties. Similarly, the explanation in terms of the patient's unconscious wish is of this "promissory" sort: similar traumatic experiences will result in a similar neurosis provided the person who suffers them is in certain as yet undiscovered respects (perhaps physiological, perhaps psychological) like the present patient. I am inclined, therefore, to regard the language of unconscious motives as having a heuristic rather than an explanatory function.

III

One may understandably ask: Why all this reluctance to speak of introspectively unobservable mental processes, mental processes which really occur and causally determine human behavior yet cannot be directly observed but only inferred? Don't the physicists, without apology to positivists or operationists, speak of perceptually unobservable physical events, like the flights of subatomic particles, bombardments of atomic nuclei, etc.? Yet, in the first place, a methodological justification of psychoanalysis by comparison with theoretical physics is out of place, because psychoanalysis is too young a science still to be in a position to lay a precise and solid theoretical foundation for its rough empirical generalizations. This may easily be overlooked because psychoanalytic jargon is, almost repulsively, replete with highly abstract terms. But the latter are, as I have suggested, more on the level of "promissory" disposition terms than on that of theoretical terms in the postulates of a partially interpreted deductive theory. Secondly, it seems to me that an uncritical acceptance of talk about unexperienced mental events arises from a tacit *objectification* of psychological language. It is impossible to believe that one is in pain without actually being in pain (if "pain" is used in a purely phenomenal sense); similarly, it would be nonsense to say "he thinks he desires to kiss that girl but he really has no such desire." But those who objectify psychological language believe that "A thinks that p" is compatible with "not p" even if "p" is a description of A's immediate experience, like a pain, a surge of hatred, or a longing. Daring to use language which is much frowned upon since the behaviorist revolution in psychology, I venture to assert that it is logically impossible for a pain or a desire to occur without the subject's being conscious of it, because pains and desires are just the sort of "private" states that are meant by the old-fashioned expression "state of consciousness."

The thesis of the infallibility of beliefs about one's own immediate experiences, perceptual or affective or conative, may be and has been criticized on the ground that *misdescription* of one's mental states is surely possible, just as it is possible to make mistakes in describing physical events or things. That I feel the desire which I feel is true enough—similarly it is beyond dispute that I see what I see. But is it not an enormous leap from this truism to the assertion that no mistakes can be made in *introspective analysis*? To illustrate, suppose that I feel a certain emotion towards a colleague in my profession which I describe honorifically as "contempt for his obvious manner of displaying his skills, calculated to impress those who are capable of promoting him." Is it not possible that this description is incorrect, that the correct description of the emotion is the less flattering one "jealousy of my colleague, on account of certain of his skills which I lack and would like to possess"? Certainly, some introspective beliefs may be mistaken, but it is important to understand why one introspective belief may be mistaken while another—like the belief that one is thirsty, or hungry (phenomenally, whatever the physiological condition of the body may be)—may not. Now, just as in the case of descriptions of perceptual data, the possibility of error arises from the predictive content of the descriptions. In describing my emotion of antipathy or even hatred more specifically as "jealousy" or as "contempt" I am not conveying any additional information about the intrinsic quality of the emotion (it may be doubted whether contempt "feels" any differently from jealousy) but am asserting a causal proposition concerning the beliefs which give rise to my antipathy. In the first case I am claiming that what makes me dislike my colleague is his manner of displaying himself, his immodesty; in the second case I humbly confess that it is the belief that he has desirable abilities which I lack that produces my antagonism. Such causal propositions can be tested by further introspective observations: if the first hypothesis is correct, then, other things being equal, I would cease to dislike my competitor if, after getting the promotion he fought for, he should adopt the kind of modest (or complacent?) reserved behavior which secure, respected people can afford. If the second hypothesis is correct, then I should continue to dislike him after the described change of personality; indeed, my antagonism should be intensified, since he got his promotion!

The objection from the possibility of misdescription of one's own mental states has served its purpose of forcing a clarification of the thesis that introspective beliefs are infallible. It must be qualified by distinguishing between *intrinsic qualities* and *causal properties* of mental states. Such conative verbs as "desiring (to go for a walk)," "fearing (to be scratched by the cat)," "liking (John)," "disliking (Bill)," as well as sensation words like "sour-tasting," "seeing red," "noisy," designate what I call intrinsic qualities of mental states. A person's belief that his present mental state has such and such an intrinsic quality can be produced only by the occurrence of a mental state with that quality. If so, it follows that it cannot be mistaken. To put it more accurately, such a belief *is* nothing else than an introspective awareness of a state characterized by that quality; and how could there be an introspective awareness of a state having a certain intrinsic quality if the subject were not in such a state? The distinction between illusory and correct belief simply does not apply here. On the other hand, when we describe our mental states by such terms as "contempt," "jealousy," "feeling sympathy (for X)," "admiring," "feeling remorse" (in contrast to "being apprehensive of the dangerous consequences for one's self of a past deed"), we make implicit assertions about the causal contexts of these states. Therefore introspective analysis can go wrong here; and because of people's notorious reluctance to admit unworthy emotions and desires to themselves, impartial spectators of manifest behavior may indeed have more reliable knowledge of such causal properties of mental states than the biased introspecting subject. As C. D. Broad has pointed out (*loc. cit.*), the word "unconscious" is often used in this sense of mistaken introspective analysis. Thus a jealous wife might say to her husband, "You claim to be aware only of a virtuous feeling of sympathy for that poor, forsaken widow; but what you really feel, though *unconsciously,* is great sexual attraction."

Her description of her husband's feelings is obviously causal: she implicitly predicts that he would still chase that woman if she turned into the happiest, most lavishly supported widow in the world. There is no reason why the word "unconscious" should not be so used if one is clear about that usage. But the confusion to be avoided is to ascribe to introspective reports of intrinsic qualities a fallibility of which only introspective reports of causal properties are susceptible. "You don't really like him, as you claim; you dislike him intensely, though unconsciously" does not make any more sense than "You are wrong in thinking that the needle hurts you; you really enjoy the sensation, though you are not conscious of the pleasure."

To "objectify" psychological language means, further, to make and consider significant such statements as "He really hates him, though he is not aware of it; he is not lying when he denies this emotion, he is just unconsciously repressing it." A good many people, some of them professional psychologists, others just educated laymen who have picked up the jargon, will be astonished that one should even raise the question whether such statements make sense. It seems, however, that a subtle ambiguity of the expression "awareness" (and the corresponding verb) is responsible here for a confusion of two different propositions, one obviously true, the other just as obviously false (hence the controversy whether there can be unconscious emotions). Consider the question "is it possible to see red without being aware of seeing red?" and compare it with the question "is it possible that lightning should occur without anyone's being aware of it?" This very comparison of awareness of a mental event with awareness of a physical event will suggest a negative answer to the first question: seeing red, it may be replied, is just the sort of event we call an act of awareness ("state of consciousness"). But it is important to understand that in saying that it is impossible to see red without being aware of it one is, if the statement is true, using "awareness" as a categorial term which does not denote a distinguishable mental state, but is related to such terms as "seeing red," "feeling bored," "hearing a dissonant chord," as "colored" is related to the determinate predicates "blue," "red," etc. In this usage "I see red" entails "I am aware of seeing red" in the same way in which it entails "I see a color." That is, the expression following "of" in "I am aware of . . ." refers, not to an object of awareness—in the sense in which a tree may or may not be an object of awareness—but to a species of awareness.[5] In a second sense, however, "awareness of seeing red" and "awareness of one's hatred of X" denote an act of introspection which need not, and often does not, accompany the introspectable state. This is so whatever the correct analysis of the concept of introspection may be (subvocal description, or something more elusive). Now, that emotions and desires may occur without any awareness of them in this latter sense is obviously true. But it does not follow that one could fail to be aware of a desire or emotion in the former sense of "aware of": this is just as impossible as seeing red without seeing a color; for, just as blue and red are species of color, so seeing red, feeling bored, desiring to pass the examination, hating the landlord, are species of consciousness. Certainly one can hate a person at a time when, oblivious of the enemy, one is in a relaxed, even loving mood. Emotion words, unlike perception words, are partly dispositional. But one cannot, in the ordinary sense of the word, fail to be aware of one's hatred, or of one's wish, when one tries to detect it introspectively. It is a conscious emotion in the sense that its owner must become aware of it *if* he introspects. One may have reasons to suspect of dishonesty the person who denies one's diagnosis, but to say he represses the emotion into the unconscious layers of his mind is to employ a spatial metaphor whose literal meaning, if it has any, has never become clear to me. And one cannot exonerate oneself of the task of empirical interpretation by citing constructs of physical theories which likewise do not denote observable phenomena; for the price to be paid for the license of merely partial interpretation of theoretical terms is the construction of a deductive theory with fairly precise postulates, but psychoanalysis has not, and cannot be expected to have, reached that advanced stage.

IV

It may be replied that inferences from observed behavior to unobservable mental causes are of just the same logical form as analogical inferences to microevents and microentities in physics, and must therefore be accepted as scientific by anybody but a narrow positivist who is hostile to all theory construction that goes beyond phenomenalistic description. The premise of the argument is true enough, but the conclusion does not follow. Consider the following example of postulation of (directly) unobservable microprocesses in physics. An experimental physicist observes that low frequencies of vibration of a string are correlated with low pitches and higher frequencies of still visible vibrations with higher pitches. As he ascends on the ladder of pitches in order to get more confirmation for the law that pitch is a monotonically increasing function of frequency of vibration, he reaches a point where the vibrations assumed to accompany still audible pitches are no more visible. If the physicist refrained from postulations that simplify the system of physical explanation, he would restrict the range of the variable "frequency of vibration" to observable values and look for different mechanical causes of the higher pitches. Instead he postulates invisible vibrations, assuming that the causes of the higher pitches are sufficiently *analogous* to the causes of the lower pitches to warrant description in terms of the same concepts "vibration" and "frequency of vibration." The situation seems to be exactly similar in the case of explanation of human behavior in terms of unconscious mental forces. In psychoanalytic child therapy, for example, it is observed that a little boy exhibits just the sort of playing behavior that could be expected if he hated his father and sought to express this hatred through fiction, like painting a man and then splashing paint all over the picture. The boy fails to be aware of such an evil emotion, so the analyst says that the emotion exists in unconscious, repressed form. But the two cases differ in an important respect. It is no part of the meaning of a physical expression like "vibration of a string" that such a process could be seen by a human observer, any more than it is implied in the meaning of "pitch corresponding to frequency n" that the described pitch is audible by the human ear. (The kind of possibility here in question is, of course, empirical possibility, i.e. compatibility with empirical laws. Logical possibility is irrelevant in this context since obviously no vibrations are asserted to be invisible in the sense that it is logically impossible that an organism should exist with vision sufficiently acute to detect such vibrations.) It follows that in the context "invisible vibration" the word "vibration" has the same meaning as in the context "visible vibration." The word "hatred," on the other hand, is ordinarily so used that empirical possibility of introspective awareness of the emotion (expressed by a conditional statement like "if he were to reflect on his feelings towards X, he would become aware of his hatred of X") is part of its meaning. If "unconscious hatred" refers, not to a momentarily unactualized disposition, but to an efficacious mental process, then it is not like "invisible vibration" but rather like "shapeless cube."

The analogical argument for unconscious mental processes derives its seductive force from its formal similarity to arguments leading to hypotheses about physical causes. Suppose that a team of detectives discovered on a just-stolen car fingerprints which exactly resembled the carefully preserved fingerprints of a criminal whom the police had been hunting for the last ten years. And suppose that subsequently convincing evidence were produced that this criminal had died eight years ago. Understandably the detectives would be inclined to question the evidence indicating the criminal's death and to stick to their causal hypothesis. Similarly, it is very common in this age of psychoanalysis that a certain form of behavior is regarded as conclusive evidence for the efficacy of specific emotions and desires, in spite of the fact that the subject's introspective report flatly refutes the causal inference. "Naturally you fail to discover your hatred (or your incestuous desire), for you are unconsciously repressing it." But such a radical departure from the ordinary use of mentalistic words is extremely confusing when it occurs unsignaled, though legitimate enough if accompanied by the announcement that words which normally connote introspectable states of consciousness are now technically used to refer, not to mental events or processes at all, but to complicated dispositions.

Notes

1. For a careful, illuminating analysis of these different meanings, see C. D. Broad, *The Mind and Its Place in Nature* (New York: 1929), Sec. C.

2. For a detailed analysis of disposition concepts, see the following publications: A. W. Burks, "Dispositional Statements," *Philosophy of Science,* July, 1955; R. Carnap, "The Methodological Character of Theoretical Concepts," *Minnesota Studies in the Philosophy of Science,* ed. Feigl and Scriven (Minneapolis: University of Minnesota Press, 1956), Vol. I; A. Pap, "Extensional Logic and Disposition Concepts" and W. Sellars, "Counterfactuals, Dispositions, and the Causal Modalities," both in *Minnesota Studies in the Philosophy of Science,* ed. Feigl, Scriven, and Maxwell (Minneapolis: U. of Minnesota Press, 1958), Vol. II.

3. I assume here the essential correctness of the analysis of causal explanation, as a special kind of deductive argument involving a lawlike universal premise, elaborated in Hempel and Oppenheim's "Studies in the Logic of Explanation," *Philosophy of Science,* XV, 1948.

4. The question of the relevance or irrelevance of therapeutic success to validation of psychoanalytic theory is beyond the scope of this discussion. I would just like to point out, however, that the fact that the patient's neurotic behavior disappears after the analyst gets him to believe that it served such and such unconscious purposes, has in my opinion no bearing on the question whether the analyst's "explanation" is correct. In the same way religious beliefs may be psychologically beneficial without having a clear cognitive meaning according to scientific standards of cognitive significance.

5. For a penetrating discussion of this distinction, see C. J. Ducasse, *Nature, Mind and Death* (La Salle, Ill.: Open Court Publishing Co., 1949), chap. 13.

19.

On the Structure of Psychoanalysis

FRANCIS W. GRAMLICH
Professor of Philosophy
Dartmouth College

MUCH discussion of the scientific status of psychoanalysis seems to proceed on the assumption that there is a definitive psychoanalytic theory, at least loosely comparable to a developed physical theory and therefore subject to questions and criteria which are applicable to such scientific theories. Such an assumption, however, appears unwarranted and any global consideration of the scientific status of psychoanalysis relatively fruitless.

An examination of classical psychoanalytic theory, as represented by such investigators as S. Freud, E. Jones, and H. Hartmann, among many others, shows it to be a highly complex structure. For classical theory is best viewed as incorporating five interrelated approaches to personality study, or five dimensions of theory: the genetic, the structural, the topographic, the economic, and instinct theory.[1]

Instinct theory is concerned with the ultimate underlying dynamics of personality functioning. At this level of theory Freud's hypotheses of sexual and ego instincts or, later, of Eros and Thanatos are relevant. The genetic approach explores the experiences of an individual from birth, under the assumption that personality patterns at any given time are functions of constitutional predispositions as shaped by previous experiences and present situational pressures. The stages of psychosexual development, including assertions about the "Oedipus complex,"

Notes to this section begin on page 304.

represent hypotheses in genetic theory. The structural approach, on the other hand, investigates the cross-sectional organization of the personality—for example, the relation of adaptive capacities and mechanisms, drives, and conscience and ideals, in their interaction with the external world. "Ego," "id," "superego" are prime examples of structural concepts. The fourth approach, the topographic, studies the qualitative status of the various aspects and processes of the self. For this point of view, the concepts of "conscious," "unconscious," and "preconscious" are of utmost importance. And finally the economic approach treats the internal quantitative relations of trends, processes, and structures in connection with the demands of the environment. "Fixation" and "trauma" are examples of economic concepts.

Perhaps because of their deep concern with individual therapy, wherein a unique personality is always totally at issue, classical analysts tend to stress the intimate relations and interdependencies obtaining among these different theoretical dimensions. Yet as a theory of personality, rather than a therapeutic practice, classical analysis is better construed as separate sets of concepts and hypotheses, related to each other with varying degrees of freedom, both as whole sets and part sets. For example, many, although not all, of the hypotheses in topography and economic theory are closely related (e.g., trauma, fixation, repressed unconscious); but both of these dimensions of theory are in general independent of instinct theory. This is indicated by the fact that the development of instinct theory, and its radical revision by Freud in later formulations, did not significantly change economic or topographic views. Or again, many hypotheses in structural theory are dependent on those within other branches of theory. The conception of the structure of the superego in classical theory, for instance, is highly dependent on genetic hypotheses concerning the oedipal situation and its resolution, as well as on those in instinct theory which formulate the basic sources of aggression. Yet other concepts in structural theory, for example, many of the mechanisms of defense or autonomous ego functions, seem independent of these other areas of theory.

Moreover, it is necessary to distinguish different orders or levels of concepts and hypotheses among those making up any one dimension of theory. The hypothesis of emotionally charged experiences in the history of an individual which he cannot identify as his experiences, indeed may vehemently deny, but which are dynamic conditions of his present behavior (part of the individual repressed unconscious) is certainly of quite a different order from that of emotionally charged experiences in the history of the human species which condition present individual behavior (the phylogenetic unconscious). Similarly, within instinct theory, one order of concept is that of a human "instinct" or drive as (1) deriving from a state of excitation within organ systems, (2) having an internal aim, namely a somatic modification through the removal of the excitation, and (3) an external aim or object determined by experience, and therefore subject to modification, shift, and replacement. But on quite a different level are the hypotheses of Eros, Thanatos, or the Nirvana principle.[2]

This view of classical theory as comprising sets of hypotheses of different levels or orders and of varying degrees of independence seems to provide an adequate base for interpreting the phenomenon of "schools of psychoanalytic thought" as well as to receive partial confirmation from them. Such "schools," of which the works of E. Fromm, K. Horney, and H. S. Sullivan may be taken as instances, are perhaps best interpreted not as totally different systems, but as alternative groupings of concepts and hypotheses, many of which are identical with those of classical theory, although excluding some credited by classical theory and including others it does not accept. There is, for instance, rather common acceptance by all schools of most of the economic and topographic concepts, even though these conceptual identities may in part be hidden by differences in language. There is also agreement on some of the structural hypotheses, as evidenced by the widespread crediting of the mechanism of defense, although other classical concepts in this area of theory are rejected. Neo-Freudian systems, however, generally exclude most of the concepts of instinct theory. Partly because of this revision, and partly because of the inclusion of different psycho-social views of the relation of the individual to society, these systems radically modify hypotheses in genetics.[3]

This interpretation of the internal character of classical theory and of the various schools of psychoanalysis implies that it is relatively fruitless to discuss the scientific status of psychoanalysis as an integrated system. There is quite literally no such system, Freudian or otherwise. Defense of psychoanalysis as a deductively elaborated, unified theory, or total rejection of it as a mythology seem equally pointless.

Many of the hypotheses of psychoanalysis are certainly relevant and testable, even outside the clinical situation in which they originated and to which they are particularly appropriate. Hypotheses relative to trauma, fixation, the unconscious, regression, the defense mechanisms, even types of character structure, among others, have been subjected to conditions of experimental design and at least partially confirmed.[4] Doubtless legitimate questions can be raised whether some of the hypotheses tested would be accepted by psychoanalysts as equivalent to those of analytic theory; but the total body of evidence seems to indicate a rather high degree of testability for specific and important tenets.

Another, and perhaps more important, issue is the explanatory power for individual behavior of any set of psychoanalytic hypotheses—their ability to predict that behavior, which is the primary concern of psychoanalysis. Therapeutic success cannot be taken as a criterion, as L. Kubie has pointed out. For the case of "little Hans" (1909), and of the "rat man" (1909) [5] are examples of successful therapy, and yet these cases far predated the later elaborations of classical theory. Moreover, therapists of different theoretical persuasions are reportedly equally successful therapeutically. Furthermore, the fact that a thoroughly trained practicing analyst of whatever school, if given sufficient material, can predict in a significant number of cases future bits of behavior of his own patients, or of the patients of analysts under his control, is insufficient. Such a situation, although in accord with the model of theoretical prediction, cannot be equated with it. It is one thing to be so imbedded in material and practically conversant with it that future issues and outcomes are intuitively foreseen, as in medieval feats of engineering and some modern business practices, but it is quite another to have an adequate theoretical predictive system.

Freud himself was clear that the predictive power of psychoanalysis was limited. In the last pages of *Leonardo da Vinci* Freud makes the point that, given a theoretically complete system of psychoanalysis and a theoretically complete knowledge of an individual's history, still psychoanalysis could not predict definitely that a person would "turn out so and not otherwise." [6] In particular, Freud maintains that the specific character and degree of repression and of sublimation in an individual cannot be determined within analytic theory. And since, according to Freud, repression and sublimation are basic conditions for large areas of later behavior, it follows that events in an individual's history falling within the predictive powers of analysis are severely limited. It is true Freud believed that the hypotheses of analytic theory were in themselves sufficient to predict some types of behavior, and that if they could be supplemented by data and hypotheses from other fields, for instance those in biology, the theory would be sufficiently powerful to explain an individual's life history. With the advance of knowledge, this position may perhaps turn out to be true in the future. But the view of analytic theory outlined in this paper implies that at present the position of Hempel and Oppenheim is sounder:

> When certain peculiarities in the work of an artist are explained as outgrowths of a specific type of neurosis, this observation may contain significant clues, but in general does not afford a sufficient basis for a potential prediction of those peculiarities. In cases of this kind, an incomplete explanation may at best be considered as indicating some positive correlation between the antecedent conditions adduced and the type of phenomenon to be explained, and as pointing out a direction in which further research might be carried on in order to complete the explanatory account.[7]

At the present time such research would certainly involve identification and clarification of concepts and hypotheses in psychoanalytic literature with the hope of attaining general agreement, if only at the level of meaning, on as many as possible of those usually held important in analytic theory. Madison's analysis of the various meanings of "repression" in Freud's works,[8] Weiss's comparative study of ego concepts in psychoanalysis,[9] or even the difference between Freud's relatively crude statement of the oedipal situation in the *Outline of Psychoanalysis* and his relatively refined statement in *The Ego and the Id* suggest that this task is not so simple as it might seem. It becomes even more complicated when hypotheses dealing with the same subject and of the same formal structure are stated in quite different empirical terms and contexts in different systems, like, for example, many that concern anxiety in Freud's *Problem of Anxiety* and in Fromm's *Escape from Freedom*.

Such identification and clarification, however, is not only a condition for the institution of procedures outside the clinical situation which would more adequately test "what is really meant" by psychoanalytic theory, but is clearly a prerequisite to discerning the various types of hypotheses and specifying the relations obtaining among them. In all branches of theory, rigorous application of criteria of order, for example those proposed by Hempel and Oppenheim, might well raise serious issues concerning the function and the requiredness of many proposed theories. In Freud's writings, for instance, anxiety in the oedipal situation is regarded as in part dependent on anxiety related to the birth situation as "prototypical"; and, furthermore, individual repression is considered as partly dependent on a phylogenetic base, which may also be taken as "prototypical." Yet the function of such "prototype" concepts and the kind of dependency involved, so far as I know, are yet to be clearly specified.[10] Distinguishing different types and orders of hypotheses and clarifying their relation, in neo-Freudian as well as classical theory, would, I suspect, show that some theses are systematically irrelevant, and in addition would shear away a mass of pseudo-scientific overlay. The ultimate goal of such an endeavor would be a progressively more systematized body of hypotheses with increasing predictive power.[11]

Notes

1. *Cf.* R. Munroe, *Schools of Psychoanalytic Thought* (New York: The Dryden Press, 1955), esp. chap. 3; O. Fenichel, *The Psychoanalytic Theory of Neurosis* (New York: W. W. Norton and Co., 1945), esp. chaps. 2 and 5; S. Freud, *A General Introduction to Psychoanalysis*, esp. chaps. 18–26; S. Freud, *New Introductory Lectures on Psychoanalysis* (New York: W. W. Norton and Co., 1933), esp. chaps. 3 and 4; S. Freud, "Analysis Terminable and Interminable," *Collected Papers* (London: Hogarth Press, 1950), Vol. V.

2. O. Fenichel, *op. cit.*, pp. 55f; S. Freud, *New Introductory Lectures on Psychoanalysis*, pp. 131f.

3. *Cf.* R. Munroe, *op. cit.*, esp. Part Three.

4. Many studies are cited in G. S. Blum, *Psychoanalytic Theories of Personality* (New York: McGraw-Hill, 1953).

5. S. Freud, *Collected Papers* (London: Hogarth Press, 1943), Vol. III.

6. S. Freud, *Leonardo da Vinci* (New York: Random House, 1947), p. 119.

7. C. G. Hempel and P. Oppenheim, "The Logic of Explanation," H. Feigl and M. Brodbeck, *Readings in the Philosophy of Science* (New York: Appleton-Century-Crofts, Inc., 1953), p. 324.

8. P. Madison, "Freud's Repression Concept," *International Journal of Psycho-Analysis*, XXXVII (1956), pp. 75–81.

9. E. Weiss, "A Comparative Study of Psychoanalytical Ego Concepts," *International Journal of Psycho-Analysis*, XXXVIII (1957), pp. 209–22.

10. *Cf.* O. Fenichel, *op. cit.*, pp. 97–98.

11. I am indebted to my colleague, Dr. T. J. Duggan, for his suggestions and criticism.

20.

Psychoanalysis and Scientific Method

ROBERT E. SILVERMAN
Associate Professor of Psychology
New York University

DR. HARTMANN'S paper and Dr. Kubie's discussion once again reaffirm the position that psychoanalysis is a scientific discipline, although not science *qua* physics. Dr. Nagel agrees that we should expect to find neither the precision of physics nor the clarity of physical models in psychoanalysis. Nevertheless, Dr. Nagel points out that psychoanalysis is deficient in many of the requirements of scientific theory, these deficiencies occurring in both the logical and empirical aspects of the theory. I agree with Dr. Nagel that the logical structure of psychoanalytic theory is not adequate. There are few if any rules of correspondence linking constructs to each other and to observables, terms are not defined, and the deductions are often vague and contradictory. However, in my opinion, the empirical deficiencies are, at the moment, more important in view of the widely held belief by both lay and professional persons that psychoanalytic theory rests on a body of empirical knowledge and is contributing further knowledge about the behavior of man.

Dr. Nagel describes three kinds of evidence which make up the empirical foundations of psychoanalysis. Of these three, clinical data, experimental findings, and anthropological observations, only the clinical findings play a significant part in the theory. If psychoanalytic theory rested largely on experimental findings or on anthropological observations, there would be no highly elaborated theory. The so-called experimental findings are usually experimental analogues demonstrating a particular phenomenon in lower animals and occasionally in man. They are not controlled experiments designed to test an hypothesis such that a negative finding would have meaning. A case in point is the experimental analogue of displacement, where the experimental setting is designed to produce a class of behaviors which can be labelled displacement in that they resemble the phenomenon described by Freud. In this case, failure to find displacement is more a testimony to a lack of ingenuity than to a lack in any theory. To find anthropological supports for psychoanalytic theory one would have to choose among a welter of observations, some objective, some subjective, some confirming psychoanalytic propositions and some refuting these same propositions. Few psychoanalytic theorists would cite anthropology as a basis for the theory.

Psychoanalytic theory is based on clinical evidence, and it is these data which must be examined in considering the empirical aspects of the theory. The question is not one of evaluating the acceptability of clinical data in general. These data can be objective, for, as Dr. Kubie stated, it would not be difficult to record clinical interviews in order to have a record open to objective scrutiny. (It should be noted that very little of this has been done.) The question is one of what constitutes a test and confirmation of an hypothesis. It is here that the views of psychoanalytic investigators depart from the established tenets of empirical science. Psychoanalysts appear either to ignore the probabilistic basis of prediction or to base their predictions on a purely rationalist theory of probability. In either case, a basic principle of empirical science is violated. In scientific endeavors, prediction is based upon the relative-frequency interpretation of probability. Predictions are made in terms of the relative frequency with which an event will occur in a specified class of events, and confirmation is in terms of agreement with observations. Perhaps it was Freud's interest in the patient, the single case, that led him to ignore empirical probability. Freud considered himself to be an empiricist, but his techniques of observing, recording, and testing propositions belie this belief. Following Freud, contemporary psychoanalysts have been content to consider their discipline as being apart from the predictive-knowledge requirements which mark all empirical science. The "predicting the past" to which Dr. Hartmann frequently refers would be an acceptable form of prediction if probability were considered. It is not sufficient to predict from an analytic session that a patient witnessed the primal scene as a young child and then accept as confirmation for the theory of repression the fact that in a later session, following an interpretation, the patient recalls the event. What is the percentage of patients who recall primal scenes during psychoanalytic treatment? Under what circumstances do these recollections occur? Given these circumstances, do all patients recall primal scenes or other so-called repressions? These and many similar questions must be considered in order to confirm or refute the theoretical proposition. It is the failure to recognize these requirements that permits psychoanalytic theorists to base their assertions on selected demonstrations rather than upon experiments, clinical or other.

21.

Psychoanalysis and Logical Positivism

PHILIPP FRANK
President
Institute for the Unity of Science

IF WE want to understand thoroughly the status of psychoanalysis within the general body of scientific knowledge, we are bound to direct our attention to those theories of knowledge which have formulated the strictest criteria of admission into the realm of legitimate science.

Since the second quarter of our twentieth century the principal advocate of strict criteria for admission has been the school of Logical Positivism which originated from the "Vienna Circle" (1920–1935).

Obviously it would be difficult to prove that the theories of Freud or Jung could satisfy the criteria of acceptance advanced by Logical Positivism and shaped according to the model of mathematical physics. However, it is a matter of fact that among the founders of Logical Positivism, the members of the Vienna Circle, there have been quite a few scientists who exhibited a certain sympathy with the teachings of psychoanalysis. There was certainly no great inclination to pass a harsh judgment upon the discrepancy between the Freudian doctrine and the strict criteria of acceptance applied to general theories. Rarely were the psychoanalytic doctrines called "meaningless" or "tautological," as representatives of Logical Positivism have often and gladly branded the doctrines of "school philosophy" like Platonism, Thomism or even Kantianism. Otto Neurath, who was one of the leading members of the Vienna Circle and one of the strictest judges on "unscientific" and "meaningless" statements, said repeatedly about psychoanalytical theories that they revealed connections between a great range of new and surprising observed facts; hence one should not discourage this kind of research, although it is far from being logically and semantically satisfactory. This has also been the opinion of Rudolf Carnap and other positivists.

It is certainly a fact that the roots of psychoanalysis and of Logical Positivism grew up in one and the same soil, the intellectual and social climate of Vienna before and after the first World War. It is also a fact that among the workers in psychoanalysis there was a considerable group who attempted to keep contact with the Vienna Circle. We have only to mention Heinz Hartmann, who has been instrumental in keeping psychoanalysis close to scientific methods.

In order to understand this situation we have to glance at the original view of the Vienna Circle on science. This view has sometimes been obscured by a crust of technicalities, and it is certainly good occasionally to give a hard look at the core.

According to the usage of terms in modern science, a theory is "scientifically confirmed" if, firstly, all facts which are derived from the theory are in agreement with actual observation, and, secondly, if there is a great number of observable facts which *can* be derived from the theory. The latter criterion is to be taken with a grain of salt. The doctrine of Logical Positivism has always and precisely emphasized the point that from the theory itself observable facts can be derived only indirectly. The theory itself is a system of axioms (e.g., the axioms of Euclidean geometry); the axioms are not statements about observable phenomena, but they state relations between abstract concepts (or symbols) like "point," "straight line," "length," "congruence," etc. In order to derive observable facts from a theory we have to connect these abstract concepts with actual observations. The term "length," for example, has to be connected with an operation by which we can actually measure the length of a body. These connecting propositions have been introduced under different names: "rules of coordination," "operational definitions," "semantical rules," "epistemic correlations," etc. These propositions contain the description of actually observable facts and are formulated partly in the language of our everyday life.

It is easy to see that the operations which define "length" or "temperature" (let alone the operations which define "energy" or similar concepts) can be carried out only under particularly "smooth" conditions. There must not be abrupt spatial or temporal changes in temperature or density of matter. Hence, concepts like "energy" or "temperature" have certainly no general meaning; they can only be applied under smooth conditions. This very important point has been made repeatedly by P. W. Bridgman, most elaborately in his book on the *Foundations of Thermodynamics*.

If we say, for example, that the law of inertia or the law of the conservation of energy is confirmed by science, we mean only that there are in nature frequently conditions which can be regarded as smooth and can be, therefore, described by those laws. We must always have in mind that the facts of human behavior which are treated by psychology or sociology can hardly be described as smooth conditions.

It is well known that a sophisticated and somewhat malicious critic of physical science could easily uphold the proposition that the law of conservation of energy is confirmed by science not generally but only under certain restricted conditions. One could even uphold the statement that this law is in general meaningless or even tautological. Such an argument has been made by men like H. Poincaré and P. Duhem; it has been used (or misused) to prove that the general laws of traditional science are not better confirmed than the principles of theology. These authors claim that the general principles of science (inertia, conservation, etc.) are nothing but disguised definitions of terms like "rectilinear motion," "uniform motion," "energy," etc. This interpretation has been widely used as a proof of the inability of science to establish the "truth" of its general statements.

Logical Positivism accepted Poincaré's doctrine that a system of axiomatic principles can neither be confirmed nor refuted by actual sense observations. A system of axioms can be tested only if operational definitions are added. The statement "A system of axioms is confirmed by observations" means exactly: We can find convenient operational definitions which convert by their additions the system of axioms into a system of propositions that actually agree with observable facts. Since the term "convenient" has a purely pragmatic meaning, the expression "confirmation of a theory by observation or experiment" is pragmatic too. We can say that one theory is more practical or convenient than another one, but it does not make scientific sense to say that one theory is completely confirmed or completely refuted. J. B. Conant says in his book *Science and Common Sense,* commenting on the phlogiston theory in chemistry, that a theory was never refuted by a single experiment or observation, but only replaced by a new theory.

Hence, the truth of Freudian or similar theories must not be understood otherwise than pragmatically. It may be convenient or not to accept them.

But the convenience of a theory like psychoanalysis depends upon a great many factors, among which agreement with observations is only one. We have always to consider the agreement with the experience of everyday life, with the general philosophy of the period, the fitness to support some ways of life, some political, moral, and religious creeds.

There has been frequently a dilemma: Should we cover rather interesting new "facts" (direct observations) by a system which is too loosely knit to satisfy the criteria of Logical Positivism? Or should we keep strictly to these criteria and exclude some stimulating new facts from systematic treatment?

If we were to formulate this dilemma in an exaggerated way, we would say: We have a choice between a perfectly logical system which covers only a small number of observed facts and a system which covers a great realm of facts but is in some respects rather vague.

The general doctrine of the Vienna Circle does not solve this dilemma but recommends a compromise which depends upon the merits of any special case. It depends upon whether one believes that a theory like that of psychoanalysis provides important practical help in life or not.

The fundamental approach of the Vienna Circle to science was essentially pragmatic.

It is formulated well in Bridgman's statement that a theory is a "program of action." There have been brilliant men in the Vienna Circle who have developed the logical and semantic components to a high degree of perfection. Philosophers and scientists have been impressed by these successes so frequently and intensively that they have disregarded altogether the pragmatic component. However, leading authors of the Circle like Rudolf Carnap and Charles Morris have always stressed the indivisible trinity of the logical, the semantic, and the pragmatic components.

In order to understand well the attitude of the Vienna Circle towards psychoanalysis it is helpful to remember its attitude towards Marxism. Research on the connection between history and economic conditions has been generally encouraged as useful, and "historical materialism" has been regarded with an attitude of approval, while "dialectical materialism" has been mostly disapproved as a typically metaphysical doctrine.

There were even scientists in the Vienna Circle who manifested some interest in parapsychological research (such as on extrasensory perception) because they believed that there is a certain (even if small) probability that by this research new phenomena may be discovered. This line was pursued even by some strict mathematicians and logicians.

According to Logical Positivism, the system of axioms and the system of observed facts are, in principle, two independent systems which have their own lives. They are connected only by operational definitions. They form together a confirmed scientific theory if they have some points of contact where their agreement can be found. The more points of contact, the better. However, how many points of contact have to exist in a theory cannot be derived by any logical argument; it is a question of convenience and practice. It has been a main thesis of Positivism, from Auguste Comte to the Vienna Circle, that the axiomatic system by itself, as an isolated system, does not tell us any "intrinsic truth" about the real world.

From all these remarks it becomes clear that in terms of the general principles of Logical Positivism there is no reason for disliking psychoanalytical theories. It is a question to be determined by actual research, by observations and logical chains, whether theories such as Freud's should be approved by Logical Positivists.

22.

Meaning and Theoretical Terms in Psychoanalysis

ARTHUR C. DANTO
Assistant Professor of Philosophy
Columbia University

I WANT to remark on two features of our discussion of psychoanalysis which seem totally unrelated to the subject of our discussion. The first is that it often resembled a debate between believers and nonbelievers. And the second is that criticisms of psychoanalysis often sounded like *ad hominem* derogations of psychoanalysts. The purpose of this paper is to show that these features of the discussion are in fact related to the subject under discussion. But this will really be just a convenient way for me to bring out certain characteristics of psychoanalytical theory.

I

It is by now a commonplace to point out that a great many of the most highly developed and powerful scientific theories employ terms that are not explicitly definable in the language of observation. The concepts that these terms represent can hardly be understood in isolation from the system of propositions which makes up the total theory—except, perhaps, through the furnishing of intuitive models for the theory. But such models are largely heuristic; and the theory applies to the world only to the degree that some set of semantic rules relates these crucial terms to experience in some way which will effect a confirming relationship between sentences in the theory and sentences whose truth is decided by direct test and experiment. Thanks to a rather extraordinary result of William Craig, it is actually possible to replace a language which satisfies certain minimal formal criteria and which contains dubious terms, with another language free of just these terms, and with no sacrifice of theorems in the original language. For reasons not yet wholly clear, Craig's theorem is oddly trivial. And it has brought cold comfort to those very philosophers whose stringent programs of reduction might be expected to find it congenial. So as matters stand, theoretical terms must be counted uneliminable, and a person who demands that every properly scientific term be redeemed (without remainder) with observational equivalents, merely betrays allegiance to a superannuated empiricism.

It is hardly damaging any longer, therefore, to accuse psychoanalysis of being unscientific by virtue of its trafficking in unobservables. Providing that the theoretical terms function in psychoanalytical theories the way they do in (say) physical theories, and providing that psychoanalytical theories come up to the mark on syntactical grounds, the two could hardly be contrasted invidiously. So far as unobservableness goes, there is little to chose as between castration complexes and psi-functions. Perhaps it is unduly charitable to admit an analogy between psychoanalytical and physical theories on the slim basis of their mutual utilization of theoretical terms, but for the moment this does not concern me. What I want to do is to point out that two different questions relating to meaning might be raised about these theoretical terms. First we can ask whether they denote. And secondly we can ask what are the semantic rules that allow them to be significantly employed. I hope that a few brief words on each of these questions will help clarify some features of psychoanalytical theory.

II

When we ask whether a theoretical term denotes, we are in effect asking whether or not there is some entity in the real world for which the term stands. And of course there is an argument, even in physics, whether there are such things as electrons, fields, and the like. Einstein wished to look at electrons the way God does—the implication being that only what is can be looked at, and that it is a contingent fact that *we* can't see electrons. But other physicists are prepared to disallow electrons as entities, viewing them as convenient artifices, integral to a theory which works well enough whether or not there are in fact electrons. And similarly, two physicists might use the Maxwell equations and yet argue over the reality of fields. But this then becomes a matter of competing ontologies and, so long as no party to the dispute has evidence lacking to the other one, the disagreement is one in faith—a disagreement in belief which resembles a disagreement in attitude. And so long as there is unanimity in practice, the issue of denotation is an indulgence in philosophical luxury.

Now exactly similar considerations bear on the denotation of psychoanalytical terms. Are we to reckon complexes ("unconscious ideas surcharged with energy") as amongst the world's stock of entities? Or as theoretical conveniences? Parity with physical theory would suggest that here too it is an option for faith. Yet I think it is part of the psychoanalyst's commitment to believe in the existence of these *essentially* covert entities. And very frequently defenses of psychoanalytical theory are in fact no more than arguments in favor of the existence of these entities. (Often the evidence consists in exactly those facts the concept is invoked to explain.) So I think it would be intolerable to them to suggest that these might be only systematically required by a theory, the main purpose of which is to predict behavior. For it is, after all, the proud claim of psychoanalysis to have *discovered* the real mechanisms of the psyche, and to have produced a revolutionary and true image of man based on these discoveries.

But surely it is possible for a theory to be true independently of whether its theoretical terms denote, the criteria for the truth of theories lying elsewhere. And surely we may discuss the adequacies of theories quite independently of the ontologies subscribed to by theorists. There is a sense in which any important theory is a picture, but not every picture is a portrait. And it is here that Freud's models, brilliant as they often are, can be misleading. But since psychoanalysts often identify the issues of adequacy and ontology, this might go a long way toward explaining why our discussion so frequently resembled a debate between believers and nonbelievers.

III

The issue of denotation is secondary, I think, to the issue of semantic rules, the rules whereby the terms embodied in a theory get related to terms embodied in directly testable sentences. This is what I now want to discuss. For I think many of the philosophers present were dissatisfied with psychoanalysis mainly on this score.

Professor Hook raised the question whether psychoanalysts would ever admit the possibility that the Oedipus complex might not be ubiquitous. The psychoanalysts answered that if they could find an adult human, or a child of the required age, who failed to have hostile and genital desires towards one parent (of the same sex as that person), and who failed, at the same time, to wish to replace that parent in the affection and esteem of the parent of the opposite sex, then indeed the proposition that the Oedipus complex is universal would be falsified. They very much doubted, however, that such an individual might be found. But what they did not realize was, I think, that they had only retranslated Professor Hook's question. For I believe Professor Hook really wanted to know whether there are observable traits which all psychoanalysts might admit to be precisely what is required if the predicate "is oedipal" is to be applied. And I suspect he was implying that the semantic rules here are so flexible and arbitrary that the predicate can be applied come what may. And this is what led Professor Black to ask whether psychoanalysts mean *anything* by the term "Oedipus complex." For unless and until the semantic rules are clarified, it is hardly worth asking whether the proposition in question is true or false or confirmed to any degree.

Now of course psychoanalysts do mean *something* by "Oedipus complex" (and not merely that it denotes an energized unconscious idea). But it is also clear that whatever are the semantic rules they employ, these must be complex to an extraordinary degree. So complex, in fact, that a statement of the rule would very likely involve an enormously long disjunction of observation predicates, with each disjunct itself highly complex. But this then means that it requires considerable training, responsibility, and experience ever to be able to apply that term (or any other theoretical term in psychoanalysis). And it probably requires a special intuition as well. So the theory may in fact be exceedingly simple, but the rules for interpreting it from case to case almost unbelievably complicated. Only an expert, then, can really even understand the theory. I think this is the way a psychoanalyst would reply ultimately to Professor Hook's query.

But then it is easy to see why a philosopher might be suspicious, might wonder, in view of these labyrinthine rules, whether the psychoanalyst is really ever *using the theory,* and not, rather, *simply* relying on intuition. And he might wonder, further, whether there can now be any sense in which the theory might be invalidated. For it sounds like this: it is like a certain land in which every citizen is claimed to be guilty, and where it is up to the lawyers of the land to show how this is true for each citizen. It sounds rather more like casuistry than science. For to ask whether the theory is true is *now* to ask whether we have confidence in its practitioners to interpret it—as though there were something like an internal relation. Which then would go a long way towards explaining why criticisms of psychoanalysis so often take the form of *ad hominem* derogations of psychoanalysts.

23.

Psychoanalysis and Suggestion: Metaphysics and Temperament

C. J. DUCASSE
Professor Emeritus of Philosophy
Brown University

MY FIRST comment on the "Psychoanalysis, Scientific Method, and Philosophy" symposium is prompted by the fact that, so far as I am able to ascertain, psychoanalysts achieve some therapeutic successes and also meet with some failures, irrespective of the particular psychoanalytic school to which they adhere; and moreover that a somewhat similar state of affairs, although as regards ailments perhaps usually different, seems to obtain in the case of the practitioners of various forms of "faith cure."

The hypothesis this brings to my mind is that *suggestion* may be what chiefly operates both in the successes and in the failures that occur, notwithstanding the diversity of the methods of treatment and of the theories on which the methods rest. Strangely, however, suggestion was hardly mentioned at all, so as far as I can remember, either in the papers presented at the symposium or in the discussions of them.

The term "suggestion" of course frequently occurs in the literature of the field of psychotherapeutics as well as outside; but, even when the process it designates plays a major role in a therapy described, explicit analysis of what suggestion essentially consists in is seldom provided. Perhaps, therefore, an attempt to define it with some precision may not be amiss here.

I submit, then, that suggestion is essentially presentation of an idea to a person in such manner that his critical apparatus is not brought to bear upon it at the time; and that a person's "critical apparatus" consists essentially of the following three things: (a) a set of ideas he somehow already believes; (b) the capacity to compare the newly presented idea with those he already believes; and (c) the capacity to perceive the compatibility or incompatibility of it with one or others of them.

According as an idea presented to a person is liked or disliked by him, he respectively believes or disbelieves it automatically (a) if *none* of his existing beliefs or disbeliefs *is relevant to* its acceptability; or (b) if it is presented in a manner, or under circumstances, that *allow no opportunity for comparison* of it with such of his beliefs or disbeliefs as are relevant to its acceptability; or (c) if, on comparison, he *fails to perceive* the compatibility or incompatibility of it with beliefs or disbeliefs of his that are relevant to its acceptability.

Thus, whereas in the process called *persuasion,* criticisms of an idea presented are invited and each in turn is then shown not to invalidate the presented idea; in *suggestion,* on the contrary, uncritical acceptance of an idea is insured by presenting it in a manner that gives criticisms no opportunity to arise.

It must be stressed that suggestion of an idea to a person need not consist of overt assertion of it. A question may suggest it more effectively. For example, the question "Did he succeed?" insinuates, i.e., suggests, that he tried. Or a prestigious or otherwise question-begging epithet may be used.

But suggestion occurs in many cases altogether without words: perception of people running away from something suggests that the thing is dangerous; seeing one person bow to another suggests that the latter deserves respect; our peering, or listening, suggests to those who watch us that something of interest is to be seen or to be heard. A particular psychoanalyst's tone, facial expression, manner, method, or professional title—even apart from what he may be saying—can strongly suggest to a patient that that analyst does (or as the case may be, that he does not) have the capacity to deal successfully with the patient's difficulties.

Again, a person's own emotions, wishes, and aversions automatically suggest to him beliefs consonant with them about their objects. And the performances of prestidigitators make evident how much of what we naively say we perceive is, *on normal occasions as well as on these contrived ones,* not actually perceived but only suggested by what we actually perceive. The difference is only that, on normal occasions, that which is suggested by what we strictly perceive is true; whereas in cases of sleight-of-hand it is false.

Lastly, observation of persons under deep hypnosis furnishes evidence that the power which a belief that is unquestioningly harbored has to influence behavior, feelings, sensations, and thoughts, and even to cause somatic effects, may well be sufficient to account for many of the results which analysts ascribe to the psychoanalytic process. Anyway, as the remarks made up to this point will have made clear, suggestion extensively occurs automatically in the course of the relation between the analyst and his patient. Hence the question is only how far the successes obtained by the analyst are due to the power of suggestion, and how far to the patient's understanding of self and to the emotional release effected by the analysis.

I turn now to Professor Lazerowitz's contention "that the philosopher, despite all appearances, does not use language to express scientific propositions but instead uses it in such a way as to create the illusion of doing so, while in fact he gives expression *only* to his unconscious fantasies."

The first comment that comes to mind is, of course, that since that statement is itself a philosophical one—belonging as it does to the philosophy of philosophy—it does not express a scientific proposition but is *only* symptomatic of Professor Lazerowitz's own unconscious fantasies!

Behind this self-stultifying character of his statement, however, there are some truths which emerge when the statement is properly qualified.

The first is that when "metaphysics" is conceived, in the Bradleyan manner, as speculation concerning the nature and the structure of "reality," then what a metaphysical statement ultimately expresses is not a *hypothesis*—which as such would either be true or be false—but a *position,* i.e., a *positing* of some characteristic which *the metaphysician concerned* tacitly or explicitly *adopts* as criterion of realness.

Then "reality" and "real," as used by him, are essentially *value terms:* they make known what in *his* view is fundamentally significant or important in the universe. And, because what they express or illustrate is thus simply *what criterion of significance or importance he has adopted,* the statements in which he uses those terms as subject or as predicate cannot without incongruity be criticized as true or as false, but only as clear or vague, or as grammatically correct or incorrect, or conceivably even as veracious or mendacious.

But what a given person takes thus as fundamental is doubtless determined in part by what one may call his "temperament"; and some of the psychological roots of his temperament doubtless are fed by the contents of the unconscious regions of his mind. Only so much of truth is contained in Professor Lazerowitz's indefensibly sweeping statement.

Another truth, to which his paper points, is that some of the disputes among philosophers are, in fact even when unawares, over proposals to alter the current usage of some particular word. But that the alterations proposed are, as Professor Lazerowitz asserts, *arbitrary,* is not true in analytical philosophy as distinguished from irresponsible metaphysical speculation.

The crucial fact he altogether ignores in this connection is that ordinary language is a very defective instrument of communication and of inference because of the vagueness and ambiguity of many of its terms, and because of the inconsistencies and incongruities that infest the actual usage of them. Ordinary language is basic only in that it is the only instrument we originally have, wherewith to purge *it* of its own innumerable defects.

Now, when alteration of the actual usage of certain words is urged, it may be urged not arbitrarily but in order to eliminate from it for instance a contradiction to which it is naively blind, but which none the less *demonstrably* infects and condemns the particular bit of actual usage concerned.

Consider for example Professor Lazerowitz's statement that "as a matter of fact, the terms 'event' and 'has a cause' are so used in everyday speech that 'is an event but lacks a cause' is a descriptive phrase." This is true enough, but does not settle the question whether what that phrase describes is, hiddenly but in fact, a contradiction. Whether it is so or not depends in part on what one takes *causality* to consist in. If, as Hume does, one takes it to consist in purely *de facto* regularity of sequence in our past experience, then there is no contradiction in the supposition that a given event had no cause.

But, irrespective of whether Hume's conception of causality was—as Professor Lazerowitz alleges in the case of Spinoza's—prompted in some way by the particular history of his childhood curiosity about sex and birth, one may object to Hume's conception of causality on the prosaically factual ground that it would require us to apply the term "cause of" to certain cases to which *actual usage* denies that name; and also would forbid us to apply it to certain cases to which *actual usage* does apply it. And it may well be that a definition of causality that would really fit actual applicative usage of "cause of" would entail that the phrase "an uncaused event" *is,* hiddenly but in fact, self-contradictory, as I have elsewhere argued is actually the case. It is well to note that, similarly, actual usage does not proscribe the phrase "is a cube and is the sum of two cubes"; yet it does imply a contradiction, although it is by no means easy to show it.

The essential point the preceding comments illustrate is the commonplace one, neglected by Professor Lazerowitz's paper, that actual usage employs a given term sometimes *indicatively* and sometimes *predicatively;* and that it is always a relevant and factual question whether an individual thing, which actual usage *indicates,* i.e., denotes, by the given term, does or does not possess the characters which actual usage also employs the same term to *predicate.* Actual usage, for example, *applies* the name "fish" to lobsters, clams, crabs, etc.: it calls them "shell fish." Yet they lack some of the characters that actual usage *implies* by the term "fish." That is, actual usage is, in this case as in many others, *demonstrably* inconsistent.

In any such case, a proposal to alter actual usage is not *arbitrary,* but *sanatory*!

24.

The Status of Freud's Ideas

CHARLES FRANKEL
Professor of Philosophy
Columbia University

FREUD'S work carries an intellectual excitement to which it is difficult not to respond. Men have always been aware that there is much not only in the external world but in their inner lives which seems to take place without a cause and to serve no clear purpose—that dreams, moods, attachments to other persons, come and go as though they had lives of their own and were independent of the individual's will. But Freud used these apparently most "irrational" and "capricious" aspects of human experience to show that the mind and emotions have a rational order. He suggested a cause for what seems to have no cause, and a purpose behind the apparently purposeless. Whether we agree with Freud's system or not, it is an impressive imaginative achievement. It exhibits the stubborn refusal to be seduced by pleasant pictures that we expect of products of the scientific mind. But it deals with things men cannot help but take most seriously of all, and it has the sweep, the emotional impact, and some of the mysteriousness, of ancient theological or poetic visions.

All this, however, does not tell us the exact status of Freud's ideas. Was Freud the Lucretius or the Newton of psychology? Did he have an embracing vision of human life which is false in its details, but which at least follows in a crude way what we take to be the right model for the study of human affairs? Or did Freud lay down the basic theories and make the fundamental observations on which a systematic science has been, or can be, logically erected? Indeed, are Freudian theories perhaps only evocative myths, which, like most myths, correlate a large and interesting group of phenomena, but at the expense of assumptions that are clearly false, superfluous, or vague? These questions remain even after we recognize Freud's genius; and, as Dr. Kubie points out, they cannot be answered by pointing to the usefulness of Freudian doctrine as an instrument of therapy. For if these questions remain unanswered we also do not know whether Freud was not just a sort of alchemist of the soul, who could produce all sorts of startling effects without ever knowing what precise effects they were or quite how he produced them.

Unfortunately, in dealing with these fundamental issues we are not carried very far by general statements to the effect that "the unconscious" is basic to the understanding of human behavior, that this is the essential concept of psychoanalysis, and that Freud must be credited with its discovery. For Freud was not the first—nor has he been the last—to assert that overt and deliberate human behavior is but a small part of a complex system of events which are mainly hidden from view, but which must be taken into account in explaining why human beings act as they do. One can be a believer in witchcraft, or, indeed, a Watsonian behaviorist, and believe that much. The crucial question is whether the specific ideas which Freud introduced—e.g., the "id," the "Oedipus complex," the "death wish," etc.—correctly describe this system of events. And to answer this question such concepts must be much more precisely defined than I believe they are in most statements of psychoanalytic theory with which I am acquainted.

An example may illustrate the difficulty. It has been suggested at this meeting that one decisive test of the doctrine of the "Oedipus complex" would be to see if there were any children who did not have murderous or incestuous fantasies about their parents. This goes a long way towards indicating the empirical conditions under which the theory of the "Oedipus complex" might be confirmed or disconfirmed. But at least two problems remain. The first is to give a meaning to terms like "incestuous" or "murderous" that is not too far removed from the meaning these terms carry in ordinary use. Similarly, the idea of "sex" needs explication, particularly as it figures in such notions as "infant sexuality" and "polymorphous perversity." Presumably, analysts use such terms in the belief that their meanings are continuous with their meanings in ordinary usage. But if this is so, if these terms are not simply old words bent to entirely new uses, the justification for using them to describe the overt phenomena analysts have in mind is not at all clear.

A second problem is to show that the phenomena in question are explicable only by the specific theory under examination. For even if we did find that all children have murderous and incestuous fantasies, this would not be sufficient to support the theory of the "Oedipus complex." For this theory argues not simply that children have such feelings, but that these feelings arise as incidents of growth, and independently of any distinctive set of circumstances. To consider an analogy, they are events like the loss by all children of their milk teeth. But to pursue this analogy, if a child falls down and loses a tooth, this is entirely independent of the biological process by which children lose their milk teeth, and the occurrence of such an event is entirely irrelevant to the thesis that such a process takes place. Similarly, it seems more than reasonable to suppose that most children—perhaps all—will have occasion to be irritated with their parents. But the discovery that they have such feelings is not by itself enough to support the theory of the "Oedipus complex."

There is in fact a fundamental sort of vagueness in most statements of psychoanalytic theory which makes objective appraisal of the theory difficult. As supporting evidence for the truth of psychoanalytic theories it is common, for example, to point to the success psychoanalysts have in predicting the future course of behavior of their patients, or in discovering items in their patients' biographies which the patients themselves have forgotten. But it would be astonishing if psychoanalysts did not have such success. They are intelligent men, and they develop a close relationship to those they treat. But most of us, given similarly close relationships, can predict the future behavior of our friends in specific circumstances, or can correctly guess that Mr. Jones had a harsh father or Mr. Smith a puritanical mother even though Messrs. Jones and Smith have never told us so. Of course, we sometimes make mistakes. But surely psychoanalysts do, too. The question, in short, is not whether men who believe in psychoanalytic theories can successfully predict human behavior. The question is whether they can make predictions which others who do not hold these theories cannot make, and whether these predictions follow logically from the theories in question. To consider this issue, a precise and orderly formulation of psychoanalytic theory is necessary. Such a formulation may well be possible. In my judgment, however, it has not been produced at this meeting.

These comments bring me to Professor Lazerowitz's speculations about the psychic sources of philosophic doctrines with which he disagrees. I cannot share Professor Lazerowitz's sense of assurance that some truths in philosophy are so clear that one must go to pathology to explain why otherwise intelligent men did not see them. And while I do not find the philosophies of Spinoza or Bradley much more convincing than he does, I am also unable to regard it as a sign of perversity in these men that they did not have at their finger tips philosophic techniques which have only been developed in the twentieth century. Regrettably, these and other features of Professor Lazerowitz's essay make it a fairly representative example of an increasingly widespread tendency in the use of Freudian ideas. These ideas have come to serve some of the traditional uses of a theology. Freudian doctrine, for example, provides a language for saying silly things in an impressive way. Professor Lazerowitz's suggestion that Spinoza's philosophic inquiries stemmed from a perplexity about what makes babies is a case in point. Again, Freudian language offers a way of inflating the importance of findings that are merely banal. Professor Lazerowitz's elaborate argument to the effect that Spinoza and Bradley had deep emotional investments in their philosophies is once more an example. One does not need Freud, after all, to make this "discovery." One need only read the perfectly explicit statements of Spinoza and Bradley themselves. Bradley says in his *Logic* that he seeks a position which satisfies the heart as well as the mind. And

Spinoza states that it is the purpose of his philosophic effort to find an object of love so perfect that it will release him from emotional bondage to what is imperfect. Is it really news that men's preferences in philosophy are likely to spring from deeper sources, and to be more passionate than their preferences in, say, dictionaries?

There is still another respect in which Freud's views have been used as a theology. They have come to be used as a generalized technique for explaining the evil ways of the opposition. Probably the most widespread use of Freudian theory, outside strictly medical contexts, is its use as an "unmasking" technique, as a way of deflating the things we dislike. This use of psychoanalytic theory does more than make dispassionate intellectual discussion difficult. It also narrows the potential bearing of the theory and obscures a fundamental issue. For if Freudian theories are true theories of human nature they can and should be invoked to explain why men discover the truth as well as why they go wrong. If Professor Lazerowitz accepts Freudian theory, for example, he should use it to explain his friends as well as his enemies. For the same general laws presumably apply to both groups. In fact, a fundamental test of Freud's doctrines is precisely whether they can be used to explain the normal or the successful in human life. They must meet this test if the general claims that are made for them are to be vindicated. I do not know whether they can or cannot meet this test. But I am sure that the use of Freud's ideas as vehicles for unharnessed speculation does not help.

25.

Psychoanalysis: Science and Philosophy

RAPHAEL DEMOS
Professor of Philosophy
Harvard University

I. Psychoanalysis and Science

THESE remarks are directed to Professor Nagel's comments, vigorously supported by Professor Scriven and others, concerning the dubious status (as Professor Nagel saw it) of psychoanalysis as a science. As I recall, Professor Nagel asserted that psychoanalysis is not predictive, that its generalizations are not adequately tested—and more particularly that its tests lack control—and also that it employs concepts which are not clear enough to be meaningful. Thus, such a concept, or theory, as the Oedipus complex is not clearly or definitely enough stated so as to be conceivably falsified. The need for the criterion of falsifiability was also stressed by Professor Hook. Such theories as the one mentioned seem to be consistent with *every* kind of behavior in a human being. When the data seem to be inconsistent with the theory, then they get reinterpreted so as to be consistent with it. A theory which explains everything, which cannot be contradicted by any sort of facts, does not deserve to be called a scientific theory.

a) Now, I agree with these criticisms but only provided they are put in perspective. Psychoanalysis is a protoscience. Not all sciences are born, like Minerva, fully armed; some sciences have to go through a process of growth. Psychoanalysis is in the stage of adolescence—a teen-ager who is perhaps mixed up—but there is no reason to suppose that it will not grow up and out of its troubles. On the other hand, it cannot be fairly criticized for undergoing the pains and possible distortions of adolescence. From a heuristic point of view it would be highly unfortunate to restrict the award of the diploma of science to those inquiries only which have attained maturity. After all, a child is a human being no less than an adult. Inevitably, there is some pure speculation in a protoscience. Darwin, for instance, propounded the theory of pangenesis—one which was a pure speculation and without a shred of evidence. In its early stages as a science, such exercise of the speculative imagination is inevitable and may be useful.

b) I doubt that even for the exact sciences, Professor Nagel's requirement of "clear and distinct ideas" (well defined theoretical concepts) is valid. Berkeley's proof that the concept of the infinitesimal was unclear and confused was decisive, yet Newton's operations with differential equations were successful. Much later, the concept of the infinitesimal was clarified; but it would have been a mistake for Newton to refrain from utilizing it until such clarification had been achieved. It seems to me that the pattern of science emerges incidentally with the development of science itself. Scientists are primarily operators; they are rational beings, if you please, but not to the point that their intellectual conduct is subjected to specified rules of procedure. Professor Bridgman has said that a scientist has no method other than that of doing his damnedest. True enough, Professor Bridgman did formulate a logic of science; but this logic came out of his practice, and my guess is that, in carrying out his experiments with high pressures, he was not governed by a conscious adherence to such a logic.

c) Moreover, there are sciences and sciences, from the most to the least exact. Take history; surely it is not predictive? Shall we say that, at least, it is explanatory? Yes, but how "scientific" are its explanations? An explanation is valid on the basis of initial conditions along with some generalizations serving as major premises. But historical generalizations have nothing like the status of established physical laws. They have not been tested in the laboratory, nor have they been subjected to controls. Rather are they hunches, reports of common sense concerning human behavior, sometimes hardly rising above the level of old wives' tales. Consider, further, all other historical sciences such as archeology; surely archeology is not predictive, and when it explains, it does so on the basis of speculations—of theories, I mean, alternatives to which are by no means excluded. So, too, with the theory of evolution—a historical theory which, so far as I know, is not seriously predictive.

d) Perhaps Professor Nagel will object that archeology, history, evolutionary theory and so on are not scientific at all. And this brings me to my final point. It seems to me that Professor Nagel implicitly assumes the validity of such a question as "What is science in general?"; I might even go further and say that he assumes that there is a universal *essence* of science applying equally and in the same manner to all inquiries which claim the name of science. Or again, Professor Nagel seems to operate with the concept of an ideal science by reference to which all actual inquiries are to be measured and tested as adequate according as they are good approximations to this ideal. This, I think, is dangerous Platonism; in fact my implied criticism of Professor Nagel is but a slight paraphrase of Aristotle's criticism of Plato's doctrine of the Idea of the Good. I suggest that our way of eliciting what science is should be empirical. Rather than start with some a priori conception of the pattern of science, we should formulate our view as an induction from the shape of actual sciences and the behavior of scientists. (It would be otiose to define science by a stipulated definition.) I think that such an empirical concept of science will be found to be not rigid but fluid, extending over a range and being modified as it moves from one portion of the range to another. I realize I have no business to be talking about science. I have no knowledge of it from the inside, and I have the highest respect for Professor Nagel's command of the subject. So it is with some trepidation that I urge Professor Nagel to put less of Plato and more of John Dewey into his cup of tea.

II. Psychoanalysis and Philosophy

Professor Lazerowitz propounded the theory that metaphysics (and, I suspect, most philosophizing) is but the conscious expression of prohibited unconscious wishes; thus, that it is not a rational enterprise. As a proof of his theory, one of the examples which he cited was Bradley's absolute idealism. Professor Lazerowitz then suggested that Bradley's doctrine that phenomena are illusions is an expression of the death wish. Later, in support of Professor Lazerowitz's contention, Professor Paul Edwards made several points. (a) Bradley's reasoning—he said—is incredibly bad, so much so that one is driven to search for deeper unconscious motivations in order to account for Bradley's reliance on such reasoning. (b) He further pointed to the fact that Bradley's style is highly dramatic and thus suggestive of underlying emotional complexes. (c) We are in possession of some direct knowledge of Bradley's personality and we know that Bradley was the youngest of a very large family of children.

In other words, Bradley was a Benjamin and subject to all the troubles attending such a status. (a) Yet—I say—we know of many other Benjamins who have developed into normal adults. (b) And how do we judge that Bradley's reasoning is incredibly bad? When I was a young graduate student, the texts in the class were largely Bradley and Bosanquet; at that time, idealism was still above the horizon. Some of my group—like T. S. Eliot, for instance—were, I think, converts to Bradley, but nearly all of us, converts or opponents, thought of Bradley's doctrine as sensible; and some of us thought of it as powerful. (I don't think that all of my fellow graduate students were fools, either.) As for the dramatic texture of Bradley's writing, one thought of it as simply good style (I still think it is very good English writing).

As Professor Flew has said, credibility and incredibility are relative to a particular time. Perhaps we were not then as sophisticated as philosophers are today; it is also possible that, now, we are not as sophisticated as the thinkers who will come after us. What is "credible" today will probably be "nonsense" tomorrow. (Tomorrow, too, perhaps we will have forgotten more.) In my fairly numerous years as a professional philosopher I have seen quite a number of movements rise above the soil, thrive, bloom, and then wither like autumn's leaves. The course of philosophical thinking is even more unpredictable than the weather. Let us use our historical imagination and wonder whether today's (including Professor Lazerowitz's doctrine) linguistic philosophy may not become "incredible" some time later (and not very much later perhaps). I suggest that such characterizations as "credible" and "incredible," and also the *complete* assurance about the truth of one's own view and about the falsity of past views, are out of place among philosophers.

Professor Alice Ambrose made the telling point in the course of the discussion that whereas in science solutions are reached and agreement is achieved, metaphysical inquiry fails on both counts. As she said, people have been arguing on metaphysical problems for two thousand years without definitively solving anything. This difference between science and metaphysics is the heart of the matter, she urged; this fact justifies one in explaining metaphysical discussion by reference to unconscious impulses. I certainly sympathize with Miss Ambrose; for I too am often exasperated by our failure to reach agreement or solution. But is her appeal to the psychoanalytical doctor necessary for the cure of the patient, and is it true that we have a patient on our hands? For consider:

(a) Miss Ambrose and I are on opposite sides of the fence and I don't see much chance that we can ever persuade one another. Does it follow that either one or both of us are neurotics? (b) Granting that science stands for perpetual peace and philosophy for perpetual war, what is there to worry about? As we know, the war between the sexes is never-ending also. Perhaps the scientists are organization-men; perhaps they have attended those newfangled schools in which they were taught how to get along with people; perhaps they are adjusted humans. But the philosophers are maladjusted, forever unregenerate, defending the last stronghold of individualism in the western world. Also, the antagonism among philosophers is the best expression of the Hegelian dialectic that I can imagine. (c) But to speak more seriously, Professor Williams explained very reasonably (I think) why the difficulties of reaching solutions in metaphysics arise. Metaphysics tries to bring everything together; it is a cognitive response to the totality of things. But science (I would add) treats of relatively simple matters, of limited and abstracted areas. Science reaches solutions because it deals precisely with that selected group of problems which can be solved. As we all know, when philosophers devise a method for solving a problem, then that problem is taken over by science. Thus the success of science is, so to speak, analytic. Conversely, metaphysics is unsuccessful in the nature of things, because its business is to deal with those problems which science lays aside as insoluble.

Incidentally, I think the present fashion of treating unanswerable questions as otiose or meaningless, and so of dismissing them, is highly unfortunate. I have in mind the view which considers a question unanswerable when, *as of the present,* we can conceive of no method by which it may be answered. When, early in the second World War, Hitler was achieving easy and sweeping victories, Mr. Churchill declared in a speech that Hitler would be beaten. Did he (Mr. Churchill) have any idea of how such a victory could be brought off by the West? I very much doubt it. Referring to Miss Ambrose's two thousand years, I will note that for over three thousand years parents and others have been trying to discover the right way to bring up children. And the theories on this subject are more numerous and more varied than those in metaphysics. We still haven't got the answer, but yet we keep trying. So with the world's evils; when one evil is removed, another one springs out like a hydra's head. Here too, as of the present, we see no prospect of the conquest of evil. Yet we keep trying. Philosophizing is more like the activity of living than it is like the doing of science. Moses, who never reached the promised land, at least had a glimpse of it. Philosophers are worse off than Moses perhaps. Nevertheless the present way of treating so-called unanswerable questions seems to me like abandoning a fortress to the enemy. Metaphysics is a tough enterprise, calling for patience, persistence, and hardihood.

By way of a limited support of Professor Lazerowitz, Professor Philipp Frank referred to the three recent or current movements: pragmatism, positivism, linguistic analysis. Then he added that, in fact, he had found himself wondering why some philosophers should have opposed these schools, so much so that he felt inclined to look favorably at an explanation of their attitude by reference to unconscious wishes—perhaps in terms of the need for security. Professor Frank's remark induces me to make the following rejoinder.

He raises the question why people should be *against* the recent movements already cited. But he does not ask the question why some philosophers should be *in favor* of these movements. Why doesn't he? Surely his demand for a nonrational explanation cuts both ways. The failure on his part to raise the second question is fraught with serious consequences. (Since these consequences are unintended, my remarks are in no way a personal reflection on anyone.) The unintended implications of the attitude I have cited are summed up in a position like this: "I (the philosopher) assume that I am a wholly rational being and that therefore my philosophical views are certainly right. Consequently, anyone who differs from my views *must* be wrong and needs to have his head examined."

It used to be that a teacher reading a Ph.D. thesis with whose views he disagreed would say to himself, "Of course, this is nonsense; what I want to know is whether it is the right kind of nonsense." Now, it seems, we are to say that an opponent is not just a fool, but a neurotic and a schizoid to boot. I suggest that in this way philosophical argument among upholders of opposing views will become trivialized. Why argue with my opponent if I have no respect for his intellect? Let us return to the honorable tradition of philosophical discussion. And if psychoanalysis is to be used, let us apply it to ourselves, searching our hearts for secret motives and vanities; but let us leave the other fellow alone.

26.

Philosophy and Psychoanalysis

JOHN HOSPERS
Associate Professor of Philosophy
Brooklyn College

I

As I TRY to get a composite picture of the results of the conference, the thing that stands out most in my mind is the lack of genuine communication between the psychoanalysts and the philosophers. Psychoanalysts are, quite understandably, too busy treating patients to have acquainted themselves with the latest guns in the arsenal of epistemology and philosophy of science, and are therefore at a loss to reply to the charges leveled at them by the philosophers in the way the philosophers want. The philosophers, for their part, are—equally understandably—ignorant of the vast amount of empirical detail garnered by psychoanalysts in the last half-century as well as the complexity of many of the theoretical concepts employed in psychoanalysis. The inevitable result is that each party to the dispute only feels confirmed in his previous suspicions, namely that the other party's remarks are either incompetent or irrelevant, given to making either scandalously overblown claims or excessively demanding systematic requirements.

The violence of the reaction to Professor Lazerowitz's paper is a case in point, accentuated perhaps by the fact that here is a philosopher who dares to cross professional boundaries and league himself with the psychoanalysts. Yet it is often not clear (at least to me) what the philosophers are attacking. Are they attacking the Freudian principles themselves? or are they attacking Professor Lazerowitz's attempt to apply these principles to the philosophers he chose as examples?

Perhaps the philosophers are denying the psychoanalytic theories to which Professor Lazerowitz was appealing in presenting his examples. But he did not use the most controversial psychoanalytic theories at all. For example: people do sometimes give reasons for holding a belief which are not the ones that actually impel them to hold it; a person may give all sorts of arguments for belief in God, but often these are not the cause of the person's believing as he does—he has a feeling of insecurity, going back perhaps to certain features of his childhood situation, and he desperately wants security in a hostile world. Are the philosophers denying that this sort of thing occurs, and that something similar to it may have occurred in Bradley's case? People have hidden wishes, reproaches, and defenses which come out in devious ways, for example through their dreams and their verbal utterances—slips of the tongue, ways of speaking, the metaphors they use, and so on. These phenomena are familiar enough to any fairly close observer of human beings who knows what to look for. If the philosophers are denying, in the face of all these facts, that people have motives of which they are not consciously aware, they have against them a tremendous weight of evidence; they must somehow explain away a vast amount of converging evidence which psychoanalysts have brought to light over the years.

But if they do not deny these Freudian principles, are they then denying the application of the principles to the philosophers in question? They might argue this more cogently if they cited facts about Bradley's life that would count against the hypothesis about Bradley which they were attacking. But no facts about Bradley's life have been adduced which might constitute such counterevidence. On what, then, do their claims rest? Professor Lazerowitz's evidence is far from conclusive, but at least he has given *some;* whereas his philosophical opponents have presented no evidence for any counterclaim. (True, they have objected with some plausibility that one can psychoanalyze patients in his office but not persons already dead, simply on the basis of their literary remains. Freud himself declared that this attempt becomes more difficult and dangerous when the patient is not there to free-associate, and that the probability of being right is considerably less with many vital links of evidence missing. Still—though this would have to be argued at length—smaller probability is not the same as guesswork, and many good "leads" are obtainable from biographies of the dead. Some dreams, some associations, some figures of speech repeatedly used, can be dead giveaways—and the evidence for *this* statement comes from experience with patients who are very much alive.)

This leads me to consider another criticism made of Professor Lazerowitz's thesis. Some of his critics apparently took him to hold that if a philosopher has one or another kind of mental disturbance, his theories (being the outcome of this disturbance) therefore cannot be true and should not be taken seriously—that they have somehow been "explained away"; and that, furthermore, if a philosopher has no such disturbance, his theories are more likely to be true, or at least cannot be dismissed as easily as in the former case. But of course absolutely no such consequence follows. A highly neurotic person may espouse a theory which is true, and a "normal" or "well adjusted" person may come up with one which is quite false. Whether it is true or false must be determined quite independently of who thought of it or under what conditions. No one can deny that Nietzsche and Kierkegaard were extremely disturbed, in fact psychotic, personalities; and it would be difficult to deny that they both gave the world very valuable insights, or at least that what they say is deserving of the most serious consideration and not to be summarily dismissed. Another example: Psychopaths typically give extremely shrewd character-analyses of other people, while usually remaining blind to crucial aspects of their own characters. If Russell, unlike Bradley, is a "normal" personality, this fact does not give any added credibility to his theories; the theories of many "normal" people contradict one another. These considerations are so obvious that I would be embarrassed to mention them if some of the participants in the discussion had not assumed that others had denied them, whereas in fact no one did, certainly not Professor Lazerowitz.

Professor Lazerowitz's main thesis, however, as I understand it, has nothing to do with the genesis of Bradley's philosophy or Spinoza's philosophy or anyone else's. The position he is primarily concerned to defend is not that Bradley and Spinoza's writings reveal certain facts about their unconscious minds, but the very different view that the real meaning of sentences uttered by them is not their apparent or literal meaning: that a sentence in Bradley may *appear* to be about X (e.g., the Absolute), but is really about Y (e.g., a wish for security). The important point here is not simply that the truth-value of a statement must be determined irrespective of its origin—which Professor Lazerowitz would not deny—but that metaphysical statements have, on the literal level, no truth-value whatever, and possess it only when they are viewed in a very different way, such as the one which Professor Lazerowitz suggests. This far more radical thesis I am not prepared to defend. In any case, a discussion of it would take me far afield into questions of meaning and truth and the nature of metaphysics, and I wish to confine myself here to remarks about psychoanalysis.

II

I want now to examine a few of the related comments and criticisms by philosophers on remarks made by members of the psychoanalytic camp.

1. The charge was often made during the meetings that psychoanalytic theory is defective because two opposite kinds of fact are taken to prove one and the same thing, and one and the same fact is made to prove two opposite things. I believe that this charge is unfounded, and would like to refer to a couple of the examples used in the discussion to illustrate this.

(a) "If you agree with the psychoanalyst's interpretation, this is taken as an indication that the interpretation is all right; but if you disagree with it, this is taken as an indication that you are (usually because of unconscious motives) resisting the true interpretation; so it's taken as true both ways."

This worn-out example has been used countless times as a

way of attacking psychoanalytic theory, often *in toto*—as if thereby the entire body of psychoanalytic theory had been disposed of. (Never before has so much been refuted by so little!) Yet the charge is entirely without foundation. There are plenty of situations in which an interpretation is attacked and no psychoanalyst would say that the attacker was "resisting." Suppose that a group of psychoanalysts are discussing which of several alternative dream-interpretations is correct, and that there are several divergent views about this; none of them would suggest that all but one were "resisting" the right interpretation. True, if one of the group became very touchy and rejected an interpretation out of hand with great energy and passion, and refused to listen to the reasons given by the other analysts, they would suspect that his rejection was not entirely impartial and that resistance was occurring; but otherwise they would not think it —as a group they are discussing the matter as dispassionately as possible in order to get at the truth. And so it may sometimes be with laymen as well: their negative reaction to an interpretation may sometimes have good grounds, and they may give such grounds. But since the analyst knows far more about the intricacies of dream-interpretation than they do, and since the materials in the dream are always repressed materials and therefore unpleasant and hard for the patient to face (else they would not have been repressed in the first place), the chances are 99.9 per cent that when the patient rejects an interpretation that the analyst suggests, he *is* resisting. It is common knowledge that "the truth hurts," and this applies more to truths in this area, which the patient cannot face up to, than any other kind. If the interpretation did not hit the patient where it hurts, he would have no reason for such an impassioned rejection, but would be willing to discuss it rationally and at length. This is so well known to analysts that it can be practically taken as a truism—not in the sense of a tautology, but in the sense of a generalization from experience that is so familiar (to analysts) that it has become a cliche. But along come the philosophers and interpret this empirical generalization as an a priori dictum, and foist it upon the analysts as a glaring and elementary logical fallacy.

(b) "If the patient is aggressive, this may be taken as an indication that he really *is* aggressive; on the other hand, it may be taken as an indication of the opposite, that he is really passive and that the aggressiveness is only a defense against the passivity."

This is taken as an example of an empirical fact that is (erroneously, the philosophers believe) used to confirm two opposed hypotheses. But it is the philosophers who are in error: (i) While I agree that the same fact cannot *prove* (conclusively establish) two different hypotheses, the same fact can *confirm* (count toward establishing) two different hypotheses, depending on what the *other* facts are. The smile on a person's face may indicate that the person is friendly, but it may also indicate that he is unfriendly; to know which it was we might have to examine his behavior over a considerable period. His smile might reveal a genuine friendly feeling, but it might be a mask concealing hatred or resentment. How absurd it would be to argue: "A smile is taken on one occasion to indicate friendliness and on another occasion to prove unfriendliness. But it is fallacious to take one and the same empirical phenomenon sometimes to confirm one hypothesis and sometimes to confirm its opposite." Yet this same error is committed by philosophers who with monotonous regularity haul out this bruised and battered argument to prove that psychoanalysts are guilty of an elementary fallacy.

In any case, (ii) in the example of aggressive behavior, it is *not* "the same fact" that is taken to confirm two opposed hypotheses; for the behavioral manifestations in the two cases are really very different. They are similar enough for both to be called "aggressiveness," and people who are not very observant may mistake the one for the other, but the analyst wouldn't be worth his salt who could not distinguish the one kind from the other in a person's behavior. "Real" aggression is stirred into action only when there is genuine provocation from the outside world;

neurotic aggression (pseudo-aggression, as it is called) is unconsciously *self-provoked.* Real aggression is roughly proportionate to the degree of provocation; pseudo-aggression lashes out at the slightest provocation, real or imaginary. Real aggression is used to harm the aggressor and to protect oneself; pseudo-aggression damages the aggressor (and according to the psychoanalysts, this is its unconscious aim, since this is the effect that it unerringly achieves). Real aggression is used only in self-defense or for personal gain; neurotic aggression is used indiscriminately, against an innocent bystander as much as against a real offender. Real aggression is ordinarily timed so as to wait till the enemy is vulnerable; pseudo-aggression is "trigger-happy"—it is characterized by an inability to wait. (Explanation: since it is used as a defense against psychic masochism, and since the reproach of psychic masochism is constantly made, the defense is also constant, and cannot wait until the enemy is vulnerable.) The theory of psychic dynamics underlying these cases would take many pages to explain; but in any case the fallacy that is charged is not committed here. What is required is an astute observation of many kinds of behavioral detail, and the analyst is the one who by training has developed a keen nose for this kind of detail, so that he can "spot" the pseudo-aggressive defense even while the less observant person may take it for the genuine article.

2. Some of the philosophers have rather naively assumed that there must be one *experimentum crucis* that would validate or invalidate a psychoanalytic theory. In fact so stringent a requirement is not even made in physics; and whatever the degree of stringency with which this can be applied in physics, it is far smaller in psychoanalytic theory. The psychoanalyst is an expert in detecting *patterns* of behavior; individual items alone taken out of context do not mean very much. *One* slip of the tongue proves nothing; but a recurring pattern of slips of the tongue (or typographical errors) all having certain general features in common—such as reference to oral intake—can weigh heavily for a theory, especially in conjunction with data from dreams, data concerning the patient's behavior in facets of life usually shielded

from public gaze, and the like. Again, very little can be established on the basis of one dream; but the analyst whose patient reports his dreams over a period of months, together with his daily moods, his objects of like and dislike, and his free-associations, is in a position to state many things about the patient's unconscious life with very considerable confidence, on the basis of literally thousands of piled-up details falling into a pattern.

Attempts to force the psychoanalyst into a logical straitjacket by asking questions like "If the small boy shows his penis to his mother, does that prove he has an Oedipus complex?" simply will not work, for no one item alone will validate or invalidate the theory. These attempts are such gross oversimplifications that the analyst can surely be excused for emitting a sigh and saying, "How can I in a few sentences or even paragraphs possibly indicate to you all the kinds of behavior I would include as oedipal?" In the first place, the antecedent and the consequent of the above hypothetical should be interchanged; the antecedent is the theoretical statement and the consequent the empirical one. But more important, the bit of small-boy behavior referred to would be only one of a vast number of bits of behavior that would be taken as confirming the theory; and accordingly the failure of the boy to exhibit *this* bit of behavior would in no way imperil the theory. In general, any sign of inordinate affection for the mother (or mother substitute) as against the father, or wish to displace the father, would be taken as oedipal. (There are even boundary-line cases where it is not clear whether the bit of behavior, taken in isolation, is to be taken as oedipal or not.) The formulation is not "If p then q" but "If p then q or r or s or . . ." followed by a finite disjunction of propositions. And since the disjunction is finite, it is emphatically *not* true that the Oedipus complex would be believed in no matter *what* the empirical facts are: if none of the items q, r, s . . . occurred, it would have to be concluded (and would be) that the individual in question had no Oedipus complex.

It is the same throughout psychoanalysis. The concepts are open, and they can subsume an amazing range and variety of empirical detail, which to the uninitiated makes the whole theoretical structure seem amorphous and the theorizing process slovenly. Let me take just one example: consider the concept "the oral (i.e., orally regressed) personality." The oral personality can be characterized in part as follows: he is sensitive and easily hurt; he is jealous and easily provoked; he retaliates intensely against small grievances; he is highly narcissistic—"the world revolves around him" and things interest him only in so far as they tend to *his* doing or undoing; he overdramatizes himself; he has delusions of grandeur, and when these are shattered he reverts to the opposite practice of "sulking in the corner and licking his wounds" (both of these opposite things are dramatic and attention-getting, as opposed to being simply matter-of-fact, which is neither); he is furious when he is crossed, but has no hesitation in crossing other people; most of his energy goes into fighting his inner battles, so that little remains for genuine interest in the outside world and its affairs (he exhibits an interest in people and the world only in so far as these enter the charmed circle of his unconscious conflicts and can be *used* by him for some unconscious purpose); he has a knack for hurting people's feelings without being consciously aware of his provocation, and is subsequently outraged at their reaction; and so on. He may not have *all* of these characteristics; but he must have some of them; and the more of them he has, and the more continuously and intensely they manifest themselves, the deeper his oral regression is considered to be. All this, and much more, is included in the concept.

One could wish that concepts such as these could be neatly pinpointed and encapsulated in one simple formula. But they cannot, and those who crave neatness and simplicity will do well to look elsewhere than to human nature for their subject matter. Still, these concepts, though difficult to master because of their richness and complexity, are workable ones and are used again and again every day by practicing psychoanalysts; with some practice the analyst can detect the "oral personality" with amazing facility, being able on the basis of one or two personality traits to predict what other ones will turn up. Moreover, there are many terms used in the psychological and social sciences—such as "intelligence"—which are almost as unpinpointed in their reference. Yet philosophers do not appear to launch virulent attacks upon them for that reason. May it not be suggested that they extend to psychoanalysis the same privilege or at least analyze in a cool hour their failure to do so?

3. Several times during the discussion philosophers seemed to take the one and only criterion for the correctness of a psychoanalytic interpretation to be its effectiveness in curing the patient. This again is a common fallacy. Therapy may be ineffective for several reasons: the theory from which it operates may be mistaken; the analyst may not recognize this individual case as one of the right kind—he may misapply his principles in this case; he may not have the knack of getting his points over to the patient effectively, perhaps through a misuse of transference or through some personal incompatibility between himself and the patient. (On this point see Richard Peters, "Cure, Cause and Motive," on page 150 of *Philosophy and Analysis,* ed. Margaret Macdonald.) Still, if an analysis based on a given set of psychoanalytic principles does not effect a cure, there is *some* reason to doubt the principles, particularly if the same results are obtained by many analysts in a large variety of different situations (since it would be unlikely that they *all* used the wrong techniques or all had transference problems with patients, etc.). If bridges built on the assumption that certain laws of physics are correct always collapsed immediately, we would first doubt the engineering, but would later doubt the physics.

Cure may fail to result, then, even if the right principles are used. Can it occur when the wrong principles are used, or no principles at all (just as a person might make successful predictions about the weather without knowledge of meteorology)? This is a debatable point, and the answer would *seem* to be yes; all the same, I think most psychoanalysts would say no. When acute alcoholism is brought to an end, not through the long and painful "working through" of repressed material based on an understanding of the genesis of the addiction, but through a form of social conditioning like that of Alcoholics Anonymous, the latter is not accepted as a "cure" by psychoanalysts even though the statistics on cure may be just as favorable to Alcoholics Anonymous as to psychoanalytic therapy. They say that the fundamental personality disturbance is still there, that the *symptom* has been warded off (often only temporarily) by an external agency, but that as long as the person has no insight into his own psyche, the seat of the difficulty remains untouched. It is like the case of a man's being prevented from engaging in blood feuds by mounting social pressures against it, or by having his attention constantly diverted to other things, but *not* by the removal of the desire to engage in it.

4. During the course of his life Freud committed to paper many assertions; some of them would still be accepted by psychoanalysts, but some of them Freud himself later rescinded, some of them he never fully worked out, some of them are unusually liable to misinterpretation unless qualified by safeguards which he never gave, and some of them are simply mistaken though he never repudiated them. The philosophers at this meeting have tended to lump all these together indiscriminately and talk as if a refutation of one of Freud's assertions, no matter which, implied a refutation of Freud's views in general. There are many Freudian statements about which even the most orthodox Freudians today are dubious; and for others to attack these and assert triumphantly that Freud was talking nonsense, while it may be an amusing indoor sport, is quite uncharitable—and quite inconsistent with what these same philosophers practice elsewhere when they are less inspired by feelings of opposition.

There are expendable and nonexpendable assertions in the Freudian corpus. The existence of material repressed into the unconscious, the occurrence of defense mechanisms, and the significance of dreams and moods and free associations as revealing unconscious conflicts—these are all nonexpendable; they could not be removed without radically altering the character of Freud's doctrines. On the other hand, the Eros-Thanatos theory (life instinct and death instinct) and the view that the id represents our racial ancestry whereas the ego represents contemporary mores, are easily expendable, and if abandoned would result in no change in either psychoanalytic theory or therapeutic practice. Yet it is on the basis of the expendable aspects of the theory that, more often than not, the philosophers at the convention have attacked Freud. We might come across similar results if we started picking holes in Newton's theological speculations, or even some of his scientific ones.

Among the assertions of Freud to which the philosophers took the most violent exception is, curiously enough, Freud's statement that the intellect is a feeble and dependent thing, acting as the individual's underlying psychic dynamics determine.

Philosophers, in general, can be influenced by rational considerations; that is, they can make the *reasons* for behaving in such and such a way the *cause* of their behaving in that way. But because of their removal from most of humanity most of the time, they tend to overestimate the occurrence of this phenomenon in other people. In my opinion, it takes only some thoughtful acquaintance with the behavior of people outside universities, coupled if possible with knowledge of a good many psychoanalytic case histories, to see how profoundly true is Freud's judgment. To take one or two examples out of thousands: People try to justify their aggression against others with all kinds of defensive arguments which do not report their real motives at all, although they may rationalize themselves into believing that these *are* their real motives; people are adept at convincing themselves that their official motives are the ones from which they really acted. Unusually intelligent people might be expected to have more insight than others into their own motives, but usually they do not; in the process of psychotherapy these people do not use their intelligence to apply psychoanalytic precepts to their own case and thus shorten the period of therapy; on the contrary—and this is a recurring and predictable phenomenon to psychoanalysts—they throw chaff into their own eyes by thinking up all manner of ingenious arguments (many of which contradict each other) to prove that the analyst is wrong, thus protracting the analysis, using their intelligence to keep the neurosis going instead of to terminate it. Freud, more than anyone else, has shown us how all-pervasive these occurrences are, and not one whit less so in people who claim to be "above" them. Accordingly I can only conclude that the people who object to this statement of Freud have not looked at the data as carefully as they should.

I said, above, that philosophers are to a large extent influenced by rational considerations. It may be that in saying this I have done them too much justice. Philosophers are, more than other men, adept at *giving reasons* and *making distinctions;* this after all is their business. But their motives are not conspicuously different from those of other people, and their insight into their own motives is not noticeably more acute. As a class, they are as outraged as other people when their hidden motives are probed or questioned; and they are about as blind as other people when it comes to insight into "what makes them tick." Even philosophers do not usually let their intellects decide what *kind* of world-view to embrace; idealists by nature will find arguments for idealism and discount all refutations even when they cannot think of cogent answers, and philosophers who are insecure are likely to be compulsive certainty-chasers, grasping at anything to introduce order and security into their world view, even if this involves the outright postulation of entities or principles (the One, the Principle of Uniformity of Nature) which can be defended in no other way.

We are all human, and we all have secret wishes and defenses which influence our actions, our thoughts, and our theories; but the people who are most nearly free from this—and most willing to admit bias where it exists—are not the philosophers but the psychoanalysts, for they have been trained for years in the long and arduous process of interpreting their own feelings and behavior, of spotting their own pet rationalizations, and viewing with a certain detached and half-humorous unconcern the feelings and foibles which it would make most philosophers squirm to have mentioned. This, of course, is not the philosophers' fault; to look down the drains of their own psyches is not their professional business; yet it is, I think, unfortunate for them, both as philosophers and as human beings, if they remain unaware of these things. One unfortunate effect is that they are too often taken in by their own dialectical maneuvers—analyzing an argument in meticulous detail while ignoring certain crucial presuppositions, or straining at a gnat and swallowing a camel, or just simply failing to take their elaborate theorizing with a humble grain of salt. Another effect is that, in a natural (but explainable) resistance to psychoanalysis, they assume the role of carping critics without giving its manifold data a sympathetic hearing, or trying fairly to see what psychoanalysis is endeavoring to do; they try it in the balance and find it wanting on the basis of a few unguarded statements by Freud, or they demand of it a schematic rigor greater than any of which it is now capable and reject it without further ado—things they would never dream of doing in fields where they were less personally involved. Most unfortunate of all, they are content to criticize from the outside, accusing the psychoanalyst of making all kinds of unprovable or a priori pronouncements, having all the while only the meagerest conception of what psychoanalysis is all about, and not bothering to familiarize themselves *in specific detail* with the vast accumulation of behavioral data upon which the conclusions of psychoanalysis are based. Though specialists in scientific method, they refuse to look through Galileo's telescope.

III

I do not deny that psychoanalytic theory needs some tidying up; but the psychoanalysts, already fully occupied with practical problems of therapy, have neither the time, the training, nor the inclination for this kind of enterprise; this is a task for psychoanalytically trained philosophers of science—rare birds indeed! There is, however, another aspect of the relation of philosophy to psychoanalysis which is, to me at least, of equal interest, and concerning which I would like to raise a few questions.

Many of the central and frequently used terms in psychoanalysis claim to be purely "objective" labels for classes of empirical phenomena; yet in their actual application they have an emotive-persuasive ring which at least in part determines their use and which ill accords with their officially neutral employment in scientific discourse.

It is often said that psychoanalysis is morally neutral. This is argued along somewhat the following lines: "We psychoanalysts don't assert, *qua* psychoanalysts, that anything is better or more desirable than anything else. We assert only that *if* you have a symptom or characteristic that you dislike and want it removed or changed, then perhaps psychoanalysis can effect this change. But this is not to commit ourselves to saying that it is *desirable* to change it—only that *if* you want it changed we shall endeavor to do so. We therapists will try to use whatever means we can to achieve the end you desire; but we do not say that you *ought* to desire this or that end. That question we leave to the moralists."

Psychoanalysts, when questioned about the moral implications of their therapy, will say this kind of thing (perhaps to escape probing value-questions) on Mondays, Wednesdays, and Fridays; yet on Tuesdays, Thursdays, and Saturdays they will talk about "improvement," "cure," "adjustment," "normal development," and the like—all of which terms have strongly valuational overtones. That is the difficulty. For my part, I am convinced that psychoanalysis is *not* morally neutral, and that analysts who say these things on Mondays, Wednesdays, and Fridays, might well use the Sabbath to ponder the matter further. If their Monday-Wednesday-Friday remarks are true, it would seem to follow that *if* psychoanalysts could remove a patient's guilt feeling after every murder he commits, and if this is what he wants, they should have no objection to doing it. The empirical fact is that they are unable to do this anyway (reasons for this could be supplied by psychoanalytic theory—the theory of the dynamic unconscious which explains why some symptoms can be removed and others cannot has been fairly well worked out); but if analysts were morally neutral, they should be as willing to remove guilt feelings for murder as they are now to remove symptoms like writer's block and compulsive handwashing.

In fact, of course, nothing could be further from being the case. Psychoanalysts have moral convictions, not only in private life, but in their professional capacity. If an analyst learns that a patient has committed murder, he feels bound to report it to the police; but if he learns that the patient is having an illicit love affair, he feels no such obligation, even though adultery is prohibited by the laws of the state in which he resides. Further: the therapist, though he does not usually give moral instruction to the patient but tries to get him to make up his own mind as rationally as possible, inevitably encourages the patient in certain directions and (at least by suggestion) holds certain ideals to be worth attaining. He discourages rape but not sexual encounter per se. He discourages a puritanical or extremely ascetic way of bringing up children and encourages a more permissive yet not entirely permissive one; he discourages rebellion (under most circumstances) and encourages adjustment to conditions as they exist, for the sake of the patient's own happiness. And this brings us back to our question: is he not accepting certain moral judgments and, at least through suggestion, urging them upon the patient?

Let us consider the term "adjustment." It is, I think, bandied about all too carelessly, more by the general public than by the psychoanalysts themselves. We speak of this or that person as adjusted, or of psychoanalytic therapy as bringing about a condition of adjustment; and the first question is, Adjusted to what? To twentieth-century civilization as it now exists? I confess that I can think of few things more ghastly. Doubtless psychoanalysts do not mean anything quite so simple-minded as this when they talk about the desirability of adjustment; but what they do mean is often not very clear. Let me suggest something like this as a possibility: a person may be extremely discontented with a social situation, an environment, a civilization in which he finds himself, but he will not be considered maladjusted as long as he is able to live in it without too much unhappiness; if he would be much happier by changing his environment he would be well advised to do so, but if he cannot do this, or if the environment he is unhappy about is world-wide, he should try to live with it as best he can—making reasonable moves to improve it bit by bit, but not in a self-damaging way, such as by sudden spurts of effort followed by relapses which anyone could have seen would result in no change whatever except to make him even more unhappy. A person might be considered adjusted to an environment he dislikes if he is in it but not of it, compromising his ideals somewhat in order not to strike his head fruitlessly against stone walls, yet not losing sight of them so far that he omits to practice them when he can do so to good result.

This might be a reasonable—albeit somewhat vague—operating definition of "adjustment." But it leaves many questions unanswered. What is to be done in an environment which is not only unpalatable but is considered to be morally revolting, such as that of Nazi Germany? If a psychoanalyst in Nazi Germany had succeeded in getting a discontented patient to adjust to the moral climate of Nazism, would he have considered his treatment of the patient (to that extent) a success? And if the patient had rebelled openly against Nazi practices and thus gotten himself killed, would this have been taken as a mark of inability to adjust? Or should one live in an environment, no matter how loathsome, trying always to make the best of a bad situation?

In whatever way these questions are answered, I want to emphasize that psychoanalysts are employing certain ideas of what is good or desirable. We ourselves may also consider them to be so; but this does not change the fact that the psychoanalyst is *not* morally neutral—he is trying to bring some things about and not others, and I doubt whether history records any case of an analyst who has endeavored to bring about in a patient a result which he (the analyst) considered undesirable. On the whole I am in agreement with what therapists are trying to achieve; if thousands more people could be treated there would be far less *waste* of time and effort and talent, less unhappiness and misery that serves no useful purpose. Yet at the same time

I am disturbed: even the psychoanalysts' ideal of an "adjusted" person (of which the popular ideal is a caricature) has certain moral limitations. It is, to be sure, the ideal of a person doing constructive work and making some contribution to society; but also it is *not* that of the *extremely* self-sacrificing person or the *extremely* noble leader of mankind. This kind of thing seems to be left to the maladjusted people. If one grants that we need, at least once in a while, persons like Socrates and Jesus Christ and Gandhi who do not hesitate to sacrifice their comfort and their very lives for an ideal (and where would civilization be today without persons of such moral vision?), where are they to come from? From the ranks of the "adjusted"? A really great degree of moral fervor, such as is required to shock mankind into a new kind of awareness in a world where moral insights quickly become fossilized, plus the tremendously strong motivation that is required to stir lethargic humanity and to face possible calumny and persecution and death—these things do not seem to be found among the "adjusted."

I am reminded of the old folk song about the Vicar of Bray. He was the only vicar to live successively with equal comfort under the Anglicans, the Protestants, and the Roman Catholics, for the very good reason that he adjusted his religious views on each occasion to the temper of the regime that was then current. He may have been a morally disreputable character, but he was about the most adjusted person there ever was; he had an unusual ability to bend with the wind, and this is always high on the list of adjustment qualities. Or we may remember Bertrand Russell's brilliant story (in *Satan in the Suburbs*) about Hamlet after his psychoanalysis: Hamlet is a much happier man now, but he can no longer utter a single profound thought. "To be or not to be"? Hamlet is asked after his analysis. "What rubbish!" he replies; "since my analysis I have never once thought of suicide." "O that this too, too solid flesh would melt"? "What rot! What a masochistic bit of infantile exhibitionism, what corny juvenile romanticism!" (This is a caricature, not an exact quotation.) And so on, through the various problems that torment him through the play.

This example is doubtless somewhat unfair, for it is perfectly possible to be "adjusted" and still be vitally concerned with questions of life and death; but not, perhaps, with the passionate involvement of a Hamlet: such involvement, almost any analyst would tell a patient, is "neurotic" or "unhealthy." An extremely saintly person like St. Francis would not be considered by psychoanalysts to be in a state of "mental health" no matter how much good he did for mankind, because there is still within him what the psychoanalyst would call an unhealthy intrapsychical state of affairs. Like all extreme ascetics, he is still (the analyst would say) paying off ransom money to his inner conscience (superego) in the form of self-abnegation for crimes committed in fantasy or even in babyhood reality—forbidden crimes of exhibitionism or voyeurism or sexual indulgence or even curiosity, for which the superego is still demanding conscience money. As long as the superego can impose the deal, "I'll permit you the id-wish you want, even if only in fantasy, and in return for my permitting you the continuation of this infantile pattern you will pay me in the coin of self-sacrifice and suffering," the psychical situation of the person thus characterized is said to be "unhealthy," no matter how much his actions may benefit mankind. And this leads me to put the question: Would it be a good thing if everyone in the world were psychically healthy in the sense which analysts are trying to achieve for their patients?

Closely associated with the terms "adjusted" and "healthy" is the word "cure." "Cure" again is an emotively tinged word, often passing as a purely descriptive one; but in fact it is used only to describe situations which the person using the word considers desirable. No matter how much a patient changed through psychoanalysis, if the analyst did not consider the change a desirable one he would not call it a cure.

> Dr. Thomas French: A young man may be extremely boastful, rebelliously aggressive, and unable to apply himself effectively to serious effort because he is so ashamed of the fact that he really has a very strong desire to be loved like a child—a fact which he is too ashamed to admit even to himself. If the analyst can make

him aware of his strong dependent cravings and can ultimately enable him to tolerate this knowledge of himself, then it will not be necessary for the young man to waste so much of his energy in vain boasting and rebellion. With the energy thus freed he may be able to apply himself more effectively to worth-while effort and ultimately to get rid of his feelings of inferiority by achieving real success. . . .

David Riesman: Let me ask you, do you think that success is always a good thing? I have had the experience—as many other doubtless have—of seeing people go into analysis as the converse of the case which you just gave. They are shy, they are timid, and they come out aggressive; and, since our society values aggression, they succeed. Society says that they are cured. They feel that they are cured. The analyst says that they are cured. Is that a good thing?

Dr. French: That may depend. After all, the real judge and the real test of whether a person is cured or not is whether he is in harmony with himself.

From "Psychoanalysis and Ethics," *University of Chicago Round Table,* No. 638, June 18, 1950, pages 2–3.

The phrase "in harmony with himself" is rather vague (is the clerk who isn't worried about the money he stole from the bank in harmony with himself?), and the man in the street doesn't mean the same thing by it (if he means anything at all) that Plato did. In psychoanalysis it does have a rather specific meaning—it has to do with an equilibrium or balance amongst the Big Three of the unconscious: id, superego, and ego, and this could be spelled out in some detail—but even there our question only presents itself once more: is the state of harmony with oneself, which psychoanalysts strive to attain for their patients, always a good thing?

Another example: If someone through psychoanalysis lost his powers of literary creation (*if;* I am not suggesting that it happens), he would hardly be said to have been "cured" of them. I am assured on good psychiatric authority that a person who already is creatively gifted does not lose this gift through psychoanalysis, since artistic creation is a successful sublimation and therefore untouchable through psychoanalytic therapy; the superego approves the sublimation, unlike the infantile exhibitionism against which it is a defense, and therefore the change from corruptible (bribable) to incorruptible superego which is the principal transformation in psychoanalysis cannot affect it. I am not questioning that this is so. But even if psychoanalytic therapy does not blunt the edge of artistic creativity—indeed, it often removes stumbling blocks to its fulfillment—*after* it is once a going concern, it does seem to me that a certain amount of discontent, maladjustment, of being out of tune with the world, and just plain misery, are often necessary in order for it to blossom in the first place. If Beethoven had been born and raised in a suburban home in Westchester County, if he had had reasonably well-to-do and "adjusted" parents who gave him a tranquil childhood and sent him to a progressive school where no inquiries were made into ultimate questions about man and the universe, and all such tendencies were viewed with disfavor, I think it extremely unlikely if not impossible that Beethoven would have become a great composer or that he would have composed anything like the kind of music that he did. Had Beethoven been able to go to a psychoanalyst in his early years, he might well have been happier, but *we* would be worse off for lacking his music. It seems as if we need a good healthy dose of unhealthy people in this world—people whose urge to do and create unusual things is so tremendously strong that no "normal" motivation could give rise to it. Perhaps they are less happy because the endlessly intricate interplay of unconscious desires, reproaches, and defenses within their psyches has thrown up into consciousness these phenomenal drives and achievements; but so it must be—the artists are sacrificial lambs on the altar of human progress and happiness. Perhaps the rank and file of "adjusted" humanity is simply banking (quite correctly, no doubt) on the fact that there will always be enough maladjusted people around to make their esthetic experiences possible.

Most "unhealthy" psychical conditions—paranoia, masochism, schizophrenia—are completely unproductive, and of no possible benefit to either their possessor or his family and friends; they simply make life miserable for everyone involved, as well as increasing the burden of public taxation in support of mental hospitals. But there *are* persons, such as the artists and saints and moral visionaries we have mentioned, who contribute enormously to the progress of mankind, and here our question becomes pressing: The psychoanalyst in dealing with his patient has a certain end in view, but is the achievement of this end always desirable? The achievement of "cure," "adjustment," "mental health" without doubt produces happiness and peace of mind that did not previously exist; but if this result were to be achieved for everyone, would it not be at a great price? Wouldn't much that is valuable and important in human achievement go down the drain with what is unproductive and wasteful? Thus we conclude with something like G. E. Moore's question: I know that X has property A, but is it therefore good? Practicing psychoanalysts are (so it would seem) committed by their behavior to the view that it *is* good. But often people are unaware of this because terms like "cure," "adjustment," "neurotic," "diseased," "normal" conceal within themselves value judgments which we might sometimes wish to question, but are often kept from questioning by the façade of empirical description officially referred to by these terms.

27.

Comments on Professor Lazerowitz's Paper

MAX BLACK
Professor of Philosophy
Cornell University

BEFORE we seek explanations of the "remarkable intellectual illusions" that Professor Lazerowitz imputes to other philosophers, it would be well to make sure that the illusions occur. To treat metaphysical propositions as if they were "truth claims" to be tested in isolation from the systems to which they belong simplifies the task of unveiling them as "fantasies." But the same treatment would be fatal to scientific principles culled from relativity theory or the latest physical cosmologies. Theoretical systems deserve appraisal by criteria of adequacy and coherence that their own makers would accept; and a negative verdict on one ontology does not foreclose the need for sympathetic criticism of others on their own merits.

If I find Lazerowitz's short way with metaphysics unpersuasive, the reason is that he, too, stretches language for his own purpose. For philosophers to be viewed as quarrelling "over some sort of language innovations" an unusual construction must be put on "language innovations." The disputants will reject the diagnosis, so we must take them to be "really" making proposals that they will refuse to consider. Now this "really" is really dangerous.

A man is free to construct whatever myths he finds illuminating; yet the psychoanalysis of metaphysics casts a murky light. The literary Freudianism that has become the opium of the intellectuals is too automatic in its application: a license to find sexuality everywhere is useless. I would not venture to explain Lazerowitz's interest in sexual explanations by lubricious speculation about his own infantile experiences. But such hypothetical biography would be as easy, as plausible, and as jejune as his own remarks about Bradley.

When the principle of causality is identified with the biological platitude that a child needs two parents, the philosophy of philosophy runs a risk of being reclassified as fiction.

28.

Misunderstanding One Another

CAMPBELL CROCKETT
Senior Research Associate in Psychiatry
Associate Professor of Philosophy
University of Cincinnati

SOMETIMES people speak in this way: "I'm glad I attended the conference on symbolism. It taught me one important thing: that conferences on symbolism are worthless." When such an announcement is delivered in a bitter, caustic tone of voice, the announcer is not genuinely glad that he attended the conference and he does not believe that he learned anything of value.

Now I am glad that I attended the New York University Conference on Philosophy and Psychoanalysis, but I am genuinely glad and I do not write these words with a caustic flourish of my pen. Yet I fear that one of the things that I learned at the conference is that the perennial philosophical maxim "Know thyself" is not self-referring so far as the philosophical speakers at the conference are concerned. What is even more of a scandal is the fact that I find it difficult to apply this maxim to the psychoanalytic speakers at the conference.

I am convinced that philosophers and psychiatrists need each other. There may well be a neurotic flavor to this need. Philosophers, more than other academicians in the liberal arts, are inclined to feel insecure about their speciality and, indeed, to wonder if they have a speciality. Has anyone ever heard a historian wonder whether there is such a study as history? Philosophers do wonder at times whether there is such a study as philosophy. What is philosophy good for? Does philosophy make

Notes to this section begin on page 364.

progress? Must philosophers disagree? "Science learns more and more about less and less, whereas philosophy learns less and less about more and more." "Philosophy is the study of two questions and their answers: What is mind? No matter. What is matter? Never mind."

Psychiatrists, more than their colleagues in the other branches of medicine, are inclined to feel insecure and defensive about their activities. Does psychotherapy produce cures? How scientific is Freud's speculative witch, metapsychology? We know how to find brain tumors. How do we find ids? What counts for confirmation or disconfirmation of the hypothesis, for example, that a given patient is an oral character?

I am suggesting that philosophers and psychiatrists may find themselves backed into the same or similar corners. This would account for a certain neurotic dependency, and the subsequent need to give rational arguments for the alignment. Perhaps this argument, not wholly convincing to me, is worthy of serious consideration.

Regardless, I am interested in pointing out some systematic relations of importance between these two disciplines, and it will be obvious, I hope, that these relations are worthy of careful exploration. Even though they *may* have a neurotic foundation, the superstructure can be examined and evaluated independently of this foundation. Some of these relations were suggested by contributors to the conference and one was exploited by Professor Lazerowitz; but I am afraid that many left the conference with the feeling that the connection between the two disciplines was contrived and abortive. How else can one account for the ridicule with which Professor Lazerowitz's paper was received? I happen to disagree with the major thesis of this paper, but it is not absurd. What is absurd is the superficiality of the hostile criticism that it evoked, accompanied by a complete lack of insight into the motivations for this criticism. So much in the way of polemics. Now for the relations that I have mentioned but have not enumerated.

Historically, philosophy has worked behind the scenes. The sciences and the arts work on the stage, and philosophy attempts to relate and synthesize, to put the blocks together in some fairly intelligible scheme. Or, to be in the mode, philosophy is a metascience, a science of sciences, and when it attempts to change its role and pass itself off as another science, observers see quickly that Zeus has not ordained this misguided behavior.

New sciences often develop within a philosophical framework. Once they achieve (if they do achieve) a reasonable maturity, they take up an independent existence. But as Gregory Zilboorg points out, psychiatry originates, not in philosophy, but in medicine.[1] From what source is the psychiatrist to find his theoretical frameworks and his guiding insights? Surely not in autopsy material and empirical physiology. Some psychiatrists have gone to philosophers for suggestions concerning such a framework: Fromm to Spinoza, Adler to Nietzsche, Sullivan to G. H. Mead, phenomenological psychiatry to Husserl, and existentialist psychiatry to Heidegger.

All this, of course, is highly speculative, and some philosophers believe that the primary, if not the exclusive, contribution of the philosopher to psychiatry is house cleaning, the transformation of a metapsychological witch into an orderly maid. The philosopher is presumably equipped uniquely with semantic, logical, and, in general, methodological strategy. He can analyze the meanings of crucial concepts and explicate the uses and misuses of models and metaphors. Important essays, too numerous to be enumerated, have been published on "unconscious anxiety," "defences," "insight," etc.

Some philosophers and psychiatrists believe that the alleged moral neutrality of the psychotherapist is a fiction. If this is so, as the present writer believes, the psychiatrists need to be acutely aware of their value orientations. I am not saying that psychiatrists should take courses in ethics (not that this would be a shameful act), but rather that a philosopher working in a Department of Psychiatry can help provide this kind of insight.

I have spoken thus far of the contribution of the philosopher to psychiatry, but, as I know from personal experience, this relation is not asymmetrical. Psychodynamics in theory and in practice has been utilized with maximum effectiveness in esthetics and art criticism. We have known for a long time that depth psychology is invaluable in the analysis of artistic creation. We are also finding it useful in contextual analyses of certain works of art, i.e., those that contain psychodynamic material, and in analyses of the appreciative response to the work of art.[2]

Psychodynamic hypotheses about our conscious and unconscious control over action are relevant to the perennial discussions of the free-will problem; and at least one philosopher believes that the Freudian theory of ego development refutes the *tabula rasa* concept of mind in epistemology.[3]

These samples are specific contributions that psychiatry can make to philosophy. More generally, some forms of speculative philosophy can be interpreted as projections of personality structures. Surely this is at least part of what Freud had in mind when he speaks of transforming metaphysics into metapsychology. Whether the material thus produced is pathological cannot be decided a priori. These decisions, as any psychotherapist knows, are individually grounded. Some philosophers give psychodynamic diagnoses, and their patients, for historical reasons, are unavailable for comment. This procedure is highly conjectural, but no more objectionable in principle than any other form of historical inference.

I do not agree with Professor Lazerowitz that *the meaning* of statements in speculative philosophy is latent as contrasted to manifest content. To maintain his thesis is, I suspect, to succumb to a new instance of old essentialism. But I do not see how one could object to the claim that one point of some philosophical statements is what those statements reveal about their owners. Perhaps the philosopher is not best equipped to explicate this point. If so, let's change the "Know thyself" adage to "Allow others to know you."

Notes

1. "The Changing Concept of Man in Present-Day Psychiatry," *Freud and the Twentieth Century*, ed. Benjamin Nelson (New York: Meridian, 1957).

2. Campbell Crockett, "Psychoanalysis and Art Criticism," *Journal of Aesthetics and Art Criticism*, Vol. XVII, No. 1 (September, 1958).

3. Abraham Kaplan, "Freud and Modern Philosophy," *Freud and the Twentieth Century*.

Index

For Product Safety Concerns and Information please contact our EU
representative GPSR@taylorandfrancis.com
Taylor & Francis Verlag GmbH, Kaufingerstraße 24, 80331 München, Germany

www.ingramcontent.com/pod-product-compliance
Ingram Content Group UK Ltd.
Pitfield, Milton Keynes, MK11 3LW, UK
UKHW022207190926
475702UK00003B/238

* 9 7 8 1 1 3 8 5 3 1 0 3 1 *